Ophthalmic Plastic Surgery of the Upper Face

Eyelid Ptosis, Dermatochalasis, and Eyebrow Ptosis

Michael A. Burnstine, MD
Clinical Professor of Ophthalmology (Part-Time)
USC Roski Eye Institute, Keck Medicine of USC
Eyesthetica, Oculofacial and Cosmetic Surgery Associates
Los Angeles, California

Steven C. Dresner, MD
Clinical Professor of Ophthalmology (Part-Time)
USC Roski Eye Institute, Keck Medicine of USC
Eyesthetica, Oculofacial and Cosmetic Surgery Associates
Los Angeles, California

David B. Samimi, MD
Adjunct Clinical Assistant Professor of Ophthalmology
USC Roski Eye Institute, Keck Medicine of USC
Eyesthetica, Oculofacial and Cosmetic Surgery Associates
Los Angeles, California

Helen A. Merritt, MD
Adjunct Clinical Assistant Professor of Ophthalmology
USC Roski Eye Institute, Keck Medicine of USC
Eyesthetica, Oculofacial and Cosmetic Surgery Associates
Los Angeles, California

538 illustrations

Thieme
New York • Stuttgart • Delhi • Rio de Janeiro

Library of Congress Cataloging-in-Publication Data is available from the publisher

Important note: Medicine is an ever-changing science undergoing continual development. Research and clinical experience are continually expanding our knowledge, in particular our knowledge of proper treatment and drug therapy. Insofar as this book mentions any dosage or application, readers may rest assured that the authors, editors, and publishers have made every effort to ensure that such references are in accordance with **the state of knowledge at the time of production of the book.**

Nevertheless, this does not involve, imply, or express any guarantee or responsibility on the part of the publishers in respect to any dosage instructions and forms of applications stated in the book. **Every user is requested to examine carefully** the manufacturers' leaflets accompanying each drug and to check, if necessary in consultation with a physician or specialist, whether the dosage schedules mentioned therein or the contraindications stated by the manufacturers differ from the statements made in the present book. Such examination is particularly important with drugs that are either rarely used or have been newly released on the market. Every dosage schedule or every form of application used is entirely at the user's own risk and responsibility. The authors and publishers request every user to report to the publishers any discrepancies or inaccuracies noticed. If errors in this work are found after publication, errata will be posted at www.thieme.com on the product description page.

Some of the product names, patents, and registered designs referred to in this book are in fact registered trademarks or proprietary names even though specific reference to this fact is not always made in the text. Therefore, the appearance of a name without designation as proprietary is not to be construed as a representation by the publisher that it is in the public domain.

© 2020. Thieme. All rights reserved.

Thieme Publishers New York
333 Seventh Avenue, New York, NY 10001 USA
+1 800 782 3488, customerservice@thieme.com

Thieme Publishers Stuttgart
Rüdigerstrasse 14, 70469 Stuttgart, Germany
+49 [0]711 8931 421, customerservice@thieme.de

Thieme Publishers Delhi
A-12, Second Floor, Sector-2, Noida-201301
Uttar Pradesh, India
+91 120 45 566 00, customerservice@thieme.in

Thieme Publishers Rio de Janeiro,
Thieme Publicações Ltda.
Edifício Rodolpho de Paoli, 25º andar
Av. Nilo Peçanha, 50 – Sala 2508
Rio de Janeiro 20020-906 Brasil
+55 21 3172 2297

Cover design: Thieme Publishing Group
Typesetting by Thomson Digital, India

Printed in USA by King Printing Company, Inc.   5 4 3 2 1

ISBN 978-1-62-623921-0

Also available as an e-book:
eISBN 978-1-62-623922-7

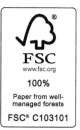

This book is dedicated to our patients (past, present, and future), to our mentors who have taught us, and to our residents and fellows who challenge us to be the best surgeons we can be. Their gifts to understanding upper facial concerns have been priceless.

Contents

3 Anatomic Considerations in the Aesthetic Surgery of the Upper Face 26
Maria Suzanne Sabundayo, Hirohiko Kakizaki

Section II Mechanical Ptosis

4 Mechanical Ptosis: Etiology and Management 32
Eric B. Hamill, Michael T. Yen

5 Upper Blepharoplasty 37
David B. Samimi

6 Double Eyelid Surgery 42
Michael A. Burnstine

Contents

Contents

Foreword

I am honored to have been invited by Dr. Michael A. Burnstine to write a foreword for this textbook. Drs. Michael A. Burnstine, Steven C. Dresner, David B. Samimi, and Helen A. Merritt have assembled a group of outstanding oculofacial plastic surgeons, to join them in the creation of an up-to-date, comprehensive publication on "the treatment of upper eyelid and brow ptosis."

There are many oculofacial plastic surgery textbooks, but most are on every aspect of the specialty. Although some of these textbooks have been on specific topics, there has been a void in blepharoptosis textbooks since the publications by Dr. Crowell Beard in the 1970s and 1980s. There have been many advancements in upper eyelid ptosis surgery since Beard's publications, so it is appropriate that Michael A. Burnstine and his associate editors fill this void.

It is important to include in a book like this the treatment of the upper eyelid dermatochalasis along with upper eyelid ptosis surgery, as these two issues have to be addressed commonly. Since, at times, the redundant upper eyelid fold is secondary to brow ptosis, it is also important to add to upper eyelid ptosis surgery the elevation of the brow to reduce the upper eyelid fold. Besides bringing us up-to-date on blepharoptosis surgery, there are two additional chapters on treatment of the upper eyelid dermatochalasis and seven chapters on treatment of brow ptosis, which has also seen many recent advancements. The focus of the textbook on upper eyelid and brow ptosis leads readers to now having one comprehensive book on ptosis that is the source of all the current knowledge in this subject.

One unique interesting chapter in this book is, "Staying Out of Trouble: Strategies Based on Recent OMIC Oculofacial Plastic Surgery Claims." Using data gathered by an ophthalmic insurance claims company provides the reader with an invaluable wealth of useful medico-legal information, an often overlooked topic in most texts.

I am proud that Michael A. Burnstine, a previous Oculofacial Plastic Surgery Fellow, has continued to be involved in adding to the scientific literature. I congratulate him and his associate editors, Steven C. Dresner, David B. Samimi, and Helen A. Merritt, on their accomplishments in assembling this comprehensive up-to-date ptosis text book.

Allen M. Putterman, MD

Preface

Management of the upper face can be challenging. The idea for this text came as a response to teaching the finer points of eyelid ptosis management and upper facial rejuvenation to our residents and fellows of ophthalmology, facial plastic surgery, plastic surgery, and oral maxillofacial surgery. In the course of our clinical practice, we find that surgeons performing blepharoplasty and brow-elevating procedures frequently miss upper eyelid ptosis and/or brow malposition. In this book, we have world-class expert oculofacial plastic surgeons break down the steps for the comprehensive evaluation and management of upper facial changes: eyelid ptosis, dermatochalasis, and eyebrow ptosis.

In the ensuing chapters, we examine the clinical assessment of patients who present with upper eyelid and eyebrow concerns and provide a useful treatment protocol to address these issues. The surgical management chapters provide a step-by-step approach for the surgeons beginning their career, with finer tips embedded for the more experienced surgeons. We have designed this text to enable health care providers to offer optimal treatment to all patients who present with upper facial concerns.

Videos

A selection of videos is available on MedOne illustrating the concepts and procedures covered in this book.

Michael A. Burnstine, MD
Steven C. Dresner, MD
David B. Samimi, MD
Helen A. Merritt, MD

Acknowledgements

We would like to thank our colleagues for their expert contributions, our families for their understanding during the creation of this book, and our Thieme editors for making this product the best that it could be.

Michael A. Burnstine, MD
Steven C. Dresner, MD
David B. Samimi, MD
Helen A. Merritt, MD

Contributors

Liat Attas-Fox, MD
Senior Oculoplastic Surgeon
Department of Ophthalmology
Meir Medical Center
Kfar Saba, Israel

Mica Y. Bergman, MD, PhD
Staff Physician, Ophthalmology
Sansum Clinic
Santa Barbara, California

Nathan W. Blessing, MD
Clinical Assistant Professor
Department of Ophthalmology
University of Oklahoma, Dean McGee Eye Institute
Oklahoma City, Oklahoma

Wesley L. Brundridge, DO
Oculoplastic and Cosmetic Surgery Fellow
EyePlasTX
San Antonio, Texas

Francesco P. Bernardini, MD
Adjunct Professor
Department of Ophthalmology and Plastic Surgery
University of Genova;
Director
Department of Oculo-Facial Plastic Surgery
Oculoplastica Bernardini
Genova, Italy

Michael A. Burnstine, MD
Clinical Professor of Ophthalmology (Part-Time)
USC Roski Eye Institute, Keck Medicine of USC;
Eyesthetica, Oculofacial and Cosmetic Surgery Associates
Los Angeles, California

Jean Carruthers, MD, FRCSC, FRC (Ophth)
Clinical Professor
Department of Ophthalmology
University of British Columbia
Vancouver, British Columbia, Canada

Jessica R. Chang, MD
Clinical Assistant Professor of Ophthalmology
Department of Ophthalmology
USC Roski Eye Institute, Keck Medicine of USC
Los Angeles, California

François Codère, MD
Associate Professor
Department of Ophthalmology
Hôpital Maisonneuve-Rosemont, Université de Montréal
Montreal, Quebec, Canada

Juan A. Delgado, MD
Fellow
Oculoplastic Surgery
Private Practice
Bogotá, Colombia

Martín H. Devoto, MD
Director
Department of Oculoplastic and Orbital Surgery
Consultores Oftalmologicos
Buenos Aires, Argentina

Steven C. Dresner, MD
Clinical Professor of Ophthalmology (Part-Time)
USC Roski Eye Institute, Keck Medicine of USC;
Eyesthetica, Oculofacial and Cosmetic Surgery Associates
Los Angeles, California

Ana F. Duarte, MD
Ophthalmologist
Orbit and Oculoplastics Unit
Department of Ophthalmology
Centro Hospitalar e Universitário de Lisboa Central;
Department of Ophthalmology
CUF Descobertas Hospital
Lisbon, Portugal

Peter J. Dolman, MD, FRCSC
Clinical Professor
Division Head of Oculoplastics and Orbit
Department of Ophthalmology and Visual Sciences
Vancouver General Hospital, University of British Columbia
Vancouver, Canada

Christopher M. DeBacker, MD
Partner
EyePlasTX
San Antonio, Texas

Jill A. Foster, MD
Associate Professor
Department of Ophthalmology
The Ohio State University
Columbus, Ohio

Robert G. Fante, MD, FACS
Clinical Professor
Department of Ophthalmology
University of Colorado Health Sciences Center;
Fante Eye and Face Center
Denver, Colorado

Alessandro Gennai, MD
Plastic and Reconstructive Surgeon
Studio Gennai
Bologna, Italy

Kimberly K. Gokoffski, MD, PhD
Assistant Professor
Neuro-Ophthalmology Division
Department of Ophthalmology
USC Roski Eye Institute
Los Angeles, California

Juliana Gildener-Leapman, MD
Oculoplastic and Reconstructive Surgery Fellow
Department of Ophthalmology
Shamir Medical Center, Tel Aviv University, Sackler School
  of Medicine
Tzrifin, Israel

Christine Greer, MD, MS
Resident
Department of Ophthalmology
USC Roski Eye Institute
Los Angeles, California

Eric B. Hamill, MD
Department of Ophthalmology
University of Southern California;
Eyesthetica, Oculofacial and Cosmetic Surgery Associates
Los Angeles, California

Hans B. Heymann, MD
Director of Oculoplastic and Reconstructive Surgery
Vold Vision
Fayetteville, Arkansas

Morris E. Hartstein, MD
Director of Ophthalmic Plastic Surgery
Department of Ophthalmology
Shamir Medical Center, Tel Aviv University, Sackler School
  of Medicine
Tzrifin, Israel

David E. E. Holck, MD, FACS
Clinical Associate Professor
Department of Ophthalmology
University of Texas Health Science Center at San Antonio;
EyePlasTX
San Antonio, Texas

John B. Holds, MD, FACS
Clinical Professor
Departments of Ophthalmology and Otolaryngology/Head
  and Neck Surgery
Saint Louis University School of Medicine
St. Louis, Missouri;
Ophthalmic Plastic and Cosmetic Surgery, Inc.
Des Peres, Missouri

Hirohiko Kakizaki, MD, PhD
Professor
Department of Oculoplastic, Orbital and Lacrimal Surgery
Aichi Medical University Hospital
Aichi, Japan

Jonathan W. Kim, MD
Professor of Clinical Ophthalmology
Director, Pediatric Oculoplastic Surgery
Children's Hospital Los Angeles
Keck Medicine of USC
Los Angeles, California

Krishnapriya Kalyam, MD
Former Clinical Instructor
Department of Ophthalmology
Washington University
St. Louis, Missouri

Wendy W. Lee, MD
Professor of Clinical Ophthalmology and Dermatology
Oculofacial Plastic and Reconstructive Surgery, Orbit and
  Oncology
Bascom Palmer Eye Institute
University of Miami Miller School of Medicine
Miami, Florida

Diana K. Lee, MD
Resident
Department of Ophthalmology
USC Roski Eye Institute
Los Angeles, California

Mark J. Lucarelli, MD, FACS
Dortzbach Endowed Professor
Director, Oculoplastic, Facial Cosmetic and Orbital Surgery
Department of Ophthalmology and Visual Sciences
University of Wisconsin–Madison
Madison, Wisconsin

Raman Malhotra, MBChB, FRCOphth
Corneoplastic Unit
Queen Victoria Hospital NHS Trust,
West Sussex, United Kingdom

John J. Martin, Jr., MD
Voluntary Assistant Faculty
Department of Ophthalmology
University of Miami
Miami, Florida

Nicholas R. Mahoney, MD
Assistant Professor of Ophthalmology
Wilmer Eye Institute
Johns Hopkins University
Baltimore, Maryland

David B. Samimi, MD
Adjunct Clinical Assistant Professor of Ophthalmology
USC Roski Eye Institute, Keck Medicine of USC;
Eyesthetica, Oculofacial and Cosmetic Surgery Associates
Los Angeles, California

Jennifer Murdock, MD
Oculo-Plastic and Orbital Reconstructive Surgery Instructor
Casey Eye Institute
Oregon Health and Science University
Portland, Oregon

John D. Ng, MD, MS
Professor
Department of Ophthalmology;
Department of Otolaryngology/Head and Neck Surgery
Casey Eye Institute
Oregon Health and Science University
Portland, Oregon

Vivek R. Patel, MD
Associate Professor
USC Roski Eye Institute
Los Angeles, California

Farzad Pakdel, MD
Professor
Department of Ophthalmic Plastic and Reconstructive
  Surgeries
Farabi Hospital, Tehran University of Medical Sciences
Tehran, Iran

Alice V. Pereira, MD
Plastic Surgeon
LMR Plastic Surgery Clinic;
Lecturer
Institute of Anatomy
Faculty of Medicine
University of Lisbon
Lisbon, Portugal

Margaret L. Pfeiffer, MD
Clinical Instructor
USC Roski Eye Institute
Eyesthetica, Oculofacial and Cosmetic Surgery Associates
Los Angeles, California

Allen M. Putterman, MD
Professor
Department of Ophthalmology
University of Illinois College of Medicine
Chicago, Illinois

Maria Suzanne Sabundayo, MD
Clinical Fellow
Department of Oculoplastic, Orbital and Lacrimal Surgery
Aichi Medical University Hospital
Aichi, Japan

Helen A. Merritt, MD
Adjunct Clinical Assistant Professor of Ophthalmology
USC Roski Eye Institute, Keck Medicine of USC;
Eyesthetica, Oculofacial and Cosmetic Surgery Associates
Los Angeles, California

Jeremy Tan, MD
Clinical Assistant Professor
Ophthalmic Plastic and Reconstructive Surgery
Dean McGee Eye Institute
Oklahoma University
Oklahoma City, Oklahoma

Magdalene Y. L. Ting, MA (Hons), MB BChir
Foundation Year 1 Doctor
Charing Cross Hospital, Imperial College Healthcare Trust
London, United Kingdom

Michael T. Yen, MD
Professor
Department of Ophthalmology
Cullen Eye Institute
Baylor College of Medicine
Houston, Texas

Katja Ullrich, BBioMedSc, BMBS, MMed (Ophthal Sc)
Corneoplastic Unit
Queen Victoria Hospital NHS Trust
West Sussex, United Kingdom

Sandy Zhang-Nunes, MD
Director, Oculofacial Plastic Surgery
Department of Ophthalmology
USC Eye Institute
Keck Medicine of USC
Los Angeles, California

Section I Introduction

1 Ptosis Classification

Michael A. Burnstine

Abstract

Ophthalmic plastic surgery of the upper face is nuanced. The surgeon must understand the anatomy of the upper face and the complex interplay between the eyebrow and the upper eyelid. In this chapter, a conceptual framework is created to classify and address a patient's upper facial concerns. While the main goal of upper facial surgery is aesthetic enhancement and functional visual improvement, protection of the health of the eye must be paramount.

Keywords: ptosis, blepharoptosis, eyebrow ptosis, dermatochalasis, ptosis classification

1.1 Introduction

It is critical for the surgeon to fully understand the patient's upper facial concerns, and to recognize and analyze the causative anatomic and aging changes. Many times, the patient is unaware of, or even surprised by, the structural changes underlying his or her undesired appearance, and it is critical that the surgeon help the patient to understand the causative mechanisms preoperatively. There is no single formula to correct eyelid and eyebrow ptosis in all patients. Preoperatively, surgeons should categorize patients into groups that respond similarly to surgical procedures. While the main goal of surgery is eyelid and/or eyebrow elevation and improved cosmesis, the protection and health of the eye must be paramount. Realistic goals and expectations are necessary to produce a happy patient and a satisfied surgeon, and the surgeon and patient must be keenly aware that there will be a need for postoperative revisions in some cases.

1.2 Ptosis Classification

Many classification systems exist for upper blepharoptosis, including congenital and acquired versus mechanistic.[1,2] Frueh divided ptosis into four major categories.[2] We expand Frueh's diagnostic categories to cover all types of ptosis (▶ Table 1.1). When ptosis is classified correctly and levator excursion (function) is assessed accurately, clear patient management follows.

Evaluation of the eyebrows also requires careful examination and attention to detail. Eyebrow ptosis can be assessed by examining photographs from a patient's youth and comparing them to the present state. Attention to the height, contour, and fullness of the eyebrow head, body, and tail is important. In general, with men, the eyebrow sits at the orbital rim and women prefer a slight temporal arch. This aesthetic norm may vary by ethnicity and age.

1.3 Preoperative Assessment

A thorough history of present illness and physical examination is necessary to adequately assess ptosis and develop a treatment plan.

1.3.1 History of Present Illness

Excellent patient care requires a thorough history of a patient's concerns. A detailed history from the patient or family members is critical. The surgeon should ask about duration, timing, severity, and variability. Photographs from youth are helpful to establish or corroborate the time of onset. An acute problem may point to a neurogenic etiology such as a Horner syndrome

Table 1.1 Ptosis types

Ptosis type	Etiology
Aponeurotic	Dehisced or disinserted levator aponeurosis
	Etiologies include age, trauma, prior surgery, blepharochalasis, and chronic eyelid edema
	Floppy eyelid syndrome
Myogenic	
• Static/ congenital	Congenital ptosis with levator maldevelopment
	Congenital fibrosis of extraocular muscles
	Double elevator palsy (monocular elevation deficiency)
	Trauma to levator muscle
	Duane's retraction syndrome
• Progressive	Oculopharyngeal dystrophy
	Chronic progressive external ophthalmoplegia
	Muscular and myotonic dystrophies
	Congenital progressive syndromic patients
Mechanical	Excessive lid weight (lid or orbital mass)
	Posterior scarring (conjunctival symblepharon)
Neurogenic	Oculomotor nerve palsy (third nerve)
	Aberrant regeneration: after third nerve palsy; Marcus Gunn; Marin Amat
	Benign essential blepharospasm and hemifacial spasm
	Horner's syndrome
	Myasthenia gravis
	Multiple sclerosis
	Ophthalmic migraine
Pseudoptosis	Enophthalmos and globe malpositions (silent sinus syndrome, orbital floor fracture)
	Contralateral exophthalmos
	Anophthalmos
	Hypotropia
	Dermatochalasis
	Contralateral eyelid retraction
	Guarding in thyroid eye disease
	Drug-induced

Table 1.2 History checklist

History of ptosis problem
Age of onset
How long has ptosis been present
Which eye
Any heralding event like trauma or surgery
Variability during the day/fatigue
Is diplopia present
Progressive or static
Any pain
Prior treatment
Family history of ptosis
Old photographs, documenting status and age of onset/progressive nature
Medical history
For children: Birth weight; developmental milestones met; any neurological issues
Surgical history
Trauma history
Drug history

Table 1.3 Eyelid measurements with contralateral eyelid elevation

Measurement	Definition
Palpebral fissure (PF)	Distance between the upper and lower eyelid in primary gaze (brow relaxed; in mm)
Palpebral fissure on downgaze (dPF)	Distance between upper and lower eyelids on downgaze (brow relaxed; in mm)
Margin reflex distance 1 (MRD1)	Distance between the pupillary light reflex and upper eyelid margin in primary gaze (in mm)
Margin crease distance (MCD)	Distance from the eyelid margin to the crease, measured on downgaze (in mm)
Margin fold distance (MFD)	Distance from eyelid margin to skin fold in primary gaze (brow relaxed; in mm)
Lagophthalmos	Eyelid opening on gentle eyelid closure (in mm)
Bell's phenomenon	Degree of upward eyeball rotation on forced eyelid closure (0–4 +)
Levator excursion (LE)	Degree of eyelid excursion from up- to downgaze (brow fixed; in mm)
Inferior limbus to brow	Distance between the inferior limbus and inferior eyebrow hair in primary gaze (in mm)
Eyebrow tail	Lateral; up/normal/down
Eyebrow head	Nasal; up/normal/down
Eyebrow body	Up/normal/down
Eyebrow fullness	

or third nerve palsy, whereas a chronic problem suggests more benign etiologies. Variability in eyelid/facial position throughout the day or concurrent double vision suggests myasthenia gravis. A history of trauma may point to a traumatic ptosis, while a history of contact lens wear may suggest aponeurotic ptosis. Obtaining thorough family, medical, surgical, trauma, and drug histories is also important (▶ Table 1.2).

Risk factor assessment prior to surgery is necessary. A history of ocular surface disease, anticoagulant use, prior eyelid or eye surgery, smoking, or other conditions like benign essential blepharospasm or snoring in sleep apnea may affect surgical decision-making.

1.3.2 Physical Examination

A complete ophthalmic examination should be performed, including visual acuity, pupillary size and response to light, extraocular motility, eyelid measurements, visual field testing, slit lamp examination focusing on the conjunctival and corneal surfaces and precorneal tear film, quantitative assessment for dry eyes by Schirmer's testing, qualitative assessment for dry eye examining tear breakup time, and dilated funduscopic examination. Noting subtle abnormalities like pupil size or lower eyelid position can aid in diagnosis and treatment. Identifying preoperative asymmetry and conveying this to the patient can help manage postoperative result expectations.

Physical examination also includes noting head position, presence or absence of chin-up posture, eyebrow and eyelid position, and examination of the conjunctiva and fornices. ▶ Table 1.3 shows eyelid measurements that are critical to the categorization of the ptosis type (also see ▶ Fig. 1.1).

Assessing for variation of ptosis with jaw or extraocular muscle movement is important to detect synkinesis in Marcus Gunn jaw-winking ptosis or aberrant regeneration syndromes after cranial nerve III and VII palsies. Further, extraocular muscle dysfunction associated with ptosis occurs in myotonic dystrophies and congenital conditions like monocular elevation deficiency (superior rectus/levator muscle maldevelopment) and congenital oculomotor nerve palsy.

At times, pharmacologic testing confirms and localizes disease such as in Horner's syndrome and in the fluctuating ptosis of myasthenia gravis. These tests are discussed in the neurogenic ptosis chapter.

Quantifying Ptosis

The vertical height of the palpebral fissures should be measured centrally with a millimeter ruler (▶ Fig. 1.2). The amount of ptosis is measured as the difference between the margin reflex distance 1 (MRD1) (distance between the upper eyelid margin and central corneal light reflex) and 4 mm (the average MRD1). This average height varies by race. Comparison should be made to eyelid and eyebrow position from older photographs, and can be helpful for discussion and documentation about patient preference for eyelid and eyebrow height and contour.

Critical to the understanding of ptosis is Hering's law of motor correspondence, which states that equal and simultaneous innervation flows to synergistic muscles concerned with the desired direction of gaze and eyelid elevation. Simply put, asymmetric bilateral upper eyelid ptosis or overcompensation for a contralateral ptosis (eyelid retraction) may be unmasked by lifting or occluding the ptotic eyelid and observing the fellow

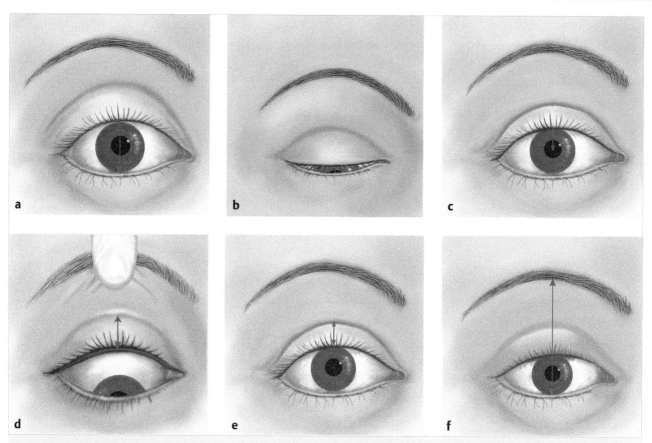

Fig. 1.1 Measurements of palpebral fissure (PF) (a), palpebral fissure on downgaze (dPF) (b), margin reflex distance 1 (c), margin crease distance (d), margin fold distance (e), and inferior limbus to brow (f). Measurements are done with the contralateral eyelid elevated, as seen in Fig. 1.2.

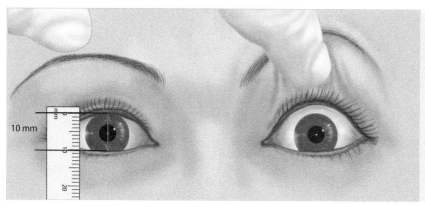

Fig. 1.2 Measuring the palpebral fissure (PF) with a ruler. Note that the contralateral eyelid is elevated while measuring the eyelid opening in primary gaze.

upper eyelid. In bilateral ptosis, the fellow eyelid will drop when lifting the more severely ptotic eyelid (▶ Fig. 1.3). In pseudoeyelid retraction, the fellow eyelid will return to normal position.

Insurance companies frequently require visual field testing prior to eyelid surgery. It is performed first with the patient gazing straight ahead while the eyelid and eyebrow are relaxed, and then with the eyelid and eyebrow taped up to a normal position. The difference in visual field between the two positions is considered the deficit produced by the eyelid and/or eyebrow malposition. Typically, a 20 to 30% upper visual field change is considered a functional deficit and is covered by

insurance. Testing with an automated perimeter or a tangent screen perimeter will document the visual field deficits.

Eye Protective Measurements

An adequate assessment of eye protective mechanisms is critical prior to surgery. The surgeon must explain to the patient that the eyelids and eyebrows are not purely decorative; they are designed to protect the cornea and preserve eye function. When lifting a ptotic eyelid, it is important to make sure that the eye remains adequately protected and can tolerate greater exposure to the outside world. The surgeon must document

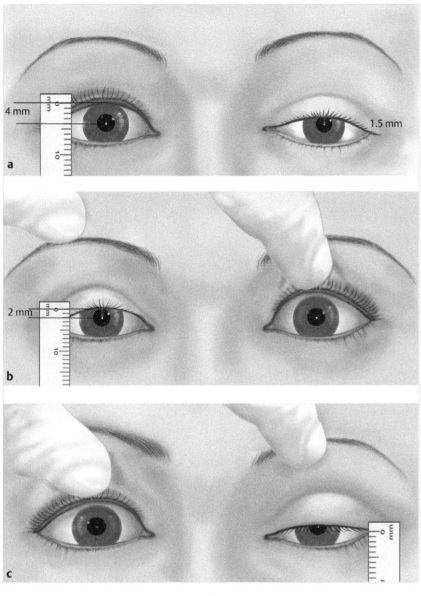

Fig. 1.3 (a–c) Bilateral ptosis unmasked when lifting the more ptotic eyelid, an example of Hering's law of motor correspondence. Here, the surgeon would report the MRD1 to be 2 mm on the right and 0 mm on the left.

measurements of ocular motility and Bell's phenomenon, tear film and dryness, orbicularis function (eyelid closure strength), lagophthalmos (eyelid opening on gentle eyelid closure), corneal sensation, and lower eyelid position and strength, each of which, if not normal, can negatively impact postoperative results. If the eyelid does not close well and there are poor corneal protective mechanisms, chronic eye pain due to exposure keratopathy or ulceration may become more likely after surgery.

Measuring Levator Excursion

Levator excursion or function is one of the most important measurements in assessing ptosis in adults and children. The surgeon measures levator function as the distance in millimeters between extreme upgaze and downgaze while the examiner is lifting the contralateral eyelid and immobilizing the ipsilateral eyebrow (▶ Fig. 1.4). Normal excursion is greater than 10 mm.

In uncooperative children and infants, this measurement may be quite difficult and multiple examinations may be necessary to get an adequate measurement.

1.4 Upper Eyelid Ptosis Classification

Once the surgeon classifies upper eyelid ptosis, defined by the appropriate eyelid measurements and measurement of levator excursion, the surgical plan follows. The authors use a modification of the classification scheme described by Frueh (▶ Table 1.4).

1.4.1 Aponeurotic Ptosis

By far, the most common type of ptosis we face is aponeurotic ptosis. Patients may have mild, moderate, or severe ptosis with good levator excursion. The ptosis arises from a stretching or dehiscence of the levator aponeurosis. The aponeurosis may become disinserted secondary to age, previous intraocular or eyelid surgery, contact lens wear, eyelid rubbing, local blunt trauma, blepharochalasis, chronic inflammation/edema, or some combination therein. The upper eyelid crease and fold are typically elevated and the eyelid may be thin (▶ Fig. 1.5). Frequently, the surgeon can observe the iris through a thin eyelid

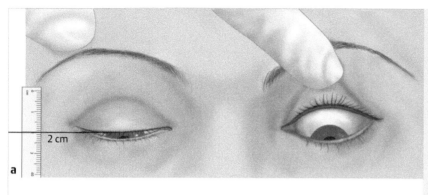

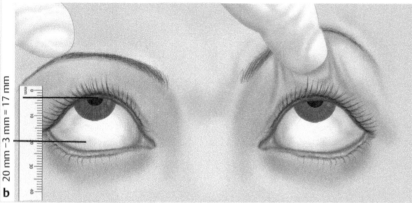

Fig. 1.4 (a, b) Measuring levator excursion between extreme downgaze and upgaze while elevating the contralateral eyelid and immobilizing the ipsilateral eyebrow.

when the levator aponeurosis has dehisced. Palpebral fissure on downgaze is diminished and correlates with difficulty reading.[3] Bell's phenomenon and levator excursion are preserved.

The surgical approach can be internal or external levator advancement. In this textbook, we describe and illustrate both approaches.

1.4.2 Myogenic Ptosis

Myogenic ptosis can either be static (congenital) or progressive. The ptosis can be from a maldeveloped levator, as seen in congenital ptosis. In progressive myopathic ptosis, a heritable disease is typically involved causing progressive muscle atrophy and dysfunction.

Static/Congenital Myopathic Ptosis

In congenital cases of myopathic ptosis, the levator muscle is typically fibrous and inelastic, thus leading to an increased palpebral fissure on downgaze (▶ Fig. 1.6). Bell's phenomenon is preserved, and levator excursion varies. The poorer the levator excursion, the greater the levator muscle is affected and the greater the lid lag (increased palpebral fissure on downgaze). If amblyopia is a risk, early surgical intervention is important. Typically, surgery is performed by age 4 to 5, when eyelid measurements are accurate and repeatable. Later in the text, there will be a more in-depth discussion on the surgical approach to these patients using methods described by Beard,[1] Berke and Wadsworth,[4] and Sarver and Putterman.[5] These methods describe repair of congenital ptosis based on degree of ptosis and levator function. In some congenital ptosis patients, examining superior rectus function is critical. If there is decreased

supraduction of the eye, the surgeon will resect more levator aponeurosis and muscle.

There are also familial inherited congenital ptoses. These include blepharophimosis ptosis syndrome and congenital fibrosis of the extraocular muscles. In the former, there is ptosis with poor levator excursion, blepharophimosis (narrowed horizontal palpebral fissure), epicanthus inversus, telecanthus, and sometimes ectropion of the lateral canthi. In the latter, the Bell's phenomenon is affected (absent) and surgical correction nuanced. These conditions and others, along with their genetics, will be discussed in later chapters.

Ultimately, the surgeon must tailor and individualize the surgical approach to the patient, based upon levator excursion and corneal protective mechanisms (ocular surface integrity, lagophthalmos, and Bell's phenomenon). The more compromised the corneal protective mechanisms, the more conservative the eyelid lift must be.

Progressive Myopathic Ptosis

By definition, this group of ptosis is progressive and usually heritable. Most patients begin life with normal eyelid height and contour and have progressive droop and extraocular muscle involvement (▶ Fig. 1.7). This group of disorders includes chronic progressive external ophthalmoplegia (CPEO), oculopharyngeal dystrophy, and muscular and myotonic dystrophies.

CPEO is bilateral and affects the extraocular muscles. As CPEO progresses, both eyes can become fixed and immobile. Heart block, pigmentary retinopathy (described as salt and pepper fundus), and some neurologic signs are reported with this syndrome; therefore, its identification is particularly critical.

Table 1.4 Ptosis classification

Ptosis type	PF (mm)	dPF (mm)	MRD1 (mm)	MCD (mm)	MFD (mm)	Lag (mm)	Bell's (present/decreased)	LE (mm)	Procedure
Aponeurotic	↓	↑	↓	←	↑	0	Present	>10 mm	Levator advancement
									If neosynephrine positive, Müller's muscle–conjunctival resection (posterior approach)
									If neosynephrine negative, external levator advancement (anterior approach)
Myogenic									
• Static/congenital	↓	Unable to look down	↓	Normal or absent	↑	0	Present	0–4 mm	Frontalis suspension if good frontalis function
								4–10 mm	Levator resection
								>10 mm	Anterior or posterior levator advancement (Neo test)
• Progressive	↓	↑	↓	Normal or increased	↑	0	Decreased	0–4 mm	Supramaximal blepharoplasty or frontalis suspension
								4–10 mm	Levator resection or supramaximal blepharoplasty
								>10 mm	Levator advancement/resection
Mechanical	↓	Normal or decreased	↓	Normal or increased	↑	0	Present	Normal or decreased	Remove the mechanical impediment or scar

Table 1.4 (*Continued*) Ptosis classification

Ptosis type	PF (mm)	dPF (mm)	MRD1 (mm)	MCD (mm)	MFD (mm)	Lag (mm)	Bell's (present/ decreased)	LE (mm)	Procedure
Neurogenic	↓	Unable to look down	→	Normal	←	0	Decreased	0	Observe. Lifting the eyelid will cause diplopia
Pseudoptosis	Normal	Normal	Normal	Normal	←	0	Present	Normal	Address primary issue (see Section 1.4.5)

Abbreviations: Bell's, Bell's phenomenon; dPF, palpebral fissure on downgaze; Lag, lagophthalmos; LE, levator excursion; MCD, margin crease distance; MFD, margin fold distance; MRD1, margin reflex distance 1; PF, palpebral fissure.
[a]MFD decreased in mechanical impediment from dermatochalasis and eyebrow ptosis.

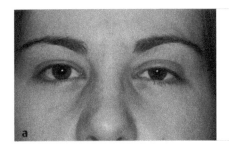 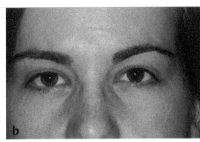

Fig. 1.5 A patient with aponeurotic ptosis with a high eyelid crease and fold. Preoperative photograph **(a)** and postoperative photograph **(b)** after left Müller's muscle–conjunctival resection.

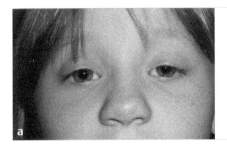 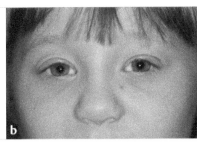

Fig. 1.6 A patient with bilateral congenital ptosis (static myopathic ptosis) and increased lid lag on downgaze. Preoperative photograph **(a)** and status post bilateral external levator resection **(b)**.

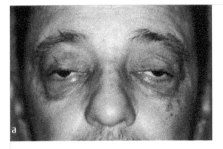 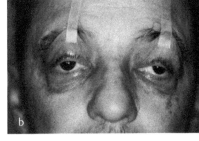
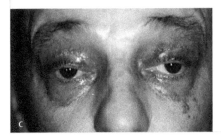 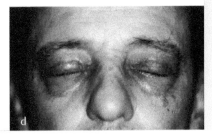

Fig. 1.7 A patient with progressive myopathic ptosis due to oculopharyngeal dystrophy. Note ptosis and ocular misalignment. Preoperative photograph **(a)**, patient compensation with eyelid taping **(b)**, status post maximal eyelid skin resection described by Burnstine and Putterman[6] **(c)**, and no lagophthalmos **(d)**.

Oculopharyngeal dystrophy is a primary myopathy that typically begins in middle age and is associated with trouble swallowing. Typically, the disease is heritable and patients may be French Canadian, Incan, or from Indian tribes in New Mexico.

Muscular and myotonic dystrophies are typically hereditable, affect many muscle groups of the head and body, and may affect the extraocular and levator muscles.

In all of these conditions, surgical intervention is based on the corneal protective mechanisms and must be conservative. Because the eye motility is limited and frequently Bell's phenomenon diminished or absent in severe disease, the surgical goals are limited to minimal eyelid elevation to clear the pupil while maintaining corneal protection. Frequently, the surgeon prescribes postoperative lubricating eye drops and ointment to stabilize the ocular surface. Due to the progressive nature of the disease, over time, the surgeon may need to repeat the surgical intervention. Typical surgical rules for static myopathic ptosis do not always apply.

1.4.3 Mechanical Ptosis

Mechanical ptosis can be caused by excessive weight on the eyelid (tumor or excess skin) or by posterior conjunctival scarring causing diminished levator excursion. Injury, prior surgery, and progressive cicatrizing processes like Stevens–Johnson syndrome can cause the latter. The palpebral fissure and MRD1 are diminished, while the palpebral fissure on downgaze is often normal or decreased. Margin crease and fold are often normal and levator excursion is normal (▶ Fig. 1.8).

Treatment is directed at the cause of ptosis. If a tumor or excess skin is present, excision is warranted. If there is a cicatrizing process, scar tissue is excised and, if need be, mucous or amniotic membrane grafting performed. In the later chapters, we will discuss the aesthetic management of ptosis caused by dermatochalasis, cicatrizing processes, and eyebrow ptosis.

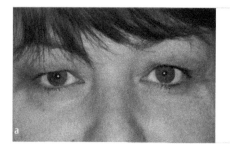
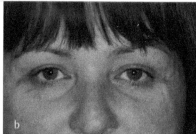

Fig. 1.8 Mechanical ptosis due to excess skin. Preoperative photograph (**a**) and status post bilateral upper eyelid blepharoplasty (**b**).

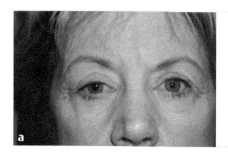
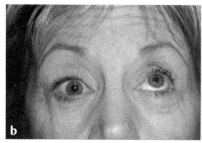

Fig. 1.9 A patient with right neurogenic ptosis due to a third nerve palsy. Note ptosis and eye deviation down and out (**a**) and poor extraocular motility with upgaze limitation and no levator excursion (**b**).

1.4.4 Neurogenic Ptosis

The most common cause of neurogenic ptosis is an oculomotor (third) nerve palsy, causing absent levator excursion (▶ Fig. 1.9). It may be peripheral, nuclear, or supranuclear. Typically, there is an associated palsy of the extraocular muscles (superior rectus, inferior rectus, and medial rectus muscles) innervated by the third cranial nerve. Palpebral fissure is diminished. The patient will have difficulty looking in most fields of gaze. The eyelid crease will be normal and the margin fold distance increased. Bell's phenomenon and levator excursion are absent.

Other causes of neurogenic ptosis include aberrant innervation syndromes, Horner's syndrome, multiple sclerosis, and ocular migraine. Horner's syndrome results from paralysis of the sympathetically innervated Müller's muscle. The ptosis is associated with miosis, anhidrosis, and reverse ptosis of the lower eyelid. The lesion may occur anywhere along the sympathetic chain. The cause must be identified by a complete medical and neurologic workup, and the underlying condition treated appropriately. In congenital cases, the presentation includes iris heterochromia. In ophthalmic migraine, oculomotor nerve paralysis tends to be recurrent, associated with a severe headache, and unilateral. Rarely is the ophthalmoplegia permanent. It is critical to differentiate a migraine from an orbital mucocele or intracranial aneurysm. These conditions will be discussed in detail in the chapter on neurogenic ptosis.

Once the primary neurologic event has stabilized, ptosis repair may be considered. The surgical management for third nerve palsies is controversial. Many argue not to perform surgery (author included). If surgery is to be performed after the palsy has stabilized (usually 6 months), the surgeon realigns the eye by strabismus surgery first, and then ptosis surgery is performed. Realigning the vertical muscles first is critical because the realignment will affect the ultimate eyelid position. Extreme care must be taken before lifting the eyelid due to a high risk of exposure keratopathy due to poor Bell's phenomenon and resultant lagophthalmos.

In patients with abnormal innervation syndromes from birth or following oculomotor nerve paralysis, treatment is not curative but aimed at cosmesis. Sometimes, the levator is excised to eliminate its function and frontalis suspension is performed (such as in Marcus Gunn jaw-winking: cranial nerve III–V synkinesis). In other circumstances, Botox may be given to the orbicularis muscle (such as in Marin Amat: cranial nerve V–VII synkinesis). These synkinetic syndromes will be discussed in later chapters.

1.4.5 Pseudoptosis

Pseudoptosis is defined as a condition resembling ptosis due to abnormalities other than in the levator muscle itself. Most of the eyelid measurements are normal, though margin fold distance may vary. The most common cause in this category is dermatochalasis. Here, the palpebral fissure is preserved, and the palpebral fissure on downgaze is normal. Levator function and Bell's phenomenon are preserved, and lagophthalmos is zero. Other causes include asymmetric upper eyelid creases, enophthalmos (orbital fracture, silent sinus syndrome, and fibrous dysplasia; ▶ Fig. 1.10), fat atrophy, anophthalmos/microphthalmos/phthisis bulbi/postenucleation or evisceration states, hypotropia of involved eye or hypertropia of contralateral eye, contralateral eyelid retraction, guarding, facial spasms, and usage of certain glaucoma drops.

Management of dermatochalasis will be discussed in the mechanical ptosis chapter. For anophthalmic and microphthalmic states, enlarging a prosthesis and adding orbital volume can obviate the need for eyelid surgery. For hypo- or hypertropia, extraocular muscle surgery typically corrects the problem. Addressing orbital tumors or floor fractures to correct a globe malposition may also be indicated. The etiologies of pseudoptosis will be discussed in detail in the pseudoptosis chapter.

1.5 Eyebrow Ptosis Classification

Eyebrow ptosis frequently accompanies upper eyelid ptosis and dermatochalasis and must be recognized as a factor that contributes to the aging periorbital area. Understanding the

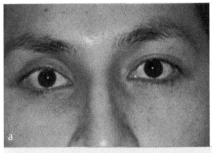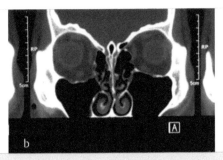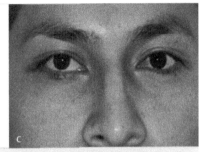

Fig. 1.10 A patient with pseudoptosis due to right medial wall and floor fractures. Note deep superior sulcus (increased MFD) in preoperative photograph **(a)**, computed tomography scan indicating right orbital floor and medial wall fractures **(b)**, and postoperative photograph after insertion of an orbital floor implant to bring the eye up and out which improved the deep sulcus and MFD **(c)**.

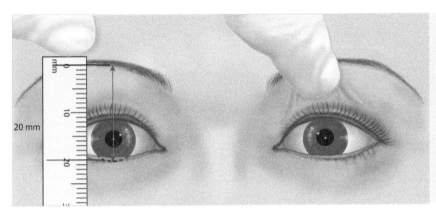

Fig. 1.11 Measuring eyebrow position while elevating the contralateral eyelid (*left*) and relaxing the ipsilateral eyebrow (*right*).

continuum between the hairline, eyebrow, and upper eyelid is critical. Chronic contracture of the frontalis muscle to compensate for eyelid or eyebrow ptosis may lead to headache, browache, and prominent transverse forehead rhytids. When eyebrow laxity is present, brow droop may frequently manifest after upper eyelid ptosis and blepharoplasty repair. This would narrow the distance between the brow and eyelashes. Crowding from postoperative brow descent then reduces the effect of upper eyelid blepharoplasty and ptosis repair. A nasal lowering of the brow accentuates glabellar folds and produces a "mean" or "worried" look. Temporal brow droop is associated with a "sad" look.

To reduce the risks of postoperative brow droop and brow droop sequelae, the surgeon must carefully assess the brow preoperatively when evaluating any patient for upper eyelid blepharoplasty or eyelid ptosis repair. It is critical to assess eyebrow laxity, position, and fullness of each portion of the eyebrow: head, body, and tail. The brow must be assessed at baseline height (inferior limbus to brow) with separate assessment of the medial, central, and temporal brow positions. To avoid compensatory eyebrow elevation from ptotic eyelids, the fellow eyebrow position should be measured when the contralateral eyelid is elevated (▶ Fig. 1.11).

Understanding the complex interplay between the brow elevators, depressors, and superficial and deep fat pads of the upper face is important. Surgical correction of temporal brow laxity and droop can be corrected by filler injection, direct brow lift, midforehead lift, indirect brow (upper blepharoplasty

incision) lift, pretricheal temporal and coronal lift, posttricheal coronal lift, or endoscopic eyebrow elevation. The surgeon corrects nasal/glabellar brow ptosis with coronal or endoscopic approaches. Direct and indirect lifts are ineffective in managing glabellar fullness and nasal eyebrow ptosis, respectively. These procedures will be discussed in more detail in the chapters on brow ptosis.

1.6 Clinical Decision-Making

Once the surgeon classifies the upper blepharoptosis and defines the eyebrow position, the surgical intervention is based on levator excursion and patient preference, respectively (▶ Table 1.4). In the ensuing chapters, the surgical preoperative considerations, detailed steps of the surgical procedure, and postoperative management, including complications, for repair of eyelid and eyebrow ptosis will be outlined.

1.7 Photographing the Patient

Photographs are helpful in preoperative discussion with the patient and as a record of the effects of surgery. These should be taken to document the case for preoperative study and be available during the case for intraoperative assessment. Photographs should be consistent in position, alignment, background, and lighting. Prior to photography, the patient removes all jewelry and eyelid makeup. The photographs are taken in primary gaze, upgaze, downgaze, and lateral views to highlight the degree of ptosis, lid lag on downgaze, overlying hooding, eyelid position, and eyebrow position. If there is change in eyelid position in directions of gaze as in Duane's syndrome, the photographer should take medial and lateral gaze photographs. If there is abnormal innervation syndrome (Marin Amat or Marcus Gunn jaw-winking), this should be documented photographically as well. Often, insurance companies will request visual fields and photographs, documenting functional compromise prior to authorizing the surgical procedure.

Documenting postoperative changes is also crucial. Patients frequently forget their preoperative appearance or become overly fixated on slight surgical changes; therefore, having a reference point is very helpful for demonstrating the improvements in appearance.

1.8 Informed Consent

In our contemporary society, it is considerate and legally necessary to provide to patients the risks associated with eyelid and eyebrow surgery. The authors mention the following risks routinely: vision loss, bleeding, bruising, swelling, infection, dry eye that may require eye lubrication, the need for a secondary surgery to address an undercorrection or overcorrection, and recurrence of eyelid or eyebrow droop over time.

1.9 Principles of Surgical Correction

My belief is that the ultimate bad result in surgery of all types is unmet patient expectations. This is especially true in surgeries that are nonurgent in nature, and painfully so when there is an element of optional, noncovered care involved. Our goal in surgery is to create an excellent patient experience to meet the patient's expectations. The surgeon should discuss with the patient that a perfect cosmetic and functional result cannot be obtained in all patients and that revision surgery may be necessary. Selecting the best ptosis procedure for each patient requires a detailed history, a thorough examination including eyelid and eyebrow assessment, and evaluation of the corneal protective measures. The result depends upon the nature of the ptosis, the type of operation selected, and the surgeon's ability and skill.

1.10 When Not to Operate

It is important to assess the patient's understanding of their complaints, management options, and the doctor–patient relationship. Most patients seek a natural and enhanced appearance from surgery that improves functionality and makes them look younger. They want to avoid the stigmata of an "overdone" or "plastic surgery appearance." Older patients should receive medical clearance from their primary care doctor. Severe medical problems should be documented and addressed prior to surgical intervention, particularly hypertension and those conditions that require anticoagulation. Both can lead to excessive bleeding.

Certain situations should give the surgeon pause about whether to perform surgery. These include procedures that would put the eye health at risk, a condition that is difficult to correct with surgery, or a patient that will never be happy. When there is a disconnect between patient expectations and what can be delivered, I suggest declining surgical intervention. Good surgeons know when to operate. Excellent surgeons know when to *not* operate.

1.11 Postoperative Complications

Complications occur in all types of ptosis surgery. Thorough understanding of the anatomy, careful preoperative history, thorough clinical examination, proper surgery selection, excellent surgical technique, and diligent postoperative care can reduce complication risk. The most common complications include undercorrection followed by overcorrection, unsatisfactory or asymmetric eyelid contour (crease and fold asymmetries), wound dehiscence or infection, scarring, and postoperative dry eye syndrome. Less common complications include orbital hemorrhage, eyelid and eyebrow contour abnormalities (entropion, ectropion, and notching), eyelash loss, lagophthalmos, lid lag, exposure keratitis, symblepharon, conjunctival prolapse, and extraocular muscle imbalance. These complications will be discussed in each subsequent chapter of surgical approaches to eyelid and eyebrow ptosis.

1.12 Aesthetic Concerns for Upper Eyelid and Eyebrow Rejuvenation

The upper facial surgeon must consider every patient a cosmetic patient. The surgical goal should be to maximize the aesthetic result while maintaining good eyelid and eyebrow function. Ultimately, a job well done results when both the patient and the surgeon are happy with the outcome.

References

[1] Beard C. The surgical treatment of blepharoptosis: a quantitative approach. Trans Am Ophthalmol Soc. 1966; 64:401–487

[2] Frueh BR. The mechanistic classification of ptosis. Ophthalmology. 1980; 87 (10):1019–1021

[3] Olson JJ, Putterman A. Loss of vertical palpebral fissure height on downgaze in acquired blepharoptosis. Arch Ophthalmol. 1995; 113(10):1293–1297

[4] Berke RN, Wadsworth JAC. Histology of levator muscle in congenital and acquired ptosis. AMA Arch Opthalmol. 1955; 53(3):413–428

[5] Sarver BL, Putterman AM. Margin limbal distance to determine amount of levator resection. Arch Ophthalmol. 1985; 103(3):354–356

[6] Burnstine MA, Putterman AM. Upper blepharoplasty: a novel approach to improving progressive myopathic blepharoptosis. Ophthalmology. 1999; 106 (11):2098–2100

2 Aesthetic Anatomy of the Upper Face

Mica Y. Bergman, Margaret L. Pfeiffer

Abstract

A detailed understanding of the anatomy of the upper face and eyelids is critical to the success of any surgeon operating in this area. In this chapter, we describe and illustrate the anatomy of the upper face and eyelids, with a particular focus on surgical relevance. This chapter outlines the layers of the face and upper eyelids, noting those structures most crucial to eyelid function, eye protection, and aesthetic rejuvenation. Subsequently, the nervous innervation to, blood supply of, and lymphatic drainage from the eyelids and upper facial structures are described and discussed in detail.

Keywords: anatomy, eyelid anatomy, eyebrow anatomy

2.1 Introduction

A thorough appreciation of the detailed anatomic relationships in the eyelids and upper face is crucial to the success of the upper facial surgeon. Here, we present functional anatomy through the surgeon's lens. We focus on those structures most important to the preoperative planning and intraoperative technique of the surgeon addressing the eyelid and eyebrow.

The layers of the face, from superficial to deep, include skin, subcutaneous and superficial fat compartments, superficial musculoaponeurotic system (SMAS), retaining ligaments, mimetic muscles, and deep fat compartments and bone (▶ Fig. 2.1). The forehead contains all of these layers. The forehead extends from the hairline superiorly to the superior orbital rim inferiorly, at which point it becomes the upper eyelid. The eyelid has both continuous and analogous structures to the forehead and some key distinct features.

The most important function of the eyelids is eye protection. The surgeon must ensure that eyelid elevation, removal of upper eyelid skin or muscle, or eyebrow elevation will not expose the ocular surface to excessive environmental factors and prevent eyelid closure. The surgeon who addresses both aesthetic and functional issues of the upper face must, therefore, be familiar with the complex interplay of multiple structures that contribute to eyelid position, eyelid opening and closing, and ocular surface protection. Lagophthalmos, the presence of eyelid opening upon gentle closure, can result from aggressive surgery. This condition can lead to chronic dry eye and corneal exposure, known as exposure keratopathy, which is uncomfortable and potentially sight-threatening.

2.2 Skin

The skin is the largest organ in the body in surface and weight. The functions of the skin include protection, temperature regulation, and sensation. It consists of two layers: the epidermis and dermis. Beneath the dermis lies subcutaneous fatty tissue. Here, we describe the unique relevant features of the skin of the upper face and eyelids.

The forehead skin contains the cilia that make up the eyebrows, perhaps the most distinctive and expressive feature of the forehead. The eyebrows sit at the superior orbital rim in males and above the rim in females. The eyebrow can be divided medially to laterally into a head, body, and tail, and the orientation of the eyebrow hairs varies by location. This is important, as incisions near the eyebrows should be parallel to the hair follicles to minimize damage. A telltale sign of aging is the descent of the eyebrows below their native, youthful position. Repair of brow ptosis is, therefore, a critical component of aesthetic facial surgery and the subject of later chapters.

The eyelid skin is the thinnest skin in the body and, in the non-Asian eyelid, is devoid of subcutaneous fat, unlike the skin of the brow and forehead. It is critical that the upper facial surgeon appreciates the transition between the thicker brow and thinner eyelid skin types, as measurement of the amount of eyelid skin is important to preoperative planning in upper eyelid blepharoplasty and external ptosis surgery. Typically, a fairly distinct transition is present between the two types of skin. At times, this transition correlates with the inferior extent of the brow hairs; at times, the brow hairs extend onto the eyelid skin itself, and therefore, this is not a useful metric. Another clue that may help the surgeon differentiate between the brow and eyelid skin is the presence, oftentimes, of a slight color difference between the two, with the eyelid skin lighter than the adjacent brow skin. The mobility and flexibility of the eyelid

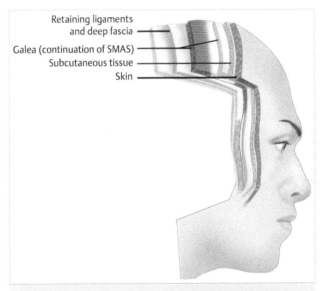

Fig. 2.1 Layers of the face. Illustration of the layers of the face. Note that the superficial musculoaponeurotic system is continuous with the galea in the forehead, the temporoparietal fascia in the temple, and the platysma in the neck. Note that the deep fat compartments are present in limited areas of the face and are not shown in this illustration. (Reproduced with permission from https://plasticsurgerykey.com/mimetic-muscles/.)

skin is crucial to allow free eyelid movement and function. Cicatrization secondary to excessive tension with wound closure, scarring, or burns carries risk of eyelid retraction or ectropion.

The eyelid crease, measured by the margin–crease distance (MCD), is an important external landmark formed by the attachment of anterior projections of the levator aponeurosis to the septae between orbicularis fibers overlying the tarsus or pretarsal orbicularis.[1] Attention to the location of the upper eyelid crease is crucial in the examination of any patient. To obtain the best aesthetic result, review of older photographs and careful discussion with the patient are critical. The normal position of the eyelid crease is approximately 8 to 10 mm above the eyelid margin in Caucasian women and approximately 6 to 8 mm above the margin in Caucasian men. In Asian individuals, it is typically a few millimeters lower.[2]

The upper eyelid fold, measured by the margin–fold distance (MFD), consists of loose upper eyelid skin and subcutaneous tissue anterior to the confluence of the levator aponeurosis and orbital septum, formed with the patient's eyes open and at rest. In patients with significant dermatochalasis (excess skin) or herniated orbital fat, the eyelid fold may overlie and obscure the eyelid crease and eyelid margin.

2.3 Subcutaneous Tissue and Fat Compartments

Throughout the face are superficial and deep fat compartments, divided by the SMAS in the face itself or by the SMAS' counterparts in the forehead (galea) and temporal region (temporoparietal fascia). The superficial fat pads lie just deep to the skin and serve protective functions. The implications of their changing morphology in the aging face are major.[3,4] The deep fat pads' principal functions are mechanical support and facial volume.[5]

From medial to lateral, the superficial fat compartments in the forehead are the central fat pad, the middle forehead fat pads, and the lateral temporal-cheek fat pads (▶ Fig. 2.2). All three are bounded superiorly by the hairline and extend inferiorly to variable degrees. The inferior boundary of the central fat pad is the dorsum of the nose, and the inferior boundary of the middle fat pad is the orbicularis retaining ligament at the superior orbital rim. The paired lateral temporal-cheek fat pads extend the farthest inferiorly, down the extent of the face to the cervical area.

There are three superficial fat compartments in the periorbital area: the superior orbital fat pad, the inferior orbital fat pad, and the lateral orbital fat pad (▶ Fig. 2.2). The superior and

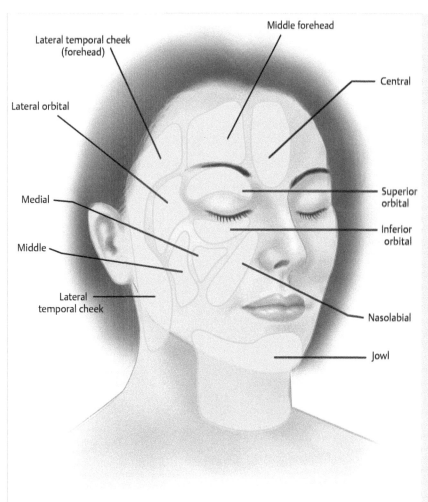

Fig. 2.2 Superficial fat pads of the face. Illustration of the superficial fat pads of the face. These fat pads lie deep to the skin and superficial to the superficial musculoaponeurotic system (SMAS). (Reproduced with permission from Prendergast.[4])

Middle forehead

Lateral temporal cheek (forehead)

Lateral orbital

Central

Medial

Superior orbital

Inferior orbital

Middle

Lateral temporal cheek

Nasolabial

Jowl

inferior orbital fat pads lie in the same plane as the superficial fat pads of the forehead but are in the upper and lower eyelid, respectively; they are deep to skin but superficial to the orbicularis oculi muscle. These are bounded laterally by the lateral canthal tendon, medially by the medial canthal tendon, and at the orbital rim by the orbicularis retaining ligament. The third orbital fat compartment is the lateral orbital fat pad, which lies lateral to the lateral canthus and is bounded laterally by the lateral temporal-cheek fat pad.

2.4 Superficial Musculoaponeurotic System

The SMAS is a complex network of layers of connective tissue that envelops and joins the skeletal muscles of the face. The SMAS is important surgically as a key target in face lifting and functionally as a distributor of facial expression. The SMAS extends from the galea aponeurotica to the platysma and is connected to the dermis via vertical septae. As mentioned above, the SMAS takes on different names in different regions: galea in the forehead, temporoparietal fascia in the temple, SMAS in the face itself, and platysma in the neck. The SMAS has little significance to the eyelid surgeon but is important to the upper facial surgeon during brow lifting in its relation to the temporal branch of the facial nerve, cranial nerve VII. The plane of dissection in brow lifting is within a loose areolar tissue layer that lies between the temporoparietal fascia superficially and the deep temporalis fascia overlying the temporalis muscle

deeply. At the zygomatic arch, the temporal branch of the facial nerve is a deep structure that courses along periosteum. As it travels superomedially toward the glabella, the nerve becomes superficial and lies within this temporoparietal fascia. Thus, it is superficial to the plane of dissection (see "Unique Considerations for the Upper Facial Surgeon: Facial Danger Zones: Avoiding Nerve Injury").

2.5 Retaining Ligaments, Canthal Tendons, and Orbital Septum

In addition to the fascial network provided by the SMAS are firmer condensations of fibrous connective tissue called true retaining ligaments. They are located in constant anatomic locations and separate fascial planes and compartments. These retaining ligaments serve as facial support structures, anchoring the dermis to the underlying periosteum of the facial skeleton and stabilizing the skin, SMAS, and underlying deep fascia. As such, they are important targets in surgery.[6]

In the lateral forehead, the deep temporal fascia, the temporoparietal fascia, and the periosteum of the frontal bone fuse together to form the conjoint tendon (also known as the conjoined tendon, superior temporal septum, frontal ligament, or temporal fusion line).[7,8] The conjoint tendon extends superotemporally from the lateral brow and inferiorly along the lateral orbital rim and zygomatic arch[6,7] (▶ Fig. 2.3). Complete release of this strong fascial attachment is critical to achieving a complete, long-lasting elevation during endoscopic browplasty.

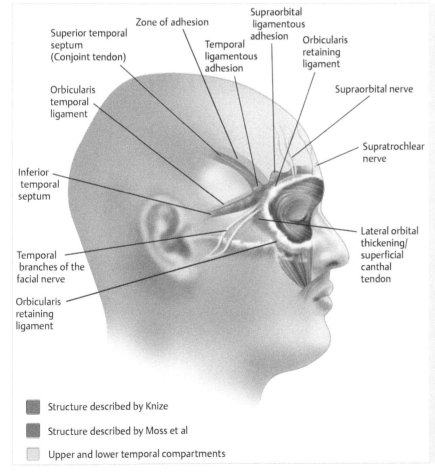

Superior temporal septum (Conjoint tendon)

Zone of adhesion

Supraorbital ligamentous adhesion

Temporal ligamentous adhesion

Orbicularis retaining ligament

Orbicularis temporal ligament

Supraorbital nerve

Inferior temporal septum

Supratrochlear nerve

Temporal branches of the facial nerve

Lateral orbital thickening/ superficial canthal tendon

Orbicularis retaining ligament

■ Structure described by Knize

■ Structure described by Moss et al

□ Upper and lower temporal compartments

Fig. 2.3 Retaining ligaments of the upper face. Illustration of the retaining ligaments of the upper face. The circumferential orbicularis retaining ligament extends between the deep orbicularis oculi muscle and the orbital rim, and condenses laterally as the lateral canthal tendon. The conjoint tendon/superior temporal septum represents the fusion of the deep temporal fascia, the temporoparietal fascia, and the periosteum of the frontal bone. (Reproduced with permission from Alghoul and Codner.[6])

The orbicularis retaining ligament extends circumferentially around the orbit along the orbital rim, inserting 2 to 3 mm outside of the rim, peripheral to the insertion of the orbital septum (▶ Fig. 2.3). The ligament extends from the fascial tissues underlying the orbicularis oculi muscle (the galea superiorly and the SMAS laterally and inferiorly) to the periosteum of the orbital rim, and its fusion with the orbital septum is known as the arcus marginalis.[9-11] In its course around the orbit, the orbicularis retaining ligament varies in thickness, length, and tautness. Of relevance to the upper facial surgeon, the ligament is relatively lax laterally compared to medially, likely contributing to the phenomenon of lateral hooding often encountered in dermatochalasis.[9]

The orbicularis retaining ligament contributes to the lateral canthal tendon, a structure that similarly anchors tissue to the periosteum. However, rather than linking superficial soft tissue to periosteum, the lateral canthal tendon anchors the tarsus to the periosteum of the lateral orbital rim at the lateral canthus, where the upper and lower eyelids meet. The tarsus is a structure that provides a majority of support to the upper and lower eyelids. In the medial canthus, the medial canthal tendon anchors the tarsus to the anterior and posterior lacrimal crests through an anterior and posterior limb, respectively (▶ Fig. 2.4). Here, the medial canthal tendon and portions of the orbicularis oculi muscle envelop the lacrimal sac in the bony lacrimal sac fossa and form the lacrimal pump.

The orbital septum is a membranous sheet that serves as the anterior boundary of the orbit. It extends from the orbital rims to the eyelids. The septum is a barrier to infection and hemorrhage within the orbit. The eyelid protractors (depressors) lie anterior to the septum, and the eyelid retractors (elevators) lie posterior to the septum.

Whitnall's ligament, or the superior transverse ligament, is an important structure in the orbit in its relationship to the levator palpebrae superioris muscle (▶ Fig. 2.5). It runs transversely from the trochlea in the medial orbital wall to the lacrimal gland in the lateral orbital wall and is thought to act as a fulcrum for the levator muscle.[12] It is white in color and often encountered in large levator advancements or resections.

False retaining ligaments are less robust bands of connective tissue that weave within the soft tissue layers of the face and are of little relevance to the upper facial surgeon.

2.6 Mimetic Muscles and Eyelid Retractors

The mimetic muscles, or muscles of facial expression, animate the face and contract to create rhytids or wrinkles. The eyelid protractor, the orbicularis oculi muscle, is responsible for eyelid closure and eye protection. The eyelid retractors, the levator palpebrae superioris and Müller's muscle, are responsible for opening the upper eyelid.

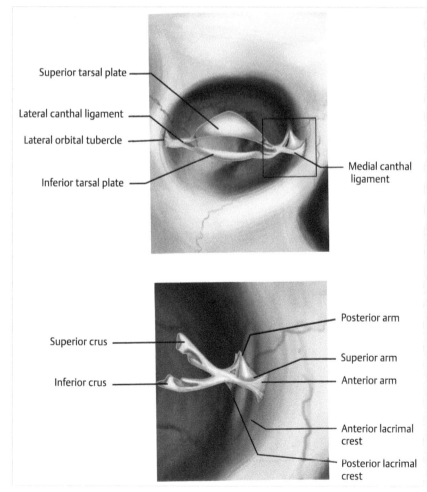

Fig. 2.4 Canthal anatomy. Anatomy of the tarsal plates, medial and lateral canthal tendons, and their connections to the orbital walls. (Reproduced with permission from Dutton.[11])

Superior tarsal plate

Lateral canthal ligament

Lateral orbital tubercle

Inferior tarsal plate

Medial canthal ligament

Superior crus

Inferior crus

Posterior arm

Superior arm

Anterior arm

Anterior lacrimal crest

Posterior lacrimal crest

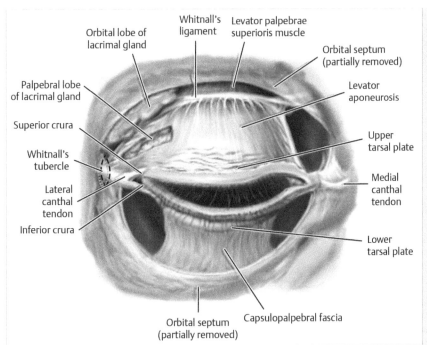

Whitnall's ligament
Levator palpebrae superioris muscle
Orbital lobe of lacrimal gland
Orbital septum (partially removed)
Levator aponeurosis
Palpebral lobe of lacrimal gland
Superior crura
Upper tarsal plate
Whitnall's tubercle
Medial canthal tendon
Lateral canthal tendon
Inferior crura
Lower tarsal plate
Orbital septum (partially removed)
Capsulopalpebral fascia

Fig. 2.5 Relationship of the levator palpebrae superioris to Whitnall's ligament and the lacrimal gland. The lateral horn of the levator muscle divides the lacrimal gland into orbital and palpebral lobes. The levator inserts on the anterior tarsal border. Whitnall's ligament runs transversely through the superior orbit to act as a fulcrum for the levator muscle. (Reproduced with permission from https://vennofem.wordpress. com/2013/10/23/lateral-canthotomy/.)

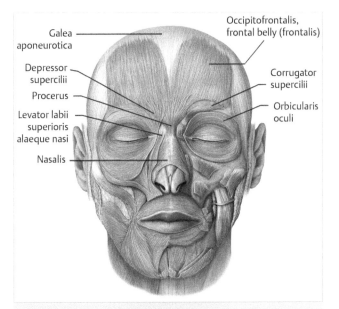

Galea aponeurotica
Occipitofrontalis, frontal belly (frontalis)
Depressor supercilii
Corrugator supercilii
Procerus
Orbicularis oculi
Levator labii superioris alaeque nasi
Nasalis

Fig. 2.6 Mimetic muscles of the upper face. Illustration of the musculature of the upper face. (Reproduced with permission from THIEME Atlas of Anatomy, Head and Neuroanatomy. © Thieme 2010, Illustrations by Karl Wesker.)

The muscles of the forehead are the frontalis, procerus, depressor supercilii, and corrugator supercilii; these are all paired muscles except the procerus, which lies in the midline (▶ Fig. 2.6). The frontalis elevates the eyebrow, and the remaining muscles depress the eyebrow. The frontalis originates from the galea and inserts into the more inferior musculature: the procerus, corrugator, and orbital orbicularis. The frontalis' lateral-most insertions do not reach the tail of the brow; as such, the tail lacks an elevator. For this reason, injection of botulinum toxin in the lateral orbicularis muscle inferior to the eyebrow can be a useful adjunct to upper facial surgery to lift the brow.

The eyebrow depressors are the procerus, depressor supercilii, corrugator supercilii, and orbicularis oculi. The procerus lies in the midline, originating at the aponeurosis of the nasalis muscle and inserting over the central forehead and medial brow, where it intersects with the frontalis muscle. The depressor supercilii and corrugator supercilii muscles cause depression of progressively more lateral portions of the brow. The depressor supercilii originates just medial to the medial canthus, from the frontal process of the maxillary bone, and extends underneath the procerus to insert on the medial brow skin. The corrugator supercilii originates quite close to the depressor supercilii, though slightly superior and on the frontal bone. This muscle then divides into two heads: the oblique courses similarly to the depressor supercilii, and the transverse assumes a more acute angle, running superolaterally. This muscle head also runs more deeply, coursing within the galeal fat pad.

The orbicularis oculi is the muscle of eyelid closure. It encircles the eye and consists of concentric muscle fibers divided into three contiguous parts: pretarsal, preseptal, and orbital. These names correspond to their anatomic location over the tarsus, orbital septum, and orbital rim, respectively. Voluntary contraction of the orbital portion of the orbicularis oculi muscle is responsible for forceful eyelid closure, and involuntary contraction of the pretarsal and preseptal portions is responsible for the spontaneous blink. The superior fibers of the orbicularis also act as eyebrow depressors, along with the muscles mentioned above. In the medial eyelid, the pretarsal orbicularis forms the lacrimal pump through attachments to the medial canthal tendon and posterior lacrimal crest of the lacrimal bone. With normal contraction and relaxation of the orbicularis oculi, tears are pumped through the canaliculi and lacrimal sac into the nasolacrimal duct. Laterally, the orbicularis inserts onto the lateral canthal tendon.

The mimetic musculature is responsible for rhytids, which run perpendicular to the direction of the muscle fibers and are popular targets for botulinum toxin injections. Thus, the vertically oriented frontalis and procerus muscles cause horizontally oriented skin wrinkles, whereas the corrugator is responsible for vertically oriented skin wrinkles (11's). The orbicularis causes horizontal wrinkles lateral to the lateral canthus (crow's feet).

The levator muscle originates in the posterior orbit from the lesser wing of the sphenoid bone and courses anteriorly. At the level of Whitnall's ligament, the posterior muscular portion becomes the more anterior fibrous aponeurotic structure, and its trajectory turns inferiorly toward the tarsus. Near the tarsus, the aponeurosis divides into anterior and posterior portions. The posterior portion inserts on the anterior aspect of the inferior third of the tarsus. The anterior portion inserts on septae between fibers of the pretarsal orbicularis and subcutaneous tissue to form the eyelid crease.[1,13] These anterior projections are less robust in the Asian eyelid, which contributes to the absence of a well-defined crease. In cases of severe aponeurotic ptosis, the levator aponeurosis may be variably disinserted and/ or attenuated and displaced superiorly, making its intraoperative identification during external levator advancement surgery challenging, as it deviates from its natural anatomic position. The identification of the preaponeurotic fat pads is again crucial, as the aponeurosis can be identified just deep to these pads. The levator aponeurosis forms a medial horn, which attaches to the medial canthal tendon, and a larger lateral horn, which inserts on the lateral canthal tendon. The lateral horn of the levator divides the lacrimal gland into orbital and palpebral lobes (▶ Fig. 2.5).

Müller's muscle is a sympathetically innervated smooth muscle that is responsible for 1 to 2 mm of upper eyelid elevation. It originates on the undersurface of the levator muscle approximately at the level of Whitnall's ligament and inserts on the superior border of the tarsus. The superior palpebral arterial arcade lies between the levator aponeurosis and Müller's muscle just superior to its insertion at the tarsus. Weak attachments exist between Müller's muscle and the overlying levator muscle. Firm attachments exist between Müller's muscle and the underlying conjunctiva. Resection of Müller's muscle in the Müller's muscle–conjunctival resection (MMCR) procedure has been shown to plicate and thus advance the levator aponeurosis.[14]

2.7 Deep Fat Compartments

The mimetic muscles overlie the deep fat pads, which serve as glide planes over which the muscles can freely move and provide additional volume to the face. In the forehead, the galea fat pad sits centrally, deep to the frontalis muscle, enveloping the procerus and corrugator muscles and separating them from the underlying frontal bone. It extends superiorly about 3 cm from the orbital rim.[4,15] The retro-orbicularis oculi fat (ROOF) pad, sub-brow fat pad, and the preaponeurotic fat pads lie in the periorbital region. The ROOF extends along the superior orbital rim along the width of the eyelid and, as the name implies, is deep to the orbital and preseptal portions of the orbicularis oculi muscle. It is continuous superiorly with the sub-brow fat pad. In the Asian eyelid, the ROOF is continuous inferiorly with a pretarsal fat pad, also deep to the orbicularis, which contributes to the fullness of the Asian eyelid.[11,16] This pretarsal fat pad is absent in the Caucasian eyelid (▶ Fig. 2.7).

Somewhat analogous to these structures, but in the anterior orbit, lie the preaponeurotic fat pads. These fat pads are deep to the orbital septum, a sheet of connective tissue that represents the anterior demarcation of the orbit, and rest on the aponeurosis or fibrous extension of the levator muscle, thus the term "preaponeurotic fat." Classically, there are two well-defined fat pads here: the lighter colored medial fat pad and the more yellow central fat pad (▶ Fig. 2.8). Fat from the medial compartment has a tendency to herniate and may be removed in upper eyelid blepharoplasty to improve the contour of the upper eyelid. The superior oblique tendon and trochlea, the cartilaginous pulley for the superior oblique muscle on the superonasal orbital wall, lie between the central and medial compartment; therefore, care must be taken when dissecting deeply to avoid these important structures and prevent postoperative diplopia. More recent cadaver and *in vivo* studies have proposed that the anatomy of the upper eyelid fat pads may be more complex, including the presence of two fat pads within the medial compartment that may be variably interconnected and an accessory lateral fat pad in approximately 20% of patients that may contribute to fullness in the lateral third of the upper eyelid.[17,18]

The lacrimal gland, which lies in a fossa in the frontal bone in the superotemporal orbit, occupies the lateral postseptal compartment adjacent to these fat pads. Surgeons must be careful to avoid resection or cautery of the lacrimal gland when removing preaponeurotic fat, which could result in postoperative dry eye. The gland is typically whiter in color than the adjacent fat pad and has a somewhat cobblestoned quality to it. In senescence, the orbital lobe of the lacrimal gland may prolapse, requiring plication, which is discussed later in this text.

2.8 Nervous Innervation to the Upper Eyelid and Forehead

2.8.1 Sensory

Sensory innervation to the upper eyelid and forehead is carried primarily by the ophthalmic division of the trigeminal nerve (cranial nerve V_1) and its branches. In the cavernous sinus, the ophthalmic nerve divides into the lacrimal, frontal, and nasociliary nerves, all of which enter the orbit through the superior orbital fissure.

The large frontal nerve is the primary mediator of sensory innervation to the upper eyelid and forehead. The nasociliary nerve mediates sensory innervation of the medial eyelids via the terminal infratrochlear nerve, which pierces the septum just superior to the medial canthal tendon.[11] The lacrimal nerve primarily innervates the lacrimal gland but provides some sensory innervation to the lateral upper eyelid via its terminal branches.[11]

Within the orbit, the frontal nerve splits into the more inferior supratrochlear and more superior supraorbital nerves, both of which play large roles in sensory facial innervation. The supraorbital nerve exits the orbit through the superomedial supraorbital notch, whereas the supratrochlear nerve continues above the superior oblique's trochlea and exits the orbit anteromedially to its counterpart.

After exiting the orbit, the supraorbital nerve branches and passes superiorly. Medially, the branches lie close to the periosteum but become more superficial as they ascend through the

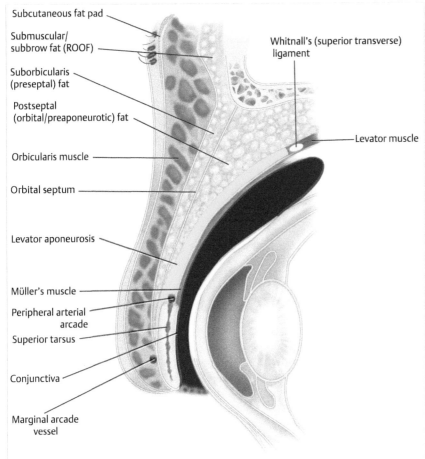

Subcutaneous fat pad
Submuscular/subbrow fat (ROOF)
Suborbicularis (preseptal) fat
Postseptal (orbital/preaponeurotic) fat
Orbicularis muscle
Orbital septum
Levator aponeurosis
Müller's muscle
Peripheral arterial arcade
Superior tarsus
Conjunctiva
Marginal arcade vessel
Whitnall's (superior transverse) ligament
Levator muscle

Fig. 2.7 Anatomy of the upper eyelids. Cross-section illustration of the upper eyelids. The posterior portion of the levator aponeurosis inserts on the anterior aspect of the inferior third of the tarsus. The anterior portion inserts on septa between fibers of the pretarsal orbicularis and subcutaneous tissue to form the eyelid crease. (Note that these anterior projections are less robust in the Asian eyelid.) Müller's muscle originates on the undersurface of the levator muscle approximately at the level of Whitnall's ligament and inserts on the superior border of the tarsus. The superior palpebral arterial arcade lies between the levator aponeurosis and Müller's muscle just superior to its insertion at the tarsus.

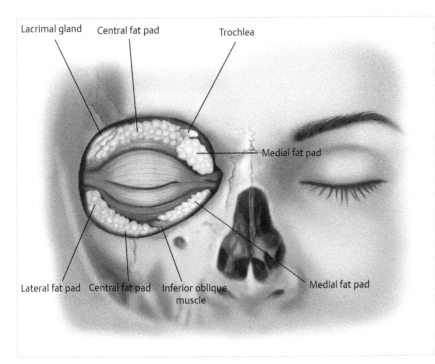

Lacrimal gland
Central fat pad
Trochlea
Medial fat pad
Lateral fat pad
Central fat pad
Inferior oblique muscle
Medial fat pad

Fig. 2.8 Preaponeurotic fat pads of the upper eyelids. Demonstration of the upper eyelid preaponeurotic fat pads. Note the whiter appearance of the medial fat pad in comparison to the more yellow appearance of the central fat pad. (Reproduced with permission from https://plasticsurgerykey.com/involutional-periorbital-changes-dermatochalasis-and-brow-ptosis/.)

corrugator and frontalis to innervate the skin just above the medial brow, the upper forehead, and the scalp. The lateral branch courses horizontally in a deep plane before turning superiorly at the lateral eyebrow. This branch remains deep until it reaches the hairline, at which point it becomes superficial to innervate the lateral scalp. The supratrochlear nerve sends branches superiorly, which pass through the corrugator and frontalis and innervate the lower forehead skin, and branches inferiorly, which innervate the anterior and posterior lamellae of the medial upper eyelid.

The maxillary division of the trigeminal nerve (cranial nerve V_2) also plays a small role in sensory innervation of the upper face; the zygomaticotemporal branch of its infraorbital nerve innervates that lateral portion of the upper eyelid and temple.

During brow surgery, appreciation of the planes in which the sensory nerves lie is critical to reduce the risk of damage. Medially, branches of the supraorbital nerve become superficial just above the brow, and are therefore at risk of injury in direct brow lifts. Laterally, supraorbital nerve branches are deeper, and thus dissection in this region may proceed more deeply. During endoscopic brow lifts, when establishing the preperiosteal or subperiosteal plane, care must be taken to avoid injuring the supraorbital nerve as it leaves its foramen. Injury to these nerves may result in upper facial paresthesia of the affected territory, though recovery over the course of months is common (see "Unique Considerations for the Upper Facial Surgeon: Facial Danger Zones: Avoiding Nerve Injury"). In eyelid surgery, there are no sensory nerves at risk of injury.

2.8.2 Motor

Motor innervation to the forehead is provided by the facial nerve (▶ Fig. 2.9**b**). The frontalis muscle is supplied on its undersurface by the temporal branch of the facial nerve, whereas the procerus, corrugator, and depressor supercilii

muscles are innervated by the temporal and zygomatic branches[4,11] (▶ Fig. 2.9**b**). It is crucial that surgeons are aware of the course of the temporal branch of the facial nerve, which, as discussed previously, is at risk for injury in upper facial surgery (see "Unique Considerations for the Upper Facial Surgeon: Facial Danger Zones: Avoiding Nerve Injury").

In the eyelid, motor innervation to each of the three muscles is distinct. The levator palpebrae superioris is innervated by cranial nerve III, the oculomotor nerve, which also innervates the superior, inferior, and medial recti and inferior oblique muscles and contains parasympathetic fibers to the iris sphincter muscle responsible for pupillary constriction. Ptosis with poor levator function, poor Bell's phenomenon, and motility deficits, with or without a dilated pupil, are key features in third nerve palsy. Surgical repair of this paralytic ptosis is controversial and will be discussed in a later chapter. Müller's muscle is innervated by sympathetic fibers, which enter the orbit running alongside the ophthalmic artery and follow branches of the long ciliary nerve into the orbit. Innervation to the orbicularis oculi muscle is provided by the zygomatic branch of the facial nerve (cranial nerve VII).

2.9 Blood Supply

2.9.1 Forehead

Blood supply to the forehead is mediated by both the internal and external carotid systems, with the primary contributor being the internal carotid artery via the ophthalmic artery (▶ Fig. 2.10). The primary contributing branches are the supraorbital, supratrochlear, and dorsal nasal arteries. The supraorbital artery is the workhorse for forehead arterial supply, providing coverage throughout the layers and extent of the forehead. The supraorbital artery branches directly from the ophthalmic artery and exits the orbit at the supraorbital notch

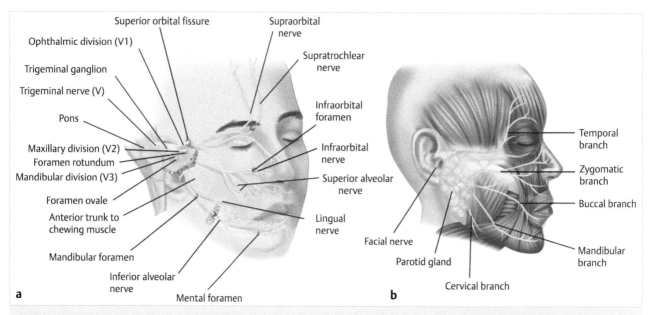

Fig. 2.9 Sensory (**a**) and motor (**b**) innervation to the upper face. Illustration of motor innervation to the face, mediated by the facial nerve, cranial nerve VII. There are five branches of the facial nerve: temporal, zygomatic, buccal, mandibular, and cervical. (a: reproduced with permission from https://healthjade.com/cranial-nerves/; b: reproduced with permission from https://doctorstock.photoshelter.com/image/I0000jnLqPxce4Rg.)

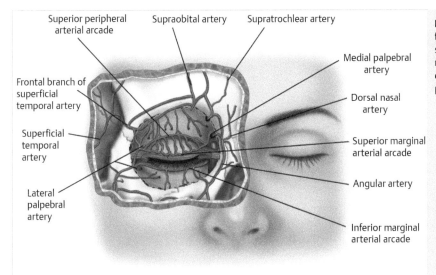

Fig. 2.10 Arterial supply to the upper eyelid and forehead. Illustration of the complex blood supply to the upper eyelid and forehead, mediated by both the internal carotid and external carotid systems. (Reproduced with permission from Dutton.[11])

with the supraorbital nerve. It then travels anteriorly to supply the corrugator before splitting into deep and superficial branches. The deep branch curves laterally, runs just superficial to the periosteum, and serves the pericranium. The superficial branch climbs superiorly to supply the muscles and skin of the brow, forehead, and scalp. The supratrochlear artery is a smaller caliber branch of the ophthalmic artery that exits the orbit just above the superior oblique trochlea with its paired nerve. The supratrochlear artery serves the medial forehead and scalp. Finally, the dorsal nasal artery exits the orbit just inferior to the supratrochlear artery and provides blood supply to the central forehead and scalp.

The external carotid system supplies the temple and lateral brow. Specifically, the superficial temporal artery, one of the terminal branches of the external carotid, supplies the skin and superficial temporal fascia in the temple, and its frontal branches course medially to supply the frontalis and its associated skin and pericranium. The superficial temporal artery anastomoses in the lateral forehead with the supraorbital artery.

2.9.2 Eyelid

Blood supply to the eyelid consists of a rich anastomotic network of vessels, also arising from the internal and external carotid arteries and terminating in arcades that span the horizontal extent of the eyelids (▶ Fig. 2.10). This extensive blood supply confers an enormous benefit to the eyelid surgeon; infection in this area is extremely uncommon. The corollary, however, is that intraoperative bleeding is common during eyelid surgery, and the surgeon must be aware of the vascular anatomy to prevent and manage it.

The ophthalmic artery serves as the root to both the medial and lateral palpebral arteries. The lateral palpebral artery is a branch of the lacrimal artery and the medial palpebral artery is the terminal branch of the ophthalmic artery. The medial palpebral artery enters the eyelid superior to the lacrimal sac. The upper eyelid branch courses between the tarsus and the orbicularis oculi about 2 mm from the eyelid margin to form the superior marginal arcade. The lower eyelid branch passes under the

medial canthal tendon and then courses between the same structures to form the lower eyelid marginal arcade. Superiorly, a branch of the medial palpebral artery gives rise to the peripheral arcade, which passes between the two upper eyelid retractors (levator aponeurosis and Müller's muscle) just above the tarsus.[11,19] Recognition of this artery can be very helpful in identifying the plane between the upper eyelid retractor muscles when performing external ptosis surgery.

After the lacrimal artery supplies the lacrimal gland, it branches into the superior and inferior lateral palpebral arteries posterior to the orbital septum.[11,19] These arteries supply the lateral part of all eyelid arcades.

The external carotid system contributes branches to the eyelid's arterial supply via the transverse facial artery and superficial temporal artery laterally and the angular artery medially.

2.10 Lymphatic Drainage

2.10.1 Forehead

Lymphatic drainage from the forehead is twofold. The medial forehead drains to the submandibular nodes, whereas the lateral forehead drains to the preauricular and parotid nodes.

2.10.2 Eyelid

Lymphatic drainage from the eyelids is divided anteroposteriorly and mediolaterally. Anteriorly, the pretarsal plexus drains lymph from the skin and orbicularis, and posteriorly the posttarsal plexus drains lymph from the tarsus and conjunctiva. The two plexuses are interconnected, and drain via two primary routes. The lateral two-thirds of the upper eyelid, the lateral one-third of the lower eyelid, and the lateral half of the conjunctiva drain laterally, whereas the medial one-third of the upper eyelid, the medial two-thirds of the lower eyelid, and the medial half of the conjunctiva drain medially. Laterally, drainage is through the preauricular node, and medially, drainage is into the submandibular nodes. Ultimately, both pathways drain into the anterior and deep cervical nodes (▶ Fig. 2.11). A 2010 study using lymphoscintigraphy suggests that this classic description may not be as universal as was once thought, and that the preauricular node may be important for medial drainage in addition to lateral drainage.[20] More work will be necessary to clarify these patterns. Clinically, these drainage patterns are important for understanding hematogenous metastatic spread of eyelid tumors, though basal cell carcinoma, the most common eyelid malignancy, tends not to spread in this way.[8,11]

2.11 Unique Considerations for the Upper Facial Surgeon: Facial Danger Zones

See ▶ Fig. 2.12 and ▶ Table 2.1.

2.12 Unique Anatomical Considerations for the Eyelid Surgeon

The structures of the eyelid are grouped into lamellae, a distinction that has important clinical and surgical implications. The anterior lamella consists of skin and the orbicularis oculi; the middle lamella consists of the orbital septum, preaponeurotic fat pads, and retractor muscles; and the posterior lamella consists of tarsus and conjunctiva. Cicatrization of any lamella results in a distinct clinical picture, and the oculofacial surgeon must recognize the results of damage to each structure during preoperative planning. For example, anterior lamella scarring or shortening can lead to eyelid eversion, or ectropion, whereas posterior lamella shortening can lead to eyelid inversion, or entropion. Middle lamella scarring can lead to difficult dissection in the ptosis reoperation patient. All of these entities can be addressed surgically by lengthening the affected lamella.

2.12.1 Anterior Lamella

The skin and orbicularis oculi muscle of the anterior lamella have been discussed. The surgeon performing blepharoplasty and external ptosis repair must remain cognizant and vigilant regarding the amount of eyelid skin to remain after resection, as discussed previously. Traditional thought is that the surgeon should leave behind 20 mm of eyelid skin between the eyelid margin and inferior eyebrow hairs to allow for proper eyelid closure. Overresection causing anterior lamellar shortening may lead to lagophthalmos and induced eyebrow ptosis.

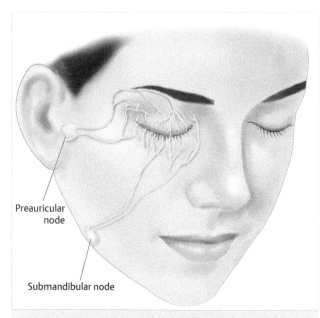

Fig. 2.11 Lymphatic drainage of the upper eyelid and forehead. Demonstration of the lymphatic drainage of the upper eyelid and forehead, showing lateral drainage to the preauricular node and medial drainage to the submandibular node. (Reproduced with permission from https://www.slideshare.net/hindalshawadify/eye-lymphatics.)

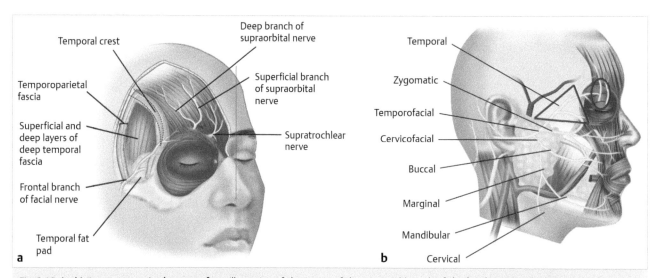

Fig. 2.12 (a, b) Danger zones in the upper face. Illustration of the course of the temporal branch of the facial nerve in the upper face and the supraorbital and supratrochlear nerves in the medial forehead and the areas in which these nerves are at particular risk for surgical damage. Note that in the temporal region, the temporal branch of the facial nerve runs in the temporoparietal fascia superficial to the deep temporalis fascia. (a: adapted from: La Trenta GS. Atlas of Aesthetic Face and Neck Surgery. Philadelphia, PA: Saunders Elsevier; 2004 (Print); Part 2: Seckel.[21])

Table 2.1 Upper facial danger zones: areas at risk of nerve damage during upper face surgery

Nerve	Sign of injury	Location	Relevant surgical anatomy
Temporal branch of the facial nerve	Paralysis of ipsilateral forehead	Within triangle formed by connecting lateral orbital rim adjacent to lateral canthus to 2 cm above tail of brow to 0.5 cm below tragus	In brow lifting, dissection must be carried out deep to temporoparietal fascia, within which nerve runs
Supraorbital and supratrochlear nerves	Numbness of upper eyelid, forehead, and scalp	Medial portion of superior orbital rim	In brow lifting, the surgeon should attempt to visualize nerves at the superior orbital rim. If dissecting corrugator muscles, the surgeon should directly visualize the supratrochlear nerve within muscle fibers

Source: Seckel.[21]

2.12.2 Middle Lamella

The orbital septum arises from the orbital rim at the arcus marginalis, a condensation of periosteum, and divides the superficial "preseptal" tissues from the "postseptal" orbital tissues. The orbital septum fuses with the levator aponeurosis 2 to 5 mm above the superior border of the tarsus in both the Caucasian and Asian eyelid.[16,22] Intraoperatively, the septum may be found deep to the orbicularis and superficial to the preaponeurotic fat pads. Sharp dissection through the septum is necessary to access the fat pads and levator muscle. Grasping the septum with forceps and pulling inferiorly will reveal a firm attachment to the orbital rim at the arcus marginalis, which may help with intraoperative identification of this structure when in question. This maneuver differentiates the orbital septum from the levator aponeurosis.

The preaponeurotic fat pads, previously discussed, lie deep to the septum. In the Asian eyelid, the preaponeurotic fat has a tendency to descend inferiorly and overhang the insertion of the septum into the levator aponeurosis, which contributes, with the pretarsal fat pad, to a "fuller" appearance to the Asian upper eyelid.[23]

The levator palpebrae superioris muscle and Müller's muscle elevate the eyelid and open the eye. The white levator aponeurosis lies deep to the preaponeurotic fat, and Müller's muscle lies deep to the aponeurosis.

2.12.3 Posterior Lamella

The tarsus is a strip of dense connective tissue that provides much of the structural support to the eyelids. The tarsus in the upper eyelid is approximately 10 mm in height and 1-mm thick. The thickness of the tarsus is important to note, and care must be taken when suturing the levator aponeurosis to the tarsus in external levator advancement surgery to ensure that suture passes are partial-thickness through tarsus. Eversion of the eyelid margin after each tarsal pass is recommended. The tarsus is firmly attached via the medial and lateral canthal tendons to the periosteum of the respective orbital walls.

The conjunctiva is a thin layer of nonkeratinized squamous epithelium that lines the inner surface of the eyelid (palpebral conjunctiva) and continues at the fornix to cover the surface of the globe (bulbar conjunctiva). The conjunctiva contains goblet cells and accessory lacrimal glands of Krause and Wolfring, which form the mucinous and aqueous components of the tear film, respec-

tively. Although ptosis surgery that includes conjunctival resection (MMCR) has been criticized for possibly risking these important tear structures, the literature and patient care have not supported this theory. Schirmer's testing does not show decreased tear production after MMCR,[24] and histologic studies of cadavers after MMCR have shown preservation of the accessory lacrimal glands located at the superior tarsus and the fornix.[14]

2.12.4 Eye Protective Mechanisms

Protection of the cornea is conferred by the eyelids, Bell's phenomenon, and the tear film. The eyelids provide mechanical protection of the cornea and, in blinking, distribute the tear film over the ocular surface. Bell's phenomenon is a reflexive movement of the eye upward upon eyelid closure. Preoperative assessment of each of these components is important to the upper facial surgeon, and a deficiency in any of these factors may require concurrent medical management or an altered surgical approach.

Eyelid Closure

Eyelid closure is mediated by the orbicularis oculi muscle. Damage to or compromise of orbicularis function may result in poor blink and lagophthalmos or incomplete passive eyelid closure. An incomplete blink fails to lubricate the cornea sufficiently, and frank lagophthalmos results in exposure of the ocular surface. Corneal damage from chronic exposure is referred to as exposure keratopathy and can be permanent and sight-threatening. Orbicularis damage and lagophthalmos may result from overly aggressive cautery or resection during eyelid surgery, overtreatment of hemifacial spasm or blepharospasm, facial nerve palsy, or trauma.

Both a weakened orbicularis and mild lagophthalmos are common in the immediate postoperative period following upper eyelid surgery as a result of disruption to the orbicularis muscle, even after orbicularis-sparing upper blepharoplasty. Fortunately, these phenomena are typically temporary and easily mitigated with the use of ophthalmic ointments, particularly at night when the exposed ocular surface is more vulnerable to desiccation. However, if too much tissue is removed during upper eyelid or brow surgery, lagophthalmos may be permanent and require intervention. In patients with preexisting dry eye disease, the corneal consequences may be more severe.

Bell's Phenomenon

Bell's phenomenon, also known as the palpebral oculogyric reflex, is a reflexive upward and outward rotation of the globes on eyelid closure mediated by cranial nerve III. While the neurobiology underlying this reflex is not well understood, the reflex is an important mechanism for protecting the cornea in the event of threat. Poor Bell's phenomenon is common in third nerve palsy and myopathic disorders such as myotonic dystrophy and chronic progressive external ophthalmoplegia. Conservative ptosis repair in these patients is important to prevent corneal exposure.

Dry Eye Disease and the Anatomy of the Tear Film

Dry eye disease is a multifactorial disorder of the ocular surface that results in symptoms of discomfort and blurry vision, "in which tear film instability and hyperosmolarity, ocular surface inflammation and damage, and neurosensory abnormalities play etiological roles," as described in a newly updated definition by the Tear Film and Ocular Surface Society's Dry Eye Workshop II (DEWS II) international committee.[25] Dry eye disease is historically thought of as aqueous deficient or evaporative, indicating a deficiency in the aqueous or lipid layers, respectively. However, our understanding of the complexity of dry eye disease has broadened more recently, as we come to understand the importance of inflammatory mediators, eyelid margin disease, and a variety of other contributing factors.

There are three components to the tear film: mucin, aqueous, and lipid. The mucin component of the tear film, which lies adjacent to the ocular surface, is secreted by the conjunctival goblet cells and helps to ensure that the tears spread and adequately cover the corneal surface. Deficiency of the mucin component is most commonly the result of vitamin A deficiency, cicatrizing conjunctival disorders, or the excessive use of particular eye drops.

The middle, aqueous component of the tear film is primarily secreted by the accessory lacrimal glands of Krause and Wolfring and supplemented by the lacrimal gland.[26] This layer is the predominant contributor to tear volume and, when deficient, is a major contributor to dry eye pathology. A wide array of systemic conditions can lead to inadequate tear production, most notably Sjögren's syndrome, though most dry eye syndrome patients do not have an identifiable, underlying systemic condition.

The outermost, lipid layer of the tear film is produced by the meibomian glands and glands of Zeiss and prevents premature evaporation of the tears. It is most commonly disrupted in meibomian gland dysfunction and blepharitis.

Given its prevalence, mention of rosacea is critical. Rosacea is a chronic inflammatory condition of the skin that primarily affects the face. Eye involvement is present in about 75% of those afflicted and manifests with many of the symptoms of dry eye disease, including burning, tearing, redness, and itching. Treatment of mild ocular rosacea is with artificial tears and eyelid hygiene, whereas more severe disease is treated with any one or more of the following: cyclosporine eye drops, metronidazole or fusidic acid gel, oral doxycycline, or light-based therapy.[27]

Dry Eye Testing and Treatment

Diagnosis and quantification of dry eye can be performed in the office setting. The Schirmer test can be performed even in the absence of a slit lamp or other specialized ophthalmologic equipment. In this test, a paper strip with millimeter markings is placed in the inferior fornix, and the moistened portion is measured after 5 minutes (▶ Fig. 2.13). The test is most commonly performed following application of a drop of topical anesthetic (e.g., proparacaine) to limit reflexive tearing, in which case it measures basal tear secretion. Less than 10 mm of moisture at 5 minutes is indicative of dry eye, and lower numbers indicate more severe pathology.

For those practitioners who have a facility with slit lamp examination, two other useful tests are fluorescein staining of the corneal surface and measurement of tear breakup time (TBUT). After instillation of fluorescein into the inferior conjunctival fornix, a cobalt blue filter is used to assess the appearance of the corneal surface. Punctate epithelial erosions, appearing as green dots, often indicate the presence of dry eye. TBUT is a measure of tear film stability; an unstable tear film is associated with more rapid breakup and a lower TBUT. To measure TBUT, after a few blinks, the patient is asked to stare forward without blinking, and the time until the appearance of the first hole in the tear film is measured. Normal TBUT is greater than or equal to 10 seconds.[28]

More specialized in office testing exists to assess tear quality and quantify the severity of dry eye disease, and many cornea and external disease specialists employ several of these techniques concurrently and in conjunction with those previously

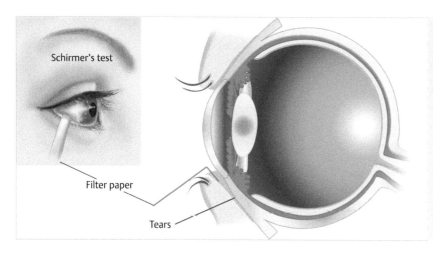

Fig. 2.13 Schirmer's testing. Illustration of the location of the paper strip during Schirmer's testing to assess eye dryness. (Reproduced with permission from https://www.health.harvard.edu/diseases-and-conditions/dry-eye-syndrome.)

mentioned to help characterize dry eye. The Ocular Surface Disease Index questionnaire is a 12-item scale on which patients rate a variety of symptoms related to dryness, providing a subjective assessment of dry eye severity that is, perhaps, the most individually relevant. There are also in-office testing systems that objectively measure different qualities of the tear film: tear osmolarity (TearLab Osmolarity System), lactoferrin (Touch Tear Microassay System) inflammatory markers such as matrix metalloproteinase 9 (InflammaDry), lipid layer thickness and quality (LipiView), tear meniscus height measured by interferometry[29] or anterior segment optical coherence tomography,[30] and meibomian gland dropout measured by infrared meibomography.[31]

Treatment of dry eye is undertaken in a stepwise fashion.[32,33] When a systemic root cause can be identified, it should be addressed directly.

Regardless of the etiology, the mainstay of dry eye treatment is with lubricating eye drops and ointments. In cases that are poorly responsive to this regimen, other topical treatments, including steroids, cyclosporine, lifitegrast, and secretagogues, may be employed. In the most severe cases, alternative topical anti-inflammatory agents or autologous serum tears may be helpful in targeting the root cause of the tear film abnormalities. Patients may also be given oral secretagogues. Nutritional supplements (e.g., omega-3 fatty acids) have been suggested for treatment of dry eye disease, but more recent evidence argues against its effectiveness.[34]

When dry eye is refractory to the aforementioned interventions or when such interventions are too difficult for patient compliance, punctal occlusion by mechanical plugging or cauterization can be helpful by reducing tear drainage. When this fails, a prosthetic replacement of the ocular surface ecosystem lens may be employed,[35] which is a scleral lens that is vaulted, so that the ocular surface is continuously bathed in tears. Upper eyelid and eyebrow surgery should be performed with caution in these refractory dry eye disease patients.

When possible, dry eye treatment should be tailored, targeting the problematic component.[32,33] For example, in patients with mucin deficiency, vitamin A ointment may also be prescribed. Patients with meibomian gland dysfunction/blepharitis should be encouraged to pursue eyelid hygiene and eyelid scrubs and may additionally use topical or oral antibiotic agents, such as doxycycline or tetracycline, primarily for their anti-inflammatory properties.

References

[1] Collin JR, Beard C, Wood I. Experimental and clinical data on the insertion of the levator palpebrae superioris muscle. Am J Ophthalmol. 1978; 85(6):792–801

[2] Saonanon P. Update on Asian eyelid anatomy and clinical relevance. Curr Opin Ophthalmol. 2014; 25(5):436–442

[3] Rohrich RJ, Pessa JE. The fat compartments of the face: anatomy and clinical implications for cosmetic surgery. Plast Reconstr Surg. 2007; 119(7):2219–2227, discussion 2228–2231

[4] Prendergast PM. Anatomy of the face and neck. In: Shiffman MA, DiGiuseppe A, eds. Cosmetic Surgery: Art and Techniques. Berlin: Springer; 2013:29–45

[5] Dumont T, Simon E, Stricker M, Kahn JL, Chassagne JF. Facial fat: descriptive and functional anatomy, from a review of literature and dissections of 10 split-faces. Ann Chir Plast Esthet. 2007; 52(1):51–61

[6] Alghoul M, Codner MA. Retaining ligaments of the face: review of anatomy and clinical applications. Aesthet Surg J. 2013; 33(6):769–782

[7] Goldberg RA. The endoscopic brow lift. In: Fry CL, ed. New Orleans Academy of Ophthalmology: Current Concepts in Aesthetic and Reconstructive Oculoplastic Surgery. the Hague: Kugler Publications; 1999:39–52

[8] Nerad JA. Techniques in Ophthalmic Plastic Surgery: A Personal Tutorial. Philadelphia, PA: Saunders Elsevier; 2010

[9] Ghavami A, Pessa JE, Janis J, Khosla R, Reece EM, Rohrich RJ. The orbicularis retaining ligament of the medial orbit: closing the circle. Plast Reconstr Surg. 2008; 121(3):994–1001

[10] Muzaffar AR, Mendelson BC, Adams WP, Jr. Surgical anatomy of the ligamentous attachments of the lower lid and lateral canthus. Plast Reconstr Surg. 2002; 110(3):873–884, discussion 897–911

[11] Dutton JJ. Atlas of Clinical and Surgical Orbital Anatomy. 2nd ed. Philadelphia, PA: Saunders Elsevier; 2011

[12] Anderson RL, Dixon RS. The role of Whitnall's ligament in ptosis surgery. Arch Ophthalmol. 1979; 97(4):705–707

[13] Kakizaki H, Zako M, Nakano T, Asamoto K, Miyaishi O, Iwaki M. The levator aponeurosis consists of two layers that include smooth muscle. Ophthal Plast Reconstr Surg. 2005; 21(5):379–382

[14] Marcet MM, Setabutr P, Lemke BN, et al. Surgical microanatomy of the müller muscle-conjunctival resection ptosis procedure. Ophthal Plast Reconstr Surg. 2010; 26(5):360–364

[15] Zide BM. ROOF and beyond (superolateral zone). In: Zide BM, Jelks GW, eds. Surgical Anatomy around the Orbit. The System of Zones. Philadelphia, PA: Lippincott Williams & Wilkins; 2006:57

[16] Meyer DR, Linberg JV, Wobig JL, McCormick SA. Anatomy of the orbital septum and associated eyelid connective tissues. Implications for ptosis surgery. Ophthal Plast Reconstr Surg. 1991; 7(2):104–113

[17] Ullmann Y, Levi Y, Ben-Izhak O, Har-Shai Y, Peled IJ. The surgical anatomy of the fat in the upper eyelid medial compartment. Plast Reconstr Surg. 1997; 99(3):658–661

[18] Persichetti P, Di Lella F, Delfino S, Scuderi N. Adipose compartments of the upper eyelid: anatomy applied to blepharoplasty. Plast Reconstr Surg. 2004; 113(1):373–378, discussion 379–380

[19] Tucker SM, Linberg JV. Vascular anatomy of the eyelids. Ophthalmology. 1994; 101(6):1118–1121

[20] Nijhawan N, Marriott C, Harvey JT. Lymphatic drainage patterns of the human eyelid: assessed by lymphoscintigraphy. Ophthal Plast Reconstr Surg. 2010; 26(4):281–285

[21] Seckel BR. Facial Danger Zones: Avoiding Nerve Injury in Facial Plastic Surgery. St. Louis, MO: Quality Medical Publishing, Inc; 1994

[22] Kakizaki H, Selva D, Asamoto K, Nakano T, Leibovitch I. Orbital septum attachment sites on the levator aponeurosis in Asians and whites. Ophthal Plast Reconstr Surg. 2010; 26(4):265–268

[23] Jeong S, Lemke BN, Dortzbach RK, Park YG, Kang HK. The Asian upper eyelid: an anatomical study with comparison to the Caucasian eyelid. Arch Ophthalmol. 1999; 117(7):907–912

[24] Dailey RA, Saulny SM, Sullivan SA. Müller muscle-conjunctival resection: effect on tear production. Ophthal Plast Reconstr Surg. 2002; 18(6):421–425

[25] Jones L, Downie LE, Korb D, et al. TFOS DEWS II Management and therapy report. Ocul Surf. 2017; 15(3):575–628

[26] Jones LT. The lacrimal secretory system and its treatment. Am J Ophthalmol. 1966; 62(1):47–60

[27] van Zuuren EJ. Rosacea. N Engl J Med. 2017; 377(18):1754–1764

[28] Lemp MA, Hamill JR, Jr. Factors affecting tear film breakup in normal eyes. Arch Ophthalmol. 1973; 89(2):103–105

[29] Savini G, Prabhawasat P, Kojima T, Grueterich M, Espana E, Goto E. The challenge of dry eye diagnosis. Clin Ophthalmol. 2008; 2(1):31–55

[30] Czajkowski G, Kaluzny BJ, Laudencka A, Malukiewicz G, Kaluzny JJ. Tear meniscus measurement by spectral optical coherence tomography. Optom Vis Sci. 2012; 89(3):336–342

[31] Chhadva P, Goldhardt R, Galor A. Meibomian gland disease: the role of gland dysfunction in dry eye disease. Ophthalmology. 2017; 124 11S:S20–S26

[32] Kent C. Three new algorithms for treating dry eye. Rev Ophthalmol. 2017; 24 (10):24–35

[33] Milner MS, Beckman KA, Luchs JI, et al. Dysfunctional tear syndrome: dry eye disease and associated tear film disorders – new strategies for diagnosis and treatment. Curr Opin Ophthalmol. 2017; 27 Suppl 1:3–47

[34] Asbell PA, Maguire MG, Pistilli M, et al. Dry Eye Assessment and Management Study Research Group. n-3 fatty acid supplementation for the treatment of dry eye disease. N Engl J Med. 2018; 378(18):1681–1690

[35] Chahal JS, Heur M, Chiu GB. Prosthetic replacement of the ocular surface ecosystem scleral lens therapy for exposure keratopathy. Eye Contact Lens. 2017; 43(4):240–244

3 Anatomic Considerations in the Aesthetic Surgery of the Upper Face

Maria Suzanne Sabundayo, Hirohiko Kakizaki

Abstract

Aesthetic management of the upper eyelids and face requires a thorough understanding of differences in anatomy, gender, and race. These differences are important to recognize to understand their clinical implications for surgery and thereby achieve good cosmetic and functional outcomes.

Keywords: aesthetic surgery, eyelids, upper face, facial beauty, race, gender

3.1 Introduction

Facial beauty is an evolving concept comprising objective, subjective, and relational aspects, broadly defined by culturally prescribed representations.[1,2] Treatment is, therefore, sought to correct underlying structural features that may produce a negative aesthetic impact.[1] The ideals of facial beauty continually change over time. Old beauty standards were determined by anthropometric data, dating back from the canons of facial aesthetics from the Renaissance era.[3,4] These, however, no longer represent the current perceptions of facial beauty.

Recent studies have reported that beauty ideals and attractiveness are broadly consistent regardless of race, age, or nationality,[5,6] yet slight differences exist in terms of specifically desired shapes and characteristics that are thought to enhance existing ethnic features.[6–8] Asians were initially perceived to undergo aesthetic surgery to achieve a "Westernized" beauty; however, the new science of beauty emphasizes the optimization of one's existing features, such as wanting to look like beautiful Asians rather than distinctly "Western."[7,8] In terms of the upper face, the current ideals for the female Asian face include a smooth, convex forehead and large eyes,[6] while Caucasian females who similarly have a relatively large forehead, small jaw, and large eyes are deemed attractive.[9] Wide-set eyes and a lower brow position are also considered attractive features regardless of race.[10] On the contrary, some contend that the current concept of facial beauty depends on dynamic features such as facial expression[1] and facial proportions rather than specific facial traits.[3,8]

The eyelids and eyebrows are the most important landmarks and distinguishing features of the upper face.[11] As such, these structures are usually the focus of aesthetic surgery. While the proper planning of surgery entails a detailed understanding of anatomy, differences exist according to race and gender. These variations, along with an adequate understanding of patient motivations and expectations, are equally important considerations for the evaluation and aesthetic treatment of the upper face.

3.2 Racial Differences

Racial differences in facial structures are well recognized in that comparative anthropometric studies have been previously done on one or more of the following principal racial groups: Caucasians (Europeans and Native Americans), Africans, and Asians.[12–17] The greatest variation is seen within the upper third of the face[18]; in fact, the two most studied facial structures in aesthetic surgery are the eyes and nose, which show the highest degree of interethnic variability.[15]

In general, Caucasian groups of Europe and North America share similar facial morphology, while similarities in the morphology of the head, mouth, and ear are observed across all ethnic groups and races.[13] Africans share identical intercanthal distance with Caucasians; however, variable patterns of eye fissure length and biocular width exist across different African ethnic groups.

Asians, on the other hand, are not a homogenous group but rather comprise many varied ethnicities that possess unique facial characteristics.[6] Farkas et al compared anthropometric measurements among different ethnic groups to normal values established on North American Whites. In their study, Indians and Middle Eastern ethnic groups shared similar orbital measurements such as intercanthal distance, eye fissure length, and biocular width with Caucasians.[13] Southeast Asians (Vietnamese, Chinese of Singapore, and Thais), on the other hand, showed both similarities and differences in upper facial morphology relative to Caucasians. Thai and Vietnamese males showed similar intercanthal distance with Caucasians, while larger measurements were observed among Singaporean Chinese of both sexes, Japanese males, and Vietnamese females. Smaller eye fissure lengths were also seen among Singapore Chinese females and Vietnamese males, while wider biocular widths were observed among Japanese of both sexes.

Asians age differently from Western populations.[7] Facial aging proceeds at a slower rate in Asians compared to their age-matched Caucasian counterparts, which is in part likely due to increased amounts of melanin that provides a higher sun protection factor in Asians. Moreover, the presence of dense fat and fibrous connections in Asians also provide a lower tendency for midfacial sagging.[19]

Most literature on the anatomy of the eyelids and upper face are focused on Caucasians (North Americans and Europeans) and Asians (Japanese, Koreans, native Chinese, or those of Chinese descent) due to the distinct differences mentioned earlier as well as the presence or absence of an upper eyelid crease. The focus of the following sections will be on these two major racial groups.

3.2.1 Eyelid Skin

Skin thickness varies across different regions of the body, and is influenced by factors such as race, age, and sex.[20] In a comparative study of skin thickness among Asians and Caucasians, the epidermis accounts for 8.3 and 4.1–4.2% of the total skin depth in these races, respectively, while dermal thickness is similar in both races.[20]

The upper eyelid has the thinnest skin in the body.[21] In Asians, the thinnest part of the upper eyelid is near the ciliary margin (320 ± 49 μm), followed by the lower tarsal area (703 ± 103 μm) and upper tarsal area (832 ± 203 μm), while the thickest part is just below the eyebrow (1,127 ± 238 μm).[22] The epidermis accounts for 11.2% of the entire skin depth near the ciliary margin compared to only 4.2 to 5.5% at other levels toward the eyebrow.[22] Although no similar study has determined skin thickness at different levels in Caucasian upper eyelids, one study measured skin thickness at different topographic areas of the face. For the upper eyelid, skin thickness was measured on the medial and lateral aspects, with the thinnest part found on the medial eyelid (799 ± 458 μm), followed by the medial canthus (883 ± 592 μm) and the lateral eyelid (1,131 ± 539 μm).[23] It was also found that dermal thickness pattern, and not epidermal thickness, dictates total skin thickness,[23] which is consistent with the finding in Asian eyelids.[22]

The skin of the upper eyelid is generally thicker in Asians (521 ± 115.8 μm)[21] than in Caucasians (380 ± 90 μm).[21,24] Consequently, too much skin removal during Asian upper eyelid blepharoplasty may result in an overhanging or full appearance of the thicker upper skin on the eyelid crease.[25] Because of this, a sub-brow skin excision is often more suitable in Asians to treat dermatochalasis with thicker upper eyelid skin. By contrast, a forehead lift or suprabrow excision is more suitable in Caucasians, as they have more prominent supraorbital rims with lower set eyebrows and less preaponeurotic fat.[26]

3.2.2 Upper Eyelid Crease

The upper eyelid crease is formed by the insertion of the posterior layer of the levator aponeurosis on the anterior aspect of the tarsal plate and subcutaneous tissue (▶ Fig. 3.1a).[27–29] On the other hand, the anterior layer of the levator aponeurosis fuses with the orbital septum.[27–29] The Asian upper eyelid has a less apparent crease and more prominent fold that lead to a fuller appearance compared to Caucasians.[27] This distinction is caused by racial differences in the location of preaponeurotic fat and thickness of the submuscular fibroadipose tissue.[27]

The junction of the orbital septum and the anterior levator aponeurosis is located above the superior tarsal border in both Asians and Caucasians.[27,30] However, preaponeurotic fat or submuscular fibroadipose tissue, which is thicker in Asians, occasionally protrudes inferiorly below the level of the superior tarsal border in Asians.[27,30,31] This interrupts the superficial fibers of the levator aponeurosis from reaching the subcutaneous tissues, resulting in a less apparent upper eyelid crease (▶ Fig. 3.1b).[32,33] In a study of eyelid structure using electron microscopy, it was observed that fibers from the levator aponeurosis penetrate the orbicularis oculi muscle (OOM) and reach the subcutaneous tissue in double eyelids, while none of the fibers pass through the OOM in nondouble eyelids.[34] Furthermore, the height of the upper eyelid tarsal plate is smaller in Asians than Caucasians,[35] which makes the preaponeurotic fat pad extend further downward.

Eyelid crease formation is also associated with the thickness of the OOM, such that a thinner OOM contributes to the formation of a double eyelid.[30] In a Japanese cadaveric study, the OOM was significantly thinner at the skin crease 10 mm from the upper eyelid margin in double eyelids compared to single eyelids, while there was no difference in thickness 3 to 5 and 15 mm from the upper eyelid margin.[30] Thickness of the skin and subcutaneous tissue, however, were not influential factors for double-eyelid formation in this report. In this regard, the surgical creation of a double eyelid entails forming a connection between the levator aponeurosis, tarsal plate, and subcutaneous tissue, as well as reducing the thickness of the OOM.[30]

3.2.3 Epicanthal Fold

An epicanthal fold or epicanthus is a vertical, semilunar fold of redundant skin of the upper eyelid that partially covers the medial canthus and lacrimal lake.[36–38] The term "epicanthus" was first coined in 1860 by Von Ammon.[39] There are four recognized types of epicanthal folds (▶ Fig. 3.2).[40] Epicanthus supraciliaris arises from the eyebrow region; epicanthus palpebralis arises from the upper eyelid; epicanthus tarsalis arises from the tarsal fold and fuses with the skin close to the inner canthus; and epicanthus inversus arises from the lower eyelid.[40] Epicanthus tarsalis is the variant commonly present in the Asian eyelid,[40,41] particularly in East Asians.[42] In fact, it is seen in 50 to 90% of Japanese and Koreans.[43]

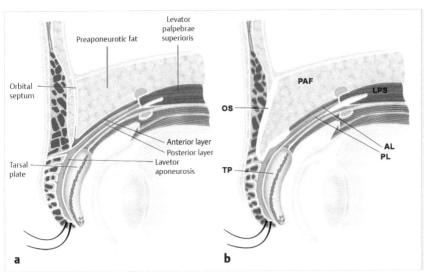

Fig. 3.1 Diagram of upper eyelid anatomy (sagittal section). The levator aponeurosis arises from the thicker superior branch of the levator superioris muscle (LPS). **(a)** The insertion of the posterior layer of the levator aponeurosis (PL) onto the anterior aspect of the tarsal plate (TP) and subcutaneous tissue forms the upper eyelid crease seen in Caucasian or double eyelids. **(b)** Preaponeurotic fat (PAF) may bulge inferiorly below the confluence of the anterior layer of the levator aponeurosis (AL) and orbital septum (OS) in Asian or single eyelids.

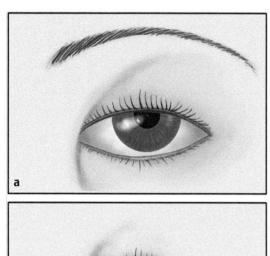

Epicanthus supraciliaris

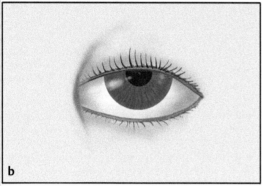

Epicanthus palpebralis

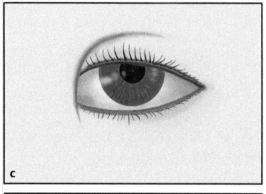

Epicanthus tarsalis

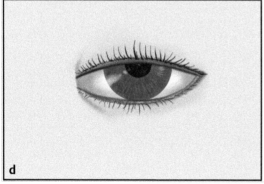

Epicanthus inversus

Fig. 3.2 Types of epicanthal folds. (a) Epicanthus supraciliaris. (b) Epicanthus palpebralis. (c) Epicanthus tarsalis. (d) Epicanthus inversus.

The formation of an epicanthal fold is influenced by the inter-muscular fibers of an obliquely directed preseptal OOM.[44] Therefore, surgical correction of this condition aims to eliminate the fold and establish a normal anatomical structure with minimal scarring by manipulating these muscle fibers.[36] In particular, dissection of deep structures above the medial canthal tendon corresponding to the intermuscular fibers of the preseptal OOM is performed.[45,46] The choice of surgical technique depends on the severity of the epicanthal fold.[45] Horizontal incision method is performed in mild cases, Z-plasty in moderate cases, and V-W plasty in severe cases.[36,45] Skin redraping and other modified techniques are also performed.[43,47]

3.2.4 Tarsal Plate

In the upper eyelid, the average tarsal plate height in Caucasians is significantly greater than in Asians, both microscopically and in vivo.[35] Microscopically, the average tarsal height is 11.3 mm in Caucasians and 9.2 mm in Asians, whereas, in vivo, measurements are 10.1 mm in Caucasians and 8.2 mm in Asians. One study on Japanese eyelids classified the tarsal plate of the upper eyelid into three morphological types.[48] Sickle type was the most common (55%), followed by triangular (29%) and trapezoid (16%) types. These are defined by round, triangular, and flat upper margins, respectively. No similar study was found among Caucasians.

The shape of the tarsal plate plays an important functional and cosmetic role in eyelid surgery. This feature should be considered when applying sutures in double-eyelid and levator suspension procedures for blepharoptosis.[48] In particular, placing sutures in a parallel fashion from the muscle to the upper margin of a trapezoid-shaped tarsus will not yield the same outcome if applied to a triangular-shaped tarsus. This is due to the varying lengths of the suspension muscles at the central and lateral portion in the latter type. Furthermore, the eyelid crease may be blunted laterally in cases of triangular-shaped tarsi because the plate does not extend to the lateral region of the eyelid. Therefore, it is prudent to evaluate the tarsal plate morphology prior to these procedures.

3.2.5 Eyebrow Height and Contour

Eyebrow thickness varies but is not significantly different among races.[11,18,49,50] Eyebrow thickness is generally greater in African Americans than Caucasians,[49] while the same is true in Chinese when compared to Indians and Whites.[18]

The brow apex or superciliare is generally located between the lateral limbus and lateral canthus across races except in Indian males where it was observed 1 to 2 mm lateral to the lateral canthus.[18] The same pattern is seen among Whites and Chinese with the apex more medial in the latter.

3.3 Gender Differences

Gender differences in eyelid and eyebrow anatomy are equally important to consider in the functional and cosmetic surgery of these areas.[51] Dimensions of the palpebral fissure, eyebrow, eyelid crease, and pretarsal skin are some of the parameters that have been compared among males and females in race-specific studies.

3.3.1 Eyelid Skin

Eyelid skin is significantly thicker in males compared to females in both Asian and Caucasian populations.[20,52] The differences between sexes are similar between the two races.[2] This can be explained by the amount of total skin collagen content as a major component of skin thickness that is found less in females.[52] Collagen content is positively correlated with androgen levels, which further justifies this gender variation.[53,54]

3.3.2 Eyelid Dimensions

Palpebral fissure height and width are generally larger in males, while crease and fold height are generally larger in females. In one study, Chinese males showed larger palpebral fissure height and width, intercanthal width, and outercanthal width than their female counterparts.[55] These findings are similar in Caucasians where males also showed significantly larger palpebral fissure width.[56] By contrast, females had slightly larger crease height and margin fold distance,[11,49,55,56] although a study on Malays showed the opposite result.[51] This gender difference was found significant in individuals 2 to 40 years of age, but not in older age groups.[51] Interestingly, these parameters strongly correlated with aesthetic ocular attractiveness among Chinese, in whom a higher eyelid crease is often considered an important representation of "beautiful" eyes.[55]

3.3.3 Eyebrow Height and Contour

The differences in eyebrow height between genders are variable. Larger eyebrow height was observed among White, Indian, and Chinese males compared to their female counterparts in one study,[18] while the opposite was true in a study among South Indians and Malaysian South Indians,[11] and in another study on African Americans and Whites.[49] Meanwhile, females have a higher eyebrow position than males.[11,49,55]

The brow apex is commonly seen between the lateral limbus and lateral canthus across sexes, except in Indian males where it is found lateral to the lateral canthus, as mentioned earlier.[18] However, the apex is seen at a more medial location in White females compared to White males, and in Chinese males compared to Chinese females.[18]

The eyebrows are the most important features of the face for sexual dimorphism and facial recognition.[57] In particular, eyebrow thickness and interbrow distance play essential roles in the identification of male and female faces[58] as well as the perception of facial attractiveness.[59] Thicker eyebrows are perceived as dominant in men,[59] while thinner eyebrows are seen as attractive in women.[60] Higher eyebrow height and greater margin fold distance are also perceived as powerful characteristics that increase facial attractiveness in women.[49] These psychological factors need to be considered in performing surgery.

3.4 Conclusions

A comprehensive and updated review of the racial and gender differences in the anatomy of the upper eyelids and face has been presented. This would facilitate the understanding of their clinical implications for surgery to attain good cosmetic results. Moreover, it is ideal to establish race-specific and gender-specific within race normative values for the dimensions of the eyelid and brow to maximize these outcomes.

References

[1] Rhee SC, An SJ, Hwang R. Contemporary Koreans' perceptions of facial beauty. Arch Plast Surg. 2017; 44(5):390–399

[2] Calogero RM, Boroughs M, Thompson JK. The impact of Western beauty ideals on the lives of women and men: a sociocultural perspective. In: Swami V, Furnham A, eds. Body Beautiful: Evolutionary and Sociocultural Perspectives. New York, NY: Palgrave Macmillan; 2007:259–298

[3] Hashim PW, Nia JK, Taliercio M, Goldenberg G. Ideals of facial beauty. Cutis. 2017; 100(4):222–224

[4] Rhee SC. Differences between Caucasian and Asian attractive faces. Skin Res Technol. 2018; 24(1):73–79

[5] Fink B, Neave N. The biology of facial beauty. Int J Cosmet Sci. 2005; 27(6): 317–325

[6] Liew S, Wu WTL, Chan HH, et al. Consensus of changing trends, attitudes, and concepts of Asian beauty. Aesthetic Plast Surg. 2016; 40(2):193–201

[7] Samizadeh S, Wu W. Ideals of facial beauty amongst the Chinese population: results from a large national survey. Aesthetic Plast Surg. 2018; 42(6):1540–1550

[8] Leem SY. Gangnam-style plastic surgery: the science of westernized beauty in South Korea. Med Anthropol. 2017; 36(7):657–671

[9] Sforza C, Laino A, D'Alessio R, Grandi G, Binelli M, Ferrario VF. Soft-tissue facial characteristics of attractive Italian women as compared to normal women. Angle Orthod. 2009; 79(1):17–23

[10] Rhee SC, Woo KS, Kwon B. Biometric study of eyelid shape and dimensions of different races with references to beauty. Aesthetic Plast Surg. 2012; 36(5): 1236–1245

[11] Packiriswamy V, Kumar P, Bashour M. Photogrammetric analysis of eyebrow and upper eyelid dimensions in South Indians and Malaysian South Indians. Aesthet Surg J. 2013; 33(7):975–982

[12] Goldstein AG. Race-related variation of facial features: anthropometric data I. Bull Psychon Soc. 1979; 13(3):187–190

[13] Farkas LG, Katic MJ, Forrest CR, et al. International anthropometric study of facial morphology in various ethnic groups/races. J Craniofac Surg. 2005; 16 (4):615–646

[14] Zhuang Z, Landsittel D, Benson S, Roberge R, Shaffer R. Facial anthropometric differences among gender, ethnicity, and age groups. Ann Occup Hyg. 2010; 54(4):391–402

[15] Fang F, Clapham PJ, Chung KC. A systematic review of interethnic variability in facial dimensions. Plast Reconstr Surg. 2011; 127(2):874–881

[16] Jagadish Chandra H, Ravi MS, Sharma SM, Rajendra Prasad B. Standards of facial esthetics: an anthropometric study. J Maxillofac Oral Surg. 2012; 11(4):384–389

[17] Gao Y, Niddam J, Noel W, Hersant B, Meningaud JP. Comparison of aesthetic facial criteria between Caucasian and East Asian female populations: anesthetic surgeon's perspective. Asian J Surg. 2018; 41(1):4–11

[18] Kunjur J, Sabesan T, Ilankovan V. Anthropometric analysis of eyebrows and eyelids: an inter-racial study. Br J Oral Maxillofac Surg. 2006; 44(2):89–93

[19] Sykes JM. Management of the aging face in the Asian patient. Facial Plast Surg Clin North Am. 2007; 15(3):353–360, –vi–vii

[20] Lee Y, Hwang K. Skin thickness of Korean adults. Surg Radiol Anat. 2002; 24 (3–4):183–189

[21] Ha RY, Nojima K, Adams WP, Jr, Brown SA. Analysis of facial skin thickness: defining the relative thickness index. Plast Reconstr Surg. 2005; 115(6):1769–1773

[22] Hwang K, Kim DJ, Hwang SH. Thickness of Korean upper eyelid skin at different levels. J Craniofac Surg. 2006; 17(1):54–56

[23] Chopra K, Calva D, Sosin M, et al. A comprehensive examination of topographic thickness of skin in the human face. Aesthet Surg J. 2015; 35(8):1007–1013

[24] Barker DE. Skin thickness in the human. Plast Reconstr Surg (1946). 1951; 7 (2):115–116

[25] Kim YS, Roh TS, Yoo WM, Tark KC, Kim J. Infrabrow excision blepharoplasty: applications and outcomes in upper blepharoplasty in Asian women. Plast Reconstr Surg. 2008; 122(4):1199–1205

[26] Lee D, Law V. Subbrow blepharoplasty for upper eyelid rejuvenation in Asians. Aesthet Surg J. 2009; 29(4):284–288

[27] Kakizaki H, Leibovitch I, Selva D, Asamoto K, Nakano T. Orbital septum attachment on the levator aponeurosis in Asians: in vivo and cadaver study. Ophthalmology. 2009; 116(10):2031–2035

[28] Kakizaki H, Prabhakaran V, Pradeep T, Malhotra R, Selva D. Peripheral branching of levator superioris muscle and Müller muscle origin. Am J Ophthalmol. 2009; 148(5):800–803.e1

[29] Kakizaki H, Zako M, Nakano T, Asamoto K, Miyaishi O, Iwaki M. The levator aponeurosis consists of two layers that include smooth muscle. Ophthal Plast Reconstr Surg. 2005; 21(5):379–382

[30] Kakizaki H, Takahashi Y, Nakano T, et al. The causative factors or characteristics of the Asian double eyelid: an anatomic study. Ophthal Plast Reconstr Surg. 2012; 28(5):376–381

[31] Miyake I, Tange I, Hiraga Y. MRI findings of the upper eyelid and their relationship with single- and double-eyelid formation. Aesthetic Plast Surg. 1994; 18(2):183–187

[32] Doxanas MT, Anderson RL. Oriental eyelids. An anatomic study. Arch Ophthalmol. 1984; 102(8):1232–1235

[33] Jeong S, Lemke BN, Dortzbach RK, Park YG, Kang HK. The Asian upper eyelid: an anatomical study with comparison to the Caucasian eyelid. Arch Ophthalmol. 1999; 117(7):907–912

[34] Cheng J, Xu FZ. Anatomic microstructure of the upper eyelid in the Oriental double eyelid. Plast Reconstr Surg. 2001; 107(7):1665–1668

[35] Goold LA, Casson RJ, Selva D, Kakizaki H. Tarsal height. Ophthalmology. 2009; 116(9):1831–1831.e2

[36] del Campo AF. Surgical treatment of the epicanthal fold. Plast Reconstr Surg. 1984; 73(4):566–571

[37] Fujiwara T, Maeda M, Kuwae K, Nishino K. Modified split V-W plasty for entropion with an epicanthal fold in Asian eyelids. Plast Reconstr Surg. 2006; 118(3):635–642

[38] Choi HL, Lee MC, Kim YS, Lew DH. Medial epicanthoplasty using a modified skin redraping method. Arch Aesthetic Plast Surg. 2014; 20:15–19

[39] Von Ammon FA. Epicanthus und das epiblepharon. Behr Hildebr J Kinder. 1860; 34:313

[40] Johnson CC. Epicanthus and epiblepharon. Arch Ophthalmol. 1978; 96(6): 1030–1033

[41] Rubenzik R. Surgical revision of the oriental lid. Ann Ophthalmol. 1977; 9(9): 1189–1192

[42] Kwon B, Nguyen AH. Reconsideration of the epicanthus: evolution of the eyelid and the devolutional concept of Asian blepharoplasty. Semin Plast Surg. 2015; 29(3):171–183

[43] Park JI. Modified Z-epicanthoplasty in the Asian eyelid. Arch Facial Plast Surg. 2000; 2(1):43–47

[44] Kakizaki H, Ichinose A, Nakano T, Asamoto K, Ikeda H. Anatomy of the epicanthal fold. Plast Reconstr Surg. 2012; 130(3):494e–495e

[45] Wang S, Shi F, Luo X, et al. Epicanthal fold correction: our experience and comparison among three kinds of epicanthoplasties. J Plast Reconstr Aesthet Surg. 2013; 66(5):682–687

[46] Jordan DR, Anderson RL. Epicanthal folds. A deep tissue approach. Arch Ophthalmol. 1989; 107(10):1532–1535

[47] Oh YW, Seul CH, Yoo WM. Medial epicanthoplasty using the skin redraping method. Plast Reconstr Surg. 2007; 119(2):703–710

[48] Nagasao T, Shimizu Y, Ding W, Jiang H, Kishi K, Imanishi N. Morphological analysis of the upper eyelid tarsus in Asians. Ann Plast Surg. 2011; 66(2): 196–201

[49] Price KM, Gupta PK, Woodward JA, Stinnett SS, Murchison AP. Eyebrow and eyelid dimensions: an anthropometric analysis of African Americans and Caucasians. Plast Reconstr Surg. 2009; 124(2):615–623

[50] Cartwright MJ, Kurumety UR, Nelson CC, Frueh BR, Musch DC. Measurements of upper eyelid and eyebrow dimensions in healthy white individuals. Am J Ophthalmol. 1994; 117(2):231–234

[51] Dharap AS, Reddy SC. Upper eyelid and eyebrow dimensions in Malays. Med J Malaysia. 1995; 50(4):377–381

[52] Shuster S, Black MM, McVitie E. The influence of age and sex on skin thickness, skin collagen and density. Br J Dermatol. 1975; 93(6):639–643

[53] Black MM, Shuster S, Bottoms E. Osteoporosis, skin collagen, and androgen. BMJ. 1970; 4(5738):773–774

[54] Shuster S, Black MM, Bottoms E. Skin collagen and thickness in women with hirsuties. BMJ. 1970; 4(5738):772

[55] Li Q, Zhang X, Li K, et al. Normative anthropometric analysis and aesthetic indication of the ocular region for young Chinese adults. Graefes Arch Clin Exp Ophthalmol. 2016; 254(1):189–197

[56] van den Bosch WA, Leenders I, Mulder P. Topographic anatomy of the eyelids, and the effects of sex and age. Br J Ophthalmol. 1999; 83(3):347–352

[57] Bashour M. Is an Objective Measuring System for Facial Attractiveness Possible? (PhD thesis). Toronto, CA: University of Toronto; 2005:291

[58] Bruce V, Burton AM, Hanna E, et al. Sex discrimination: how do we tell the difference between male and female faces? Perception. 1993; 22(2):131–152

[59] Keating CF. Gender and the physiognomy of dominance and attractiveness. Soc Psychol Q. 1985; 48:61–70

[60] Johnston VS, Solomon CJ, Gibson SJ, Pallares-Bejarano A. Human facial beauty: current theories and methodologies. Arch Facial Plast Surg. 2003; 5 (5):371–377

Section II Mechanical Ptosis

4 Mechanical Ptosis: Etiology and Management

Eric B. Hamill, Michael T. Yen

Abstract

Mechanical ptosis is the inferior displacement of the upper eyelid due to the mass or restrictive effect of an acquired eyelid lesion. The cause of mechanical ptosis is usually readily identifiable on clinical examination. Because the eyelid's neuromuscular retraction system remains intact, treatment for mechanical ptosis is directed at the underlying mass or restrictive disease process. This chapter highlights several common causes of mechanical ptosis and treatment options for the underlying conditions.

Keywords: mechanical ptosis, restrictive ptosis, cicatricial ptosis, eyelid mass, orbital mass, orbital trauma

4.1 Introduction

Mechanical ptosis is the inferior displacement of the upper eyelid due to the mass or restrictive effect of an acquired eyelid or orbital lesion. The eyelid's neuromuscular retraction system remains intact but is unable to overcome an opposing force generated by the mass or restrictive process. Mechanical ptosis is often readily identifiable on clinical examination and easy to differentiate from more common causes of ptosis such as involutional, myogenic, or neurogenic etiologies. Medical or surgical treatment for mechanical ptosis is directed at the underlying disease process.

4.2 Benign Eyelid Lesions

Any space-occupying lesion of the eyelid has the potential to cause mechanical ptosis. The amount of ptosis depends on the location and size of the lesion. Examples of benign eyelid lesions that may cause mechanical ptosis include infantile hemangiomas, chalazia, and plexiform neurofibromas.

Infantile hemangiomas are benign proliferations of capillary endothelial cells that frequently occur on the face and periocular region. They typically present in the first few months of life as a rapidly enlarging vascular lesion commonly involving the superomedial or medial aspect of the upper eyelid of an infant (▶ Fig. 4.1). After an initial proliferative phase of approximately 6 months, these lesions often stabilize and spontaneously regress at 1 year of age. Small, clinically insignificant eyelid hemangiomas may be observed without intervention. Larger lesions causing ocular morbidity, such as mechanical ptosis, visually significant astigmatism, or occlusion of the visual axis, should prompt the clinician to consider intervention. Treatment in these cases is aimed at improving cosmesis and preventing refractive or occlusion amblyopia.

First-line therapy for patients with an infantile hemangioma is oral propranolol at a dose of 1 to 3 mg/kg/day through the proliferative phase or approximately 4 to 6 months.[1] Topical timolol maleate is a viable alternative for superficial eyelid lesions. Both propranolol and timolol maleate are well tolerated and highly effective at inducing tumor regression. A thorough cardiac evaluation should be performed prior to initiation of β-blocker therapy and the infant should be monitored for cardiac events throughout treatment. Treatment options for lesions refractory to β-blocker therapy include surgical excision or intralesional corticosteroids.

Chalazia are a common cause of mechanical ptosis (▶ Fig. 4.2). If large enough to affect the eyelid's position, visual dysfunction usually results not from occlusion of the visual axis but induced corneal astigmatism. Initial treatment consists of warm compresses and gentle pressure to promote drainage of the lesion. If noninvasive therapy fails, intralesional injections of triamcinolone or curettage may be indicated. Intralesional corticosteroids are best reserved for those with small chalazia and fair skin. Incision and curettage is a better option for those with larger lesions or darker skin types. Recurrent chalazia warrant biopsy to rule out an occult malignant neoplasm.

Plexiform neurofibromas of the eyelid occur almost uniformly in association with neurofibromatosis type 1. This diffusely infiltrating lesion tends to involve the lateral aspect of the upper eyelid margin, giving it a characteristic **S**-shaped contour. Large eyelid plexiform neurofibromas may cause mechanical ptosis, corneal astigmatism, occlusion amblyopia, or psychosocial morbidity from poor cosmesis and low self-esteem (▶ Fig. 4.3). Minimizing the risk of amblyopia and improving

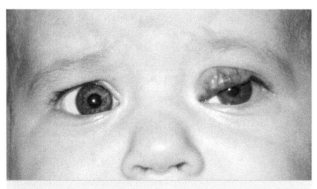

Fig. 4.1 Infantile hemangioma of the medial left upper eyelid with mechanical ptosis encroaching on the visual axis.

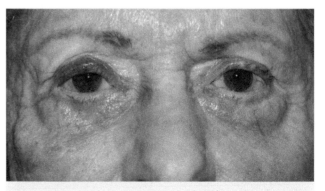

Fig. 4.2 Chalazion of the right upper eyelid resulting in mechanical ptosis.

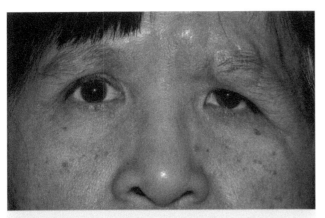

Fig. 4.3 Plexiform neurofibroma of the left upper eyelid causing significant ptosis of the eyelid.

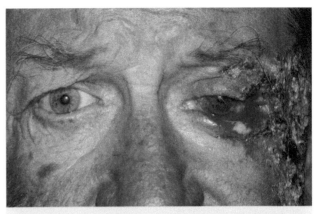

Fig. 4.4 Extensive neglected basal cell carcinoma of the left face causing ptosis of the left upper eyelid along with ulceration of the lateral canthus and lower eyelid.

physical appearance are the most common indications for intervention. Treatment involves surgical debulking, though their infiltrative nature and lack of encapsulation make plexiform neurofibromas challenging to manage. At the time of surgery, levator dehiscence and lateral canthal tendon disinsertion are frequently encountered and often require repair.[2] Long-term complications are usually related to tumor recurrence, particularly in children under 10 years of age.[3]

4.3 Malignant Eyelid Lesions

Cutaneous malignancies, such as basal cell carcinoma, squamous cell carcinoma, sebaceous carcinoma, and melanoma, may present on the eyelid with mechanical ptosis. Of these, basal cell carcinoma is the most common and accounts for more than 90% of all periorbital skin cancers. Morbidity is almost always due to local invasion into adjacent structures. Tumors large enough to cause mechanical ptosis typically have been present for many years and may have already invaded the orbit (▶ Fig. 4.4). Because basal cell carcinoma occurs most commonly in the elderly, younger patients presenting with basal cell carcinoma should raise suspicion for basal cell nevus syndrome, xeroderma pigmentosum, or an immunosuppressed state.[4]

Squamous cell carcinoma of the eyelid occurs much less frequently than basal cell carcinoma. This lesion has a tendency to spread via perineural or lymphatic invasion. If an eyelid squamous cell carcinoma is large enough to cause mechanical ptosis, it is important to palpate regional lymph nodes and consider perineural spread.[5]

Sebaceous carcinoma is a rare but highly lethal neoplasm of the eyelid's sebaceous glands. It occurs more commonly in the upper eyelid, likely due to a greater number and concentration of sebaceous glands as compared to the lower eyelid (▶ Fig. 4.5). Sebaceous carcinoma is known as a great masquerader, and its presentation may mimic chronic blepharitis, chalazia, or nonspecific inflammatory changes. Consequently, the diagnosis is often missed or delayed.[6] Rarely, other cutaneous malignancies, such as melanoma and Merkel cell carcinoma, present with mechanical ptosis. Like sebaceous carcinoma, these lesions have a high mortality rate and portend a poor prognosis.

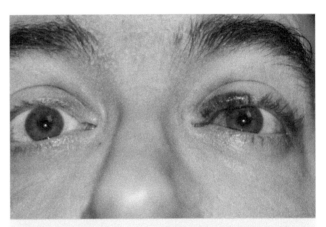

Fig. 4.5 Sebaceous cell carcinoma of the left upper eyelid resulting in mechanical ptosis. There is also pagetoid spread of the malignancy to the medial bulbar conjunctiva.

The management for most malignant eyelid neoplasms is complete surgical excision with eyelid reconstruction. In contrast to medical therapy, excision allows for histologic confirmation of the diagnosis and definitive tumor clearance at the margin. Lesions large enough to cause mechanical ptosis typically require extensive tissue removal. Reconstructions are often challenging and require rotational flaps or skin grafts. The particular reconstructive procedure should be tailored to the size and location of the deficit. With regard to the mechanical ptosis, the upper eyelid position may elevate after lesion excision; however, residual ptosis may persist due to secondary mechanical ptosis from the bulk of the reconstructed flaps or grafts, cicatrization to the levator aponeurosis and muscle, or levator dehiscence after surgery.

Not all neoplastic eyelid lesions causing mechanical ptosis are primary tumors. Breast, lung, gastric, and prostate carcinoma as well as both cutaneous and uveal melanomas have been reported to metastasize to the eyelid.[7,8] These lesions are typically small, solitary nodules but may become large enough to cause mechanical ptosis. Biopsy often reveals the diagnosis. Lymphoma, though classically associated with orbital disease, may also present with a facial mass or regional lymphatic obstruction producing periocular edema and a mechanical ptosis.[9] Treatment in all cases of systemic malignancy is aimed at the underlying disease and should be coordinated with an oncologist.

4.4 Orbital Lesions

Mechanical ptosis may be a presenting sign or complaint in patients with an anterior orbital lesion. Examples of such lesions include dermoid cyst, lacrimal gland tumors, lymphoproliferative malignancies, rhabdomyosarcoma, and orbital metastases. In addition to mechanical ptosis, clinical examination of these patients often shows nonspecific findings such as periorbital fullness, a palpable mass, chemosis, or skin discoloration.

Orbital dermoid cysts are benign choristomas, containing skin and dermal appendages. They most commonly occur at the frontozygomatic suture but may also be found at the frontonasal suture (▶ Fig. 4.6). These lesions typically present as a slowly progressive, painless mass in the superotemporal or superonasal quadrant of the orbit in a child. Intervention is usually performed to improve cosmesis, though rarely these lesions may become large enough to cause mechanical ptosis and occlude the visual axis. Orbital dermoid cysts are usually readily accessible through an eyelid crease incision and should be completely excised.

Rhabdomyosarcoma is a highly malignant mesenchymal tumor associated with significant morbidity and mortality if untreated. When arising in the orbit, the classic presentation is a new, rapidly progressive unilateral proptosis with globe displacement in a child. Mechanical ptosis is a presenting sign in 30 to 50% of patients, typically with overlying skin changes such as edema and erythema (▶ Fig. 4.7). After establishing the diagnosis, the mainstay of treatment is radiation and systemic chemotherapy. If detected early, these tumors have a relatively good prognosis. Small, encapsulated lesions may be surgically excised in conjunction with radiation and chemotherapy.[10]

Adult patients with a history of malignancy presenting with an orbital lesion causing mechanical ptosis should elicit a high suspicion for metastatic disease (▶ Fig. 4.8a, b). Breast and lung carcinomas are the most common primary malignancies to metastasize to the orbit (▶ Fig. 4.9). Orbital metastases from breast carcinoma may show a unique scirrhous reaction in which orbital soft tissues fibrose and retract, often causing enophthalmos, ptosis, and restricted ocular motility. The clinician should consider metastatic disease in any patient with a history of breast cancer presenting with this triad or any of its permutations. Treatment of orbital metastases is usually palliative and may involve local radiation therapy.

4.5 Periorbital Infections and Inflammation

Both preseptal and orbital cellulitis commonly present with mechanical ptosis. Eyelid changes include edema, erythema, and warmth; the edema is often significant enough to cause inferior displacement of the upper eyelid (▶ Fig. 4.10). Medical management includes treating the underlying infectious process with the appropriate antimicrobials. If an eyelid abscess is

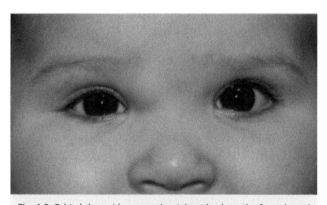

Fig. 4.6 Orbital dermoid cyst on the right side along the frontal-nasal suture line resulting in mechanical ptosis of the right upper eyelid.

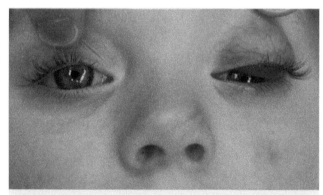

Fig. 4.7 Orbital rhabdomyosarcoma of the left superior orbit causing mechanical ptosis of the left upper eyelid. The overlying skin of the left upper eyelid is erythematous, and there is also tumor protruding into the superior fornix.

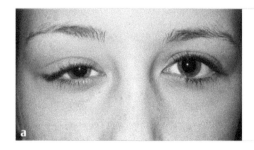

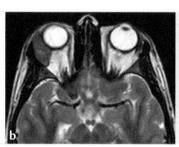

Fig. 4.8 (a) Leukemic infiltrate of the right lacrimal gland causing mechanical ptosis of the right upper eyelid with an S-shaped configuration to the eyelid. (b) Axial cut of the orbital magnetic resonance imaging (MRI) show significant enlargement of the right lacrimal gland.

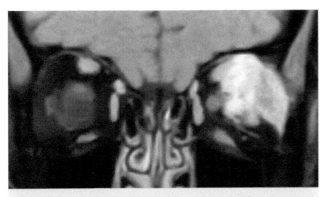

Fig. 4.9 Coronal cuts of an orbital MRI in a patient with metastatic breast carcinoma to the superior orbit.

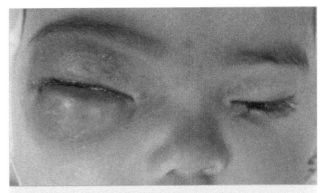

Fig. 4.10 Preseptal cellulitis of the right upper eyelid with significant erythema and edema resulting in mechanical ptosis.

present, surgical drainage may facilitate the resolution of the infection. Corticosteroids may also aid the resolution of eyelid inflammation and mechanical ptosis.[11]

Blepharochalasis is a rare and particularly challenging cause of mechanical ptosis. This condition is characterized by chronic and recurrent episodes of idiopathic angioedema localized to the eyelids, usually in a child or adolescent. Patients often present during an acute episode with marked eyelid edema and complaints of mechanical ptosis. Recurrent episodes lead to loss of dermal elastic tissue, wrinkled and discolored periorbital skin, and atrophy of the periorbital fat pads. Notably, levator function is preserved. Though many different triggers have been reported to cause flares, the etiology of disease remains unknown.

Treatment options for mechanical ptosis caused by blepharochalasis are limited. There is currently no effective medical management for the acute episode of eyelid angioedema; rather, treatment involves supportive care until the angioedema subsides, which usually occurs in 3 to 5 days. In chronic relapsing–remitting disease, stretching or disinsertion of the levator aponeurosis may occur at which time the ptosis is managed as aponeurotic ptosis.[12] Surgical repair should be performed during a quiescent phase of the disease.

Autoimmune and postoperative inflammatory changes may also lead to mechanical ptosis. Mucous membrane pemphigoid, Stevens–Johnson syndrome, trachoma, and chemical burns frequently cause cicatrization of the ocular surface, keratinization and thickening of the tarsal conjunctiva, and symblepharon formation. Adhesions between the palpebral and bulbar conjunctiva may result in an inferiorly displaced eyelid and a mechanical restriction to elevation (▶ Fig. 4.11). Eyes with multiple prior anterior segment surgeries may also present with similar findings.

4.6 Other Considerations

Sometimes, postoperative mechanical ptosis is intentional, as in the case of weighted eyelid implants for paralytic lagophthalmos. Special care is taken to choose a weight that provides adequate lid closure while blinking without excessively obscuring the visual axis in primary gaze. Obscured vision from excessive mechanical ptosis is a known side effect of such procedures and

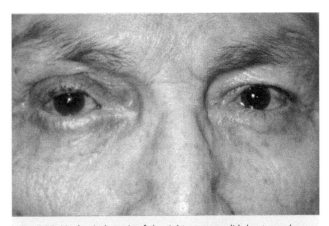

Fig. 4.11 Mechanical ptosis of the right upper eyelid due to ocular cicatricial pemphigoid with resulting conjunctival scarring limiting the excursion of the upper eyelid.

can usually be avoided with careful preoperative planning as well as intraoperative assessment of eyelid position and excursion.

Rarely, orbital and adnexal amyloid may cause mechanical ptosis (▶ Fig. 4.12**a**, **b**). These lesions are typically found within the superior palpebral conjunctiva; however, these lesions may be more extensive and infiltrate the levator complex. Despite the amyloid subtype, most cases of conjunctival amyloid are a primary localized disease without systemic involvement.[13] Cutaneous involvement of the eyelid skin, in contrast, has a much higher association with systemic disease. Curettage and debridement of the amyloid infiltrate with a spooned curette is often effective at debulking the lesion, though additional tightening of the levator aponeurosis may be necessary to fully correct the mechanical ptosis.[14]

Ocular trauma, both blunt and penetrating, are relatively common causes of mechanical ptosis. Blunt trauma to the periorbital region frequently produces mechanical ptosis from eyelid edema. Patients with more extensive craniofacial injuries may have mechanical ptosis from a superiorly located intraorbital foreign body, such as glass or metallic shrapnel, or bone fragment from the orbital roof impinging on the levator complex (▶ Fig. 4.13). Penetrating trauma causing partial or complete transection of either the levator or levator aponeurosis may

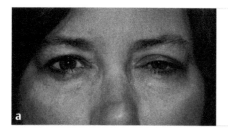
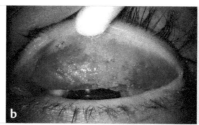

Fig. 4.12 (a) Mechanical ptosis of the left upper eyelid caused by amyloid deposition and infiltration. (b) Eversion of the upper eyelid reveals thick, infiltrative depositions in the palpebral conjunctiva.

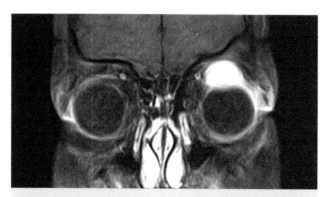

Fig. 4.13 Coronal cuts of an orbital MRI in a patient with a retained orbital foreign body in the superior orbit causing mechanical ptosis.

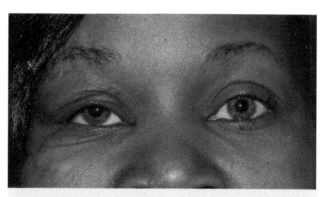

Fig. 4.14 Mechanical ptosis of the right upper eyelid due to previous reconstructive surgery of the eyelid with full-thickness skin graft.

lead to ptosis, depending on the extent of the injury. Surgical exploration of the orbit and levator complex is necessary to remove any impinging material and allow direct visualization and repair of the levator aponeurosis. Iatrogenic trauma, such as from eyelid surgery or postoperative scarring, can also result in mechanical ptosis (▶ Fig. 4.14).

4.7 Summary

Mechanical ptosis refers to the inferior displacement of the upper eyelid due to the mass or restrictive effect of an acquired eyelid lesion. There are many possible underlying causes for mechanical ptosis. Treatment is usually directed at the underlying etiology.

References

[1] Drolet BA, Frommelt PC, Chamlin SL, et al. Initiation and use of propranolol for infantile hemangioma: report of a consensus conference. Pediatrics. 2013; 131(1):128–140

[2] Lee V, Ragge NK, Collin JR. Orbitotemporal neurofibromatosis. Clinical features and surgical management. Ophthalmology. 2004; 111(2):382–388

[3] Avery RA, Katowitz JA, Fisher MJ, et al. OPPN Working Group. Orbital/periorbital plexiform neurofibromas in children with neurofibromatosis type 1. Ophthalmology. 2017; 124(1):123–132

[4] de Imus GC, Arpey CJ. Periorbital Skin Cancers: A Dermatologist's Perspective [eBook]. 2006 Focal Points Collection. American Academy of Ophthalmology; 2006

[5] Faustina M, Diba R, Ahmadi MA, Esmaeli B, Esmaeli B. Patterns of regional and distant metastasis in patients with eyelid and periocular squamous cell carcinoma. Ophthalmology. 2004; 111(10):1930–1932

[6] Shields JA, Demirci H, Marr BP, Eagle RC, Jr, Shields CL. Sebaceous carcinoma of the ocular region: a review. Surv Ophthalmol. 2005; 50(2):103–122

[7] Ahmad SM, Esmaeli B. Metastatic tumors of the orbit and ocular adnexa. Curr Opin Ophthalmol. 2007; 18(5):405–413

[8] Bianciotto C, Demirci H, Shields CL, Eagle RC, Jr, Shields JA. Metastatic tumors to the eyelid: report of 20 cases and review of the literature. Arch Ophthalmol. 2009; 127(8):999–1005

[9] Smith LB, Pynnonen MA, Flint A, Adams JL, Elner VM. Progressive eyelid and facial swelling due to follicular lymphoma. Arch Ophthalmol. 2009; 127(8):1068–1070

[10] Shields JA, Shields CL. Rhabdomyosarcoma: review for the ophthalmologist. Surv Ophthalmol. 2003; 48(1):39–57

[11] Yen MT, Yen KG. Effect of corticosteroids in the acute management of pediatric orbital cellulitis with subperiosteal abscess. Ophthal Plast Reconstr Surg. 2005; 21(5):363–366, discussion 366–367

[12] Koursh DM, Modjtahedi SP, Selva D, Leibovitch I. The blepharochalasis syndrome. Surv Ophthalmol. 2009; 54(2):235–244

[13] Hamill EB, Thyparampil PJ, Yen MT. Localized immunoglobulin light chain amyloid of the conjunctiva confirmed by mass spectrometry without evidence of systemic involvement. Ophthal Plast Reconstr Surg. 2017; 33(5):e108–e110

[14] Patrinely JR, Koch DD. Surgical management of advanced ocular adnexal amyloidosis. Arch Ophthalmol. 1992; 110(6):882–885

5 Upper Blepharoplasty

David B. Samimi

Abstract

Age-related descent and deflation of the upper eyelid and eyebrow often leads to the perception of "saggy upper eyelid skin." Surgical treatment with upper blepharoplasty is described here, with an emphasis on safe and natural-appearing results by orbicularis muscle and preaponeurotic fat preservation, and maintenance of an appropriate upper eyelid crease and fold height.

Keywords: blepharoplasty, upper eyelid blepharoplasty, eyelid lift

5.1 Introduction

Along with being the aesthetic centerpiece of the face, the eyelids are responsible for protecting and framing one's vision. Aging changes related to skin quality and upper facial volume often result in skin descent and potential obstruction of one's visual field (▶ Fig. 5.1a).

Nonsurgical treatment options for upper eyelid skin descent include eyebrow depressor muscle botulinum toxin and hyaluronic acid fillers to lift and fill the upper eyelid–brow complex and are addressed elsewhere in this book. This chapter focuses on the most common surgical procedure for improvement of upper eyelid skin descent, upper blepharoplasty, a technique centered around the artful removal and shaping of upper eyelid skin and soft tissue.

Traditional goals of blepharoplasty have been the elimination or minimization of excess eyelid tissue. This led to a largely subtractive procedure, removing skin, orbicularis muscle, and orbital fat, and placement of a relatively high eyelid crease, resulting in a postsurgical appearance (▶ Fig. 5.2). Upper blepharoplasty technique has evolved in parallel with our understanding of the etiologies of the aging face. The importance of soft tissue volume in the youthful face supports the preservation of upper eyelid preaponeurotic fat during blepharoplasty surgery. The relative prominence of medial fat in the aging upper eyelid has been shown in observational studies and may be related to a higher concentration of stem cells[1,2] (▶ Fig. 5.1). This finding supports selective medial fat removal or repositioning. With the intent of minimizing worsening preexisting dry eye symptoms, in 2007, Dresner et al revealed that upper blepharoplasty with preservation of the orbicularis muscle did not lead to an increase in dry eye symptoms.[3] The patients were also found to have an improvement in postsurgical cosmetic appearance and eyelid blink function. Minimizing trauma or excision to the orbicularis muscle remains one of the most important components of modern upper blepharoplasty surgery.

Failure to identify concurrent blepharoptosis secondary to malfunction or malposition of the levator aponeurosis or eyebrow descent may limit the success of upper blepharoplasty. Treatment of blepharoptosis and eyebrow ptosis can be performed concurrent with upper blepharoplasty as described here and is addressed in other chapters of this book.

5.2 Goals of Treatment

- Functional improvement of superior field of vision when the excess skin causes field loss.
- Improved cosmesis.
- Preservation of a natural appearance.
- Preservation of normal blink and eyelid function.
- Relief from frontalis contraction and compensatory eyebrow elevation.

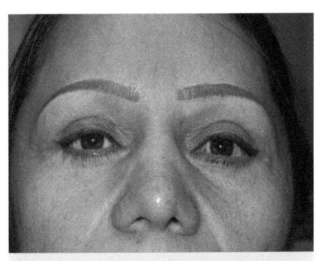

Fig. 5.2 Unnatural-appearing postblepharoplasty result secondary to removal of preaponeurotic fat and orbicularis, and placement of a relatively high eyelid crease.

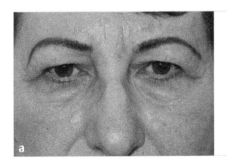
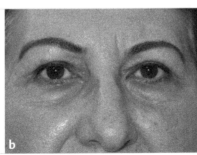

Fig. 5.1 Typical upper blepharoplasty candidate before (a) and after surgery (b).

- Patient satisfaction, optimized by preoperative expectation management.

5.3 Risks

- Vision loss from orbital hemorrhage.
- Temporary lagophthalmos.
- Temporary eyelid edema.
- Worsening dry eye.
- Undercorrection.
- Overcorrection.
- Visible scar.
- Wound dehiscence.
- Acute or delayed infection.[4]

5.4 Benefits

When performed correctly, patients undergoing upper eyelid blepharoplasty can expect an improvement in their superior visual field, improvement in the sensation of heaviness from upper eyelid skin, lessened need for chronic frontalis and eyebrow elevation, and improved cosmesis.

5.5 Informed Consent

All patients should be informed of the risks as described above and that, as with any surgery, every patient may heal differently and results are never guaranteed. Surgery should never proceed without a signed consent from the patient or guardian acknowledging an understanding of the risks, benefits, and alternatives to surgery.

5.6 Indications

- Upper eyelid skin resting on or below eyelashes.
- Superior visual field obstruction that improves with elevation of eyelid skin.
- A displeasing facial aesthetic.

5.7 Contraindications

- Upper eyelid skin deficiency from previous blepharoplasty.
- Suspicion for cutaneous periocular malignancy and need for possible rotation flap or skin graft.
- Upper eyelid descent secondary to levator aponeurosis dehiscence and minimal upper eyelid skin (▶ Fig. 5.3).
- Unrealistic patient expectations.

5.8 The Procedure

It can be performed in an office-based procedure room or surgery center.

5.8.1 Preoperative Checklist

- Signed consent in chart.
- Documentation of symptoms and signs of preoperative dry eye:
  ○ Dry eye complaints.
  ○ Ocular surface examination.
  ○ Schirmer's testing in patients with dry eye.
- Blood thinners have been stopped at an appropriate interval before surgery.
- Sterile instrumentation on hand.
- Preoperative photographs documenting the eyelid malposition, primary and oblique angles.

5.8.2 Instruments Needed (▶ Fig. 5.4)

- Sterile marking pen.
- Skin ruler or Jameson caliper (Bausch & Lomb E2410).
- Scalpel and #15 blade or diamond knife.
- Skin hook (single).
- Skin rake: three-prong or four-prong.
- Toothed forceps (0.5 Castroviejo or other but should avoid larger Adson-like teeth on delicate eyelid skin).
- Blunt-tip Westcott scissors.
- Castroviejo needle drivers.
- Cautery: Bovie, needle tip (Colorado type) or bipolar.

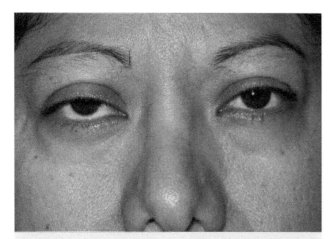

Fig. 5.3 Poor candidate for upper blepharoplasty alone as the patient's eyelid descent is related to involutional blepharoptosis and not redundancy of upper eyelid skin.

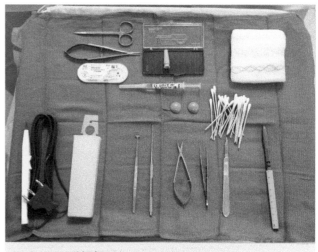

Fig. 5.4 Upper blepharoplasty surgical instrumentation.

5.8.3 Sutures Used

A 6–0 Prolene or 6–0 plain gut.

5.8.4 Operative Technique: Step by Step

Skin Marking

- It is useful to have an upright, preoperative photograph hanging in the room to aid the surgeon assess anatomic variation while marking and during surgery.
- Marking can be performed with the patient sitting up, but for convenience and efficiency, the author performs with the patient in supine position.
- Use caliper to mark central lid crease height appropriate for the patient.
  - Female: ~7 to 10 mm.
  - Male: ~6 to 8 mm.
  - Typically lower in the Asian eyelid and described elsewhere in this book.
- Set superior extent of marking to correlate with 10 mm from the upper eyelid–brow skin transition. Place upward curve to medial and lateral aspect of lower incision to minimize dog-ear when eventually closing the eyelid (▶ Fig. 5.5). Use caliper to confirm accuracy and symmetry of markings.
- If the patient is awake, have patient look straight ahead and adjust markings with an eye toward a similar pattern of skin removal with patient in primary gaze. This step provides an additional checkpoint to compensate for less tangible factors, such as orbital volume asymmetry, thereby increasing the probability of postoperative eyelid crease symmetry (▶ Fig. 5.6).

Anesthesia

Instill one drop of ophthalmic topical anesthetic such as propar-acaine to ocular surface of each eye. Inject ~2 mL of a 1:1 dilution of 1% lidocaine and 0.5% bupivacaine, both with 1:100,000 epinephrine, into upper eyelids in a subdermal/preorbicularis plane; 0.5 mL can be added to deeper area of medial fat, with concurrent digital lateral displacement globe to avoid the risk of needle contact with eye (▶ Fig. 5.7).

Procedure

- Periocular area and face prepped in normal sterile fashion with 5% povidone-iodine.
- A #15 blade is used to cut along skin markings.
- With forceps elevating skin perpendicular toward the ceiling, use the needle-tip Bovie on cutting mode, Westcott scissors, or #15 blade to remove a skin-only flap. Appropriate countertension and careful lateral to medial subdermal plane dissection are used to preserve and minimize trauma to orbicularis muscle (▶ Fig. 5.8a, b). Needle-tip Bovie can be used for hemostasis.
- Assistant holds four-prong rake in the superomedial aspect of the wound and use Westcott scissors to sharply dissect through exposed medial orbicularis along longitudinal muscle fiber direction. Reveal anterior medial orbital fat with careful posterior Westcott scissor blunt dissection. If the patient is awake, 0.5 mL of local anesthetic is injected into the fat, orienting needle away from the globe. Bovie cautery is

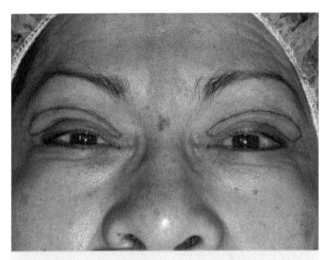

Fig. 5.6 Examination of marking accuracy and symmetry by having patient look at surgeon in primary gaze to facilitate fine adjustments of marking before injection of local anesthetic.

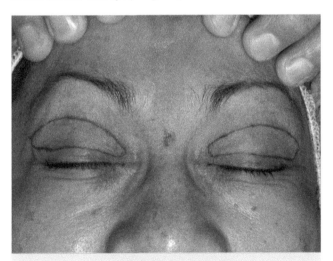

Fig. 5.5 Typical preoperative blepharoplasty marking.

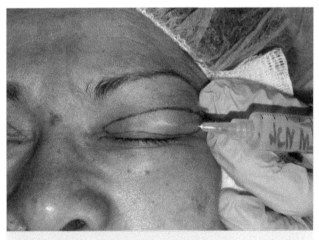

Fig. 5.7 Injection of local anesthetic in a subdermal plane to facilitate hydrodissection of dermis from orbicularis.

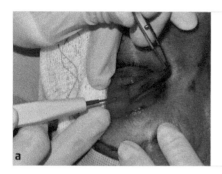 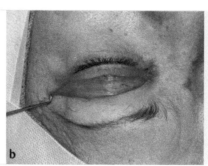

Fig. 5.8 Multidirectional countertraction and skin flap elevation facilitates (a) creation of skin-only flap with minimal hemorrhage and (b) preservation of healthy orbicularis with undisturbed vascularity and innervation.

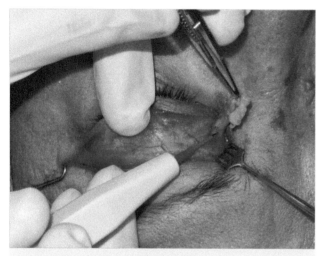

Fig. 5.9 Selective medial orbital fat excision.

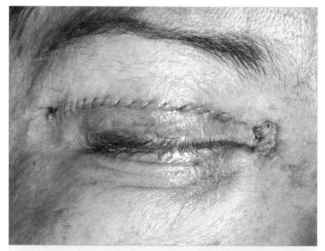

Fig. 5.10 Sutured wound with air knot medially for ease of postoperative removal.

used to cauterize the base of the pedicle, and cutting cautery is used for excision (▶ Fig. 5.9).

- Although beyond the scope of this chapter, any adjunctive procedures such as medial or preaponeurotic fat pedicle repositioning, fat grafting, or brow stabilization suture can be performed here.
- Placement of a single skin hook at the lateral apex of the wound facilitates easier wound orientation for closure that minimizes risk or poor skin alignment or dog-ear (▶ Fig. 5.8b). The wound is closed with a running 6–0 Prolene or 6–0 plain suture. If Prolene suture is used, an air knot can be placed at the beginning of the wound, and the suture can be tied onto itself at the end of the wound to facilitate ease of removal at the postoperative appointment (▶ Fig. 5.10).
- The face and wound are cleaned with sterile saline-soaked gauze and ophthalmic antibiotic ointment is placed on the incision site.
- In the recovery area, the head of bed is elevated 30° and ice compresses are placed over the upper eyelids.
- Typical pre- and postoperative results are shown in ▶ Fig. 5.1a, b.

5.8.5 Expert Tips/Pearls/ Suggestions

- Local anesthetic pearls:

  - Place commercially available or compounded lidocaine topical anesthetic cream on the upper eyelid skin 15 minutes before marking to dull the discomfort from the needle stick during injection. Cream should be wiped off well before marking.
  - The addition of sodium bicarbonate 8.4% to the local anesthetic mixture buffers the medication closer to physiologic pH, which minimizes burning during injection. Add the equivalent of approximately 0.5 mL of bicarbonate to every 10 mL of anesthetic solution.
  - The addition of hyaluronidase to the local anesthetic aids in hydroenzymatically dissecting skin from tightly adherent underlying orbicularis in preparation for preserving orbicularis during the procedure.
- Management of the deflated eyebrow:
  - Patients with preoperative brow deflation and descent are at higher risk of postoperative dissatisfaction with the appearance of residual hooding after upper eyelid blepharoplasty alone. Telltale signs of predisposed brows include the lack of brow convexity on side profile view and the presence of "brow whiskers," which are noticeable rhytids oriented superotemporally throughout the lateral half of the brow (▶ Fig. 5.11a, b).
  - Management of these patients include:
    1. Preoperative education on the limitation of results from blepharoplasty alone.
    2. Consideration for concurrent temporal browlift with possible fat grafting.

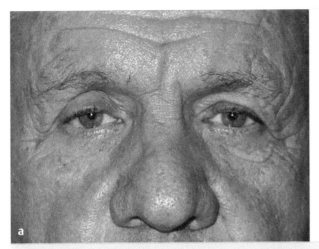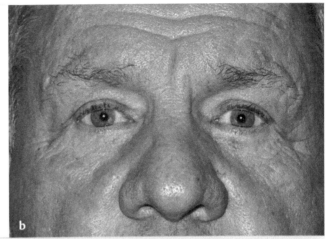

Fig. 5.11 Example of patient with preoperative **(a)** eyebrow deflation and skin degeneration exhibiting lack of eyebrow projection and superotemporal rhytids, which the author describes as "eyelid whiskers" putting the patient at higher risk for dissatisfaction with skin removal alone. This patient also exhibits concurrent involutional blepharoptosis and asymmetry of superior sulcus volume. Postoperative photograph **(b)** 3 months after bilateral upper eyelid blepharoplasty, including adjunctive preaponeurotic fat advancement pedicle on the right upper eyelid for improvement in volume asymmetry, bilateral Müller's muscle–conjunctival resection ptosis repair, direct temporal browlift, and lower eyelid cosmetic skin pinch blepharoplasty.

3. Postoperative soft tissue filler and neurotoxin, to lift and fill.

5.8.6 Postoperative Care Checklist

- Topical antibiotic ophthalmic ointment placed on wound three times per day for 1 week.
- Keep head elevated above the heart as much as possible and ice compress over the eyes 20 minutes every hour for the first 48 hours.
- Postoperative appointment for suture removal at days 6 to 9.

5.9 Complications and Their Management

- Postoperative hemorrhage: Oozing from the wound on postoperative days 1 to 2 is to be expected; however, patients who report extreme pain and vision loss with signs of anterior and inferior globe displacement should be taken immediately back to the operating room for drainage of retrobulbar hematoma and cautery, where necessary. Consideration should be made in regard to hematologic coagulation status and blood pressure.
- Wound dehiscence: When occurring between postoperative days 1 and 6, the wound should be debrided and

reapproximated with suture. Dehiscences after 1 week that are less than one-third of wound length usually heal well by secondary intention.
- Wound infection: Acute infections after upper blepharoplasty are rare, given the robust vascularity of the eyelid. Any acute infection should be cultured and treated with appropriate antibiotics. Nodular erythema occurring 3 weeks or later after surgery should raise suspicion for atypical mycobacteria infection.[4] Management typically involves wound debridement with fresh tissue culture, long-term antimicrobial therapy, and consultation with infectious disease.

References

[1] Oh SR, Chokthaweesak W, Annunziata CC, Priel A, Korn BS, Kikkawa DO. Analysis of eyelid fat pad changes with aging. Ophthal Plast Reconstr Surg. 2011; 27(5):348–351
[2] Korn BS, Kikkawa DO, Hicok KC. Identification and characterization of adult stem cells from human orbital adipose tissue. Ophthal Plast Reconstr Surg. 2009; 25(1):27–32
[3] Saadat D, Dresner SC. Safety of blepharoplasty in patients with preoperative dry eyes. Arch Facial Plast Surg. 2004; 6(2):101–104
[4] Mauriello JA, Jr, Atypical Mycobacterial Study Group. Atypical mycobacterial infection of the periocular region after periocular and facial surgery. Ophthal Plast Reconstr Surg. 2003; 19(3):182–188

6 Double Eyelid Surgery

Michael A. Burnstine

Abstract

Double eyelid surgery, also known as Asian blepharoplasty, is one of the most common facial procedures performed on the Asian face. The desired outcome is based on the patient's facial anatomy and personal preference for final outcome. Double eyelid surgery may be performed to relieve a functional superior visual field loss or address dissatisfaction in the upper eyelid crease such as absent eyelid crease, partial eyelid crease, multiple eyelid creases, and tapering eyelid creases. Additional reasons for aesthetic and functional double eyelid surgery are many and include: enhancing the face and creating a more aesthetically pleasing vertical and horizontal eyelid palpebral fissure, relieving eyelash ptosis, creating a greater eyelid platform (margin fold distance) for the application of cosmetic products (eyeliner and eyeshadow), and relieving nonsurgical applications to improve the eyelid height and contour. Some patients may spend a significant amount of time using adhesive glues and tapes to create an eyelid appearance that they desire. Clear discussion of a patient's goal in single or double eyelid surgery is critical to ensure total patient satisfaction.

Keywords: single eyelid, double eyelid, Asian blepharoplasty

6.1 Introduction

This chapter focuses on the anatomical differences between Asians and Caucasians and the unique surgical considerations in double eyelid surgery. Asian eyelids refer to the varied eyelid morphologies on the continent of Asia, including those of Chinese, Korean, Japanese, Indian, Middle Eastern, South East Asia, and other descent. In the past, for surgeons and patients, the goal of Asian eyelid surgery was the western Caucasian look. However, the western look makes the patient appear unnatural. As a result, a frameshift has occurred toward the unique and beautiful ideals of an Asian aesthetic. The surgical discussion with the patient should inform the patient about his/her own periorbital anatomy with particular attention to the eyelid relationship to the eyebrow and forehead, the eyelid crease, and the medial and lateral canthal areas. Frequently, Asian patients will have an overactive brow prior to blepharoplasty. Listening and responding to a patient's concerns and personal preference is mission critical.

The upper facial surgeon must help the patient understand what can and cannot be achieved. Discussions must be frank and include items such as current eyelid crease and fold positions as well as concomitant aponeurotic ptosis, eyebrow ptosis, and eyelid skin hooding when indicated. Careful documentation in the chart of the patient's response to the discussion and preferences is critical. When a plan is agreed, a thorough discussion on patient financial expectations and pre- and postoperative care is needed. Preoperatively, this discussion includes smoking cessation and avoidance of blood thinners such as aspirin, nonsteroidal anti-inflammatories, warfarin, heparin, and herbal remedies. The postoperative discussion includes downtime needed for recovery, use of ice and warm compresses, bruising expectations, and when a patient can return to work.

6.2 Anatomical Considerations

6.2.1 The Eyelid Crease and Fold

About half of all Asians have some form of an eyelid crease; therefore, there are half that do not have an eyelid crease and fold.[1] In Asians of Chinese, Korean, and Japanese descent, the upper tarsal plate is smaller (6.5–8 mm) than that of Americans and Europeans (9–11 mm).[1-3] The importance of this difference lies in where to judiciously place the upper eyelid crease in designing a patient's surgical plan. It is thought that the upper eyelid crease results from the presence of subcutaneous internal interdigitations of the levator aponeurosis in the pretarsal and superior tarsal border.[4] Further, in Asians without an upper eyelid crease, there is a thicker skin–orbicularis oculi–fat complex.[5] Kakizaki et al found that the distance from the orbital septum attachment site to the superior tarsal border is similar in Asians and Whites; however, there was a tendency to a lower extension of the preaponeurotic fat pads in Asians.[6,7] Taken together, a smaller tarsal plate and more inferior fat extension in the upper eyelid may account for the differences in the Asian and White eyelids.

The relationship of the fat pads may also contribute to the presence or absence of the upper eyelid crease.[8] These fat pads include subcutaneous, pretarsal, preseptal/postorbicularis, postseptal (preaponeurotic or orbital), and submuscular or subbrow area (▶ Fig. 6.1).[9] The submuscular fat is superficially located under the orbicularis muscle and is contiguous with the retro-orbicularis oculi fat (ROOF) of the brow. In Asians without an eyelid crease, the fat pads intertwine and comingle in a way not seen in Asians and Caucasians with a crease.[10,11] It must be noted that these racial differences are generalizations and are not 100% specific to individuals of various ethnicities. Further, when most Asians request a double eyelid from a single one, they wish to look Asian and not have a higher eyelid crease and fold.

Careful documentation of crease presence, crease asymmetry between sides, segmented crease, and multiple creases is important to preoperative surgical planning. Careful preoperative photographs should be taken of the patient, including frontal view, oblique side views, upgaze, and downgaze. If a patient has had prior surgery, this should be documented.

6.2.2 The Medial Canthal Area

Most Asians have a medial canthal fold. The fold may be tapered into the medial canthus or parallel (▶ Fig. 6.2). Some Asians request a change in the medial canthal fold area from a tapered crease to a parallel one. The discussion to change the medial canthal fold appearance must be frank; changing the epicanthal fold from a tapered fold to a parallel one will induce a change in the face appearance.

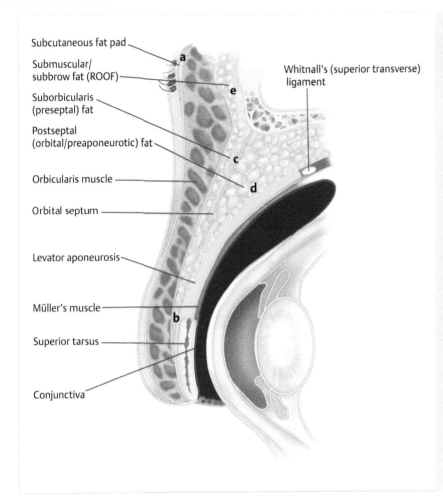

Subcutaneous fat pad

Submuscular/
subbrow fat (ROOF)

Suborbicularis
(preseptal) fat

Postseptal
(orbital/preaponeurotic) fat

Orbicularis muscle

Orbital septum

Levator aponeurosis

Müller's muscle

Superior tarsus

Conjunctiva

Whitnall's (superior transverse)
ligament

Fig. 6.1 The five upper eyelid fat pads: subcutaneous (**a**), pretarsal (**b**), suborbicularis (preseptal) (**c**), postseptal (orbital/ preaponeurotic fat) (**d**), and submuscular/ subbrow fat (**e**). Note the continuum in **b**, **c**, and **e**.

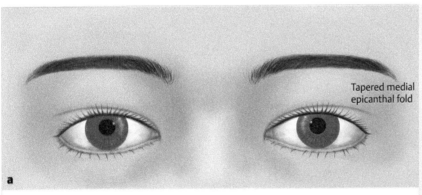

Tapered medial
epicanthal fold

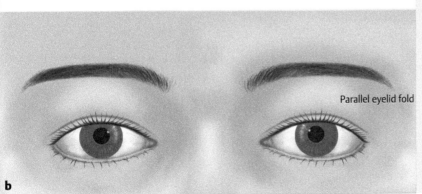

Parallel eyelid fold

Fig. 6.2 Examples of a tapered epicanthal fold (**a**) and parallel eyelid fold (**b**).

6.2.3 The Lateral Canthal Area

In blepharoplasty, it is important to consider the lateral eyelid and orbit. The levator aponeurosis spans the lacrimal gland, creating orbital and palpebral lobes. Documenting the lateral fullness and defining how a patient prefers the lateral angle are critical in double eyelid surgery. Rarely, some patients request a slight upward widening over the lateral segment of the eyelid rather than a leveled configuration.

6.3 Goals of Intervention/ Indications

The main goal of upper blepharoplasty in the Asian patient is to meet the patient's desires.
- Improvement in the superior field of vision.
- Enhancement of the face by creating a more aesthetically pleasing vertical and horizontal eyelid palpebral fissure.
- Relief of eyelash ptosis.
- Creation of a greater eyelid platform (margin fold distance) for the application of cosmetic products (eyeliner and eyeshadow).
- Relief from nonsurgical applications to improve the eyelid height and contour.

6.4 Risks of the Procedure

- Bleeding.
- Infection.
- Asymmetric eyelid crease and fold.
- Regression of the eyelid crease back to a single eyelid.

6.5 Benefits of the Procedure

- Improvement of superior field of vision.
- Aesthetic enhancement of the upper face, including widened vertical and horizontal palpebral fissures.
- Improvement of eyelash ptosis.
- Ability to wear makeup.
- Avoidance of nonsurgical preparations to create the desired eyelid height and contour.

6.6 Informed Consent

- Include risks and benefits (as above).
- Discussion of the need for enhancement to equalize the eyelid crease and folds if a resultant asymmetry occurs.

6.7 Contraindications

None.

6.8 The Procedure

The procedure described can be done in an outpatient surgery center or in an office-based setting.

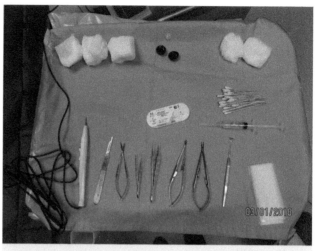

Fig. 6.3 Instrumentation utilized for double eyelid surgery.

6.8.1 Instruments Needed (▶ Fig. 6.3)

- Surgical marking pen.
- Ruler.
- Local anesthesia:
  ○ Two percent lidocaine with 1:100,000 U epinephrine (5 mL).
  ○ Marcaine 0.75% (4 mL).
  ○ Bicarbonate (8.4%) 1 mL.
  ○ Vitrase 1 mL/20 mL local.
- Castroviejo needle holder.
- Bishop Harmon forceps.
- Colorado needle tip with monopolar cautery.
- Hemostat.
- Sutures: 6–0 Prolene suture for wound closure.

6.8.2 Preoperative Checklist

- Informed consent.
- Instrumentation on hand.
- Clear discussion with the patient on the desired eyelid crease and fold height, medial canthal fold position, and lateral eyelid show (margin fold distance).
- Preoperative photographic documentation.

6.8.3 The Operative Technique

This procedure can be done under local, monitored, or general anesthesia in an office-based procedure room, ambulatory operating room, or hospital-based setting. To achieve a natural look, this author believes minimal tissue dissection and tissue debulking is needed. Some authors believe in eyelid crease fixation to ensure crease position and prevent ptosis from undetected levator injury as an integral step in double eyelid surgery. This author does not. However, if ptosis is present, it should be addressed concurrently.
- Premedication with lorazepam 1 mg and acetaminophen/ hydrocodone 5 mg/325 mg may be given 30 minutes before the procedure.
- The blepharoplasty incisions are marked. *This is the most important step!*

- The eyelid crease is set based on the patient's wishes, usually at 4 to 7 mm, based on the patient's preference for eyelid crease (▶ Fig. 6.4).
  1. Usually, the eyelid crease is set at or slightly below the maximum tarsal height.
- A decision is made with the patient about the preservation of the medial canthal fold.
  1. For a parallel crease, a more level and equidistant crease is demarcated.
  2. For a medial canthal tapered incision, the incision should fall into the fold medially.
  3. To change a medial epicanthal fold to a parallel eyelid crease, a Z-plasty may need to be performed.
- A decision is made as to how much eyelid skin to be shown (margin fold distance) postoperatively.
- A preoperative decision is made as to how to shape the lateral canthal incision.
  1. Whether the patient wishes to have an upward widening of the margin fold distance or a leveled configuration.
- Local anesthesia is injected and massaged into place, waiting 5 to 10 minutes for the full anesthetic and hemostatic effect.
  - Hyaluronidase is used to help spread the local anesthetic with minimal injection sites.
- A traction suture may or may not be placed.
- An incision is made with a #15 blade or diamond knife (▶ Fig. 6.5).
- A skin-only blepharoplasty is performed, preserving orbicularis muscle using the Colorado needle tip, Westcott scissors, or diamond blade (▶ Fig. 6.6). Some subdermal tissue (subcutaneous fat) may be removed.
  - By preserving the orbicularis muscle, eyelid closure is not affected.
  - Orbicularis excess may be sculpted with gentle cautery of the Colorado needle tip.
- A 2- to 3-mm strip of pretarsal orbicularis is removed above the incision line—no septum (▶ Fig. 6.7).
- If there is fatty prominence, a small amount of fat may be removed or sculpted by buttonholing through orbicularis and the nasal and central septum with Westcott scissors.
  - Typically, in the Asian eyelid, minimal fat is removed.

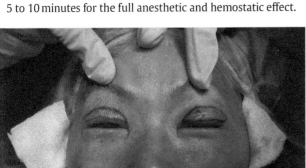

Fig. 6.4 An example of eyelid crease placement for double eyelid surgery.

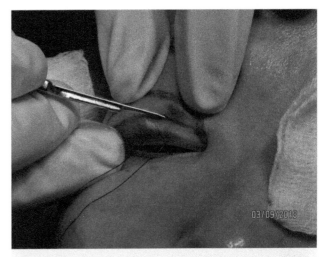

Fig. 6.5 The incision is made with a #15 blade, preserving the medial epicanthal fold.

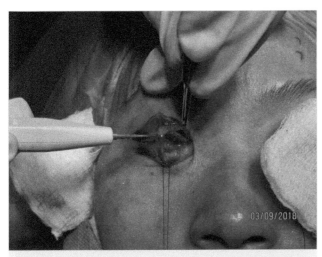

Fig. 6.6 Dissection of a skin and subcutaneous fat plane in double eyelid surgery; orbicularis muscle is preserved.

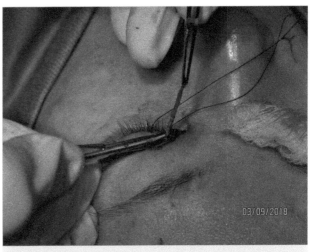

Fig. 6.7 Removal of a 2-mm strip of pretarsal orbicularis muscle.

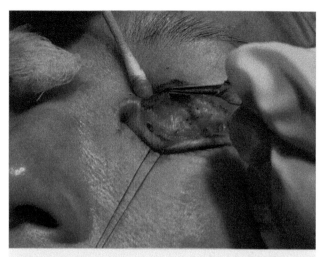

Fig. 6.8 An example of orbital fat removal. Entry to the orbital fat compartment is done in the suborbicularis space. Typically, minimal fat is removed.

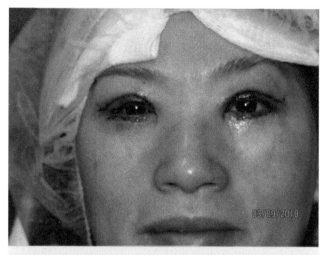

Fig. 6.9 Closure of the wound may be done with or without supratarsal fixation. The harder the crease, the greater supratarsal fixation. In this case, a subcuticular closure was performed to achieve a softer crease.

- The fat pad is removed in a controlled fashion with monopolar cautery (▶ Fig. 6.8).
  - Occasionally, in patients with very full upper eyelids, significant central and nasal fat is removed.
  - Rarely, fat may need repositioning to help define the upper eyelid crease.
- Lacrimal gland repositioning is done if there is lacrimal gland prolapse (see Chapter 26).
  - If a patient wishes lateral elevation of the eyelid crease, the crease is tapered up, and more skin and subcutaneous fat is removed.
- The wound is closed with a running 6–0 Prolene suture (▶ Fig. 6.9).
  - By avoiding crease-forming sutures from skin to tarsus to levator to skin, a hard crease is not observed on downgaze.
  - A softer crease is created by alternating skin closure with skin-to-skin followed by skin–tarsus–skin (supratarsal fixation). On downgaze, this will create a softer crease.
  - If a very soft crease is desired, no supratarsal fixation is performed (▶ Fig. 6.10).

6.8.4 Expert Tips/Pearls/Suggestions

- Ensure no other conditions exist prior to performing upper blepharoplasty such as ptosis, eyebrow ptosis, and lash ptosis.
- The lower line of the blepharoplasty incision will determine the height and contour of the newly formed upper eyelid crease.
- In general, most women prefer a higher eyelid crease than men. A clear discussion must be had before the procedure.
- Measure twice and cut once.
- The formation of the eyelid crease is critical.
  - Taper into the fold for a nasally tapered crease.
  - Reposition the nasal crease higher (but not angled up) for a parallel medial eyelid crease.
  - For modification of a tapered medial epicanthal fold to a parallel fold, a Z-epicanthoplasty may be performed.

- Laterally, the crease should not be placed past the lateral angle unless there is an unaddressed component of eyebrow ptosis. If so, the incision should travel with a rhytid of facial expression (crow's feet).
- The incision should be deep but not too deep. It should remove skin and subcutaneous fat.
- Always remove fat with the tips of Westcott scissors pointed upward in the orbit to avoid damage to the levator muscle or its aponeurosis.
- Minimal rather than aggressive fat dissection is needed to form a double eyelid.
  - Frequently, no fat removal is necessary in double eyelid surgery.
- Always watch out for the prolapsed lacrimal gland. If present, it should be sculpted or reanchored to the orbital rim superiorly (see Chapter 26).
- Pretarsal fat and orbicularis can be removed if a defined crease formation is threatened. Frequently, it will lead to prolonged healing time and postoperative edema.
- To enhance and make a harder crease, crease-forming sutures may be applied: skin–tarsus–levator–skin. A 6–0 Vicryl suture with an S-14 needle may be utilized.
- Before leaving the surgical operating room, ensure symmetry between sides.

6.8.5 Postoperative Care Checklist

- Ice is applied to the operative sites for 48 hours, 15 minutes on/off while awake.
- The patient is advised to sleep with the head of the bed elevated.
- The patient may shower the next day.
- The wound should be kept clean with tepid water, and the bacitracin eye ointment is applied four times daily.
- Postoperative medications are given:
  - Antibiotic eye ointment (bacitracin preferred) to the wounds.
  - Oral pain medication, typically acetaminophen/ hydrocodone, 5 mg/325 mg.

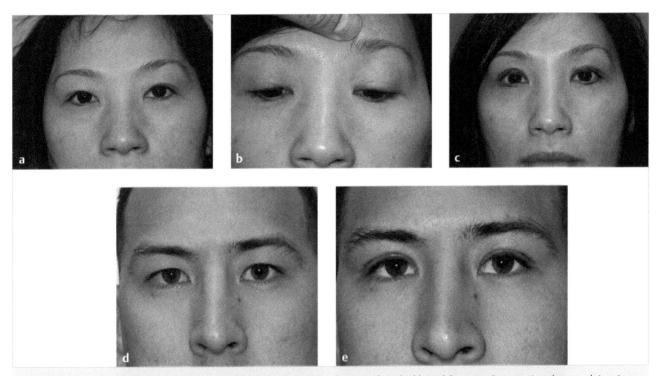

Fig. 6.10 Typical pre- and postoperative photographs from revision of another provider's double eyelid surgery. Preoperative photograph in primary gaze (a), preoperative photograph of asymmetric eyelid creases on downgaze (b), and 2 weeks' postoperative photograph in primary gaze (c). Preoperative (d) and postoperative photographs (e) after double eyelid surgery in an Asian male with no supratarsal fixation and subcuticular eyelid closure.

- Workouts and strenuous exercise should be avoided for 1 week.
- Blood thinners like aspirin and nonsteroidals should be avoided for 1 week.
- No eye or eyelid exercises are needed to maintain the created eyelid crease.
- Suture removal is performed at week 1.

6.9 Complications and Their Management

In my experience, most suboptimal results in double eyelid surgery stem from poor communication between the patient and the surgeon. The preoperative preferences are not illuminated and discussed in a clear fashion. In addition, the surgeon unaware of the anatomical differences between races and the nuances in surgical technique like crease placement may inadvertently cause suboptimal results. Should an enhancement (touch-up) be necessary, the revision may happen at week 6. Usually, the crease is lowered to match the fellow side in patients with asymmetric crease placement.

6.10 Alternative Approaches to Double Eyelid Surgery

Other individuals advocate the use of sutures to fixate an eyelid crease or perform the blepharoplasty through a subbrow approach.[12-16] The former may cause an unstable eyelid crease,

can only be used in a youthful patient due to redundant and lax skin development with age, and may be complicated by ocular foreign body sensation, suture granuloma formation, and absence of a dynamic crease on downgaze. The subbrow approach may correct lateral hooding and revise eyebrow contour and tattoo, avoids a long lateral scar and dog-ear formation, enables thinning of the ROOF, and allows for internal brow suspension. However, the subbrow approach may leave an unsightly scar in the subbrow region and can only be used on those patients that have had a double eyelid before tissue redundancy developed. Addressing a patient's desired changes to the medial crease formation is not possible through the subbrow approach.

References

[1] Chen WP. Asian blepharoplasty. Update on anatomy and techniques. Ophthal Plast Reconstr Surg. 1987; 3(3):135–140

[2] Chen WP, Park JD. Asian upper lid blepharoplasty: an update on indications and technique. Facial Plast Surg. 2013; 29(1):26–31

[3] Kim YS, Hwang K. Shape and height of tarsal plates. J Craniofac Surg. 2016; 27(2):496–497

[4] Collin JR, Beard C, Wood I. Experimental and clinical data on the insertion of the levator palpebrae superioris muscle. Am J Ophthalmol. 1978; 85(6): 792–801

[5] Saonanon P, Thongtong P, Wongwuticomjon T. Differences between single and double eyelid anatomy in Asians using ultrasound biomicroscopy. Asia Pac J Ophthalmol (Phila). 2016; 5(5):335–338

[6] Kakizaki H, Leibovitch I, Selva D, Asamoto K, Nakano T. Orbital septum attachment on the levator aponeurosis in Asians: in vivo and cadaver study. Ophthalmology. 2009; 116(10):2031–2035

[7] Kakizaki H, Selva D, Asamoto K, Nakano T, Leibovitch I. Orbital septum attachment sites on the levator aponeurosis in Asians and whites. Ophthal Plast Reconstr Surg. 2010; 26(4):265–268

[8] Galatoire O, Touitou V, Heran F, et al. High-resolution magnetic resonance imaging of the upper eyelid: correlation with the position of the skin crease in the upper eyelid. Orbit. 2007; 26(3):165–171

[9] Uchida J. A surgical procedure for blepharoptosis vera and for pseudo-blepharoptosis orientalis. Br J Plast Surg. 1962; 15:271–276

[10] Saonanon P. Update on Asian eyelid anatomy and clinical relevance. Curr Opin Ophthalmol. 2014; 25(5):436–442

[11] Jeong S, Lemke BN, Dortzbach RK, Park YG, Kang HK. The Asian upper eyelid: an anatomical study with comparison to the Caucasian eyelid. Arch Ophthalmol. 1999; 117(7):907–912

[12] Fan J, Low DW. A two-way continuous buried-suture approach to the creation of the long-lasting double eyelid: surgical technique and long-term follow-up in 51 patients. Aesthetic Plast Surg. 2009; 33(3):421–425

[13] Kim YS, Roh TS, Yoo WM, Tark KC, Kim J. Infrabrow excision blepharoplasty: applications and outcomes in upper blepharoplasty in Asian women. Plast Reconstr Surg. 2008; 122(4):1199–1205

[14] Lee D, Law V. Subbrow blepharoplasty for upper eyelid rejuvenation in Asians. Aesthet Surg J. 2009; 29(4):284–288

[15] Kim YS. Subbrow blepharoplasty using supraorbital rim periosteal fixation. Aesthetic Plast Surg. 2014; 38(1):27–31

[16] Osaki MH, Osaki TH, Osaki T. Infrabrow skin excision associated with upper blepharoplasty to address significant dermatochalasis with lateral hooding in select Asian patients. Ophthal Plast Reconstr Surg. 2017; 33(1):53–56

7 A Guide to Eyebrow Contouring Options

David B. Samimi

Abstract

Eyebrow shape and position play a powerful role in expression of mood, youth, and, at times, the ability to maintain superior field of vision. Advances in our understanding of facial aging have shifted the focus on brow enhancement surgery from altering vertical position with a browlift to conceptual considerations for the shape of the brow in three dimensions. This book includes a description of several modern approaches to eyebrow rejuvenation. Incisionless approaches include muscular denervation with neurotoxin and volume replacement with synthetic filler or autologous fat. Surgical rejuvenation may be approached through an incision in the eyelid crease, above eyebrow cilia, in central forehead rhytids, and at or behind the superior forehead hairline. A focused history and physical exam should be performed to choose the optimal procedure. This chapter helps the reader understand how to integrate a patient's goals and anatomy to choose the optimal eyebrow rejuvenation approach.

Keywords: browlift, eyebrow lift, forehead lift, facial rejuvenation

7.1 Introduction

The eyebrow region is an integral functional and aesthetic component of the upper face. Position and shape powerfully convey one's mood and youth (▸ Fig. 7.1). Any alterations in the form of the brow should take into account a patient's gender, age, and harmony with the rest of the face. Anatomic understanding of the upper face and brow region is critical to performing many of the procedures safely and is covered in Chapter 2.

Surgical rejuvenation has classically focused on vertical eyebrow elevation. Recently, there has been an appreciation for the three-dimensional orientation of the eyebrow and focus on facial proportions. This chapter aims to provide the reader with a framework for understanding the "when and why" of eyebrow rejuvenation procedures described in the subsequent chapters, including the use of nonsurgical adjuncts such as hyaluronic acid gel fillers for soft tissue inflation and botulinum toxin placement for relaxation of eyebrow depressor and elevator muscles.

7.2 Evolving Trends in Brow Beauty

The desired eyebrow aesthetic has evolved over time. To understand where we are now, it is important to appreciate aesthetic trends over time, volume loss and tissue descent, and ideal eyebrow height associated with facial proportions.

7.2.1 History of Eyebrow Aesthetics

The ideal eyebrow and upper facial appearance is fluid, mirroring changes in fashion and ideal body aesthetics. The most notable shifts in the brow aesthetic occur with the feminine eyebrow and are associated most commonly with shape and cilia density. During the roaring 1920s, female celebrities preferred a pencil thin, downward sloping eyebrow tail that provided the moody appearance that was chic at the time. Eyebrows stayed thin in the 1930s but incorporated a round arch with the highest point closer to center. Evolving styles of grooming and makeup application following World War II brought further changes. In the 1950s, Marilyn Monroe exhibited a thicker brow, filled in with makeup, with its arch at the lateral third, closer to what we see today. Trends in brow shape and contour have continued to alternate throughout more recent decades, mirroring desires for a more natural upper facial aesthetic in the 1980s (e.g., Brooke Shields) and a more groomed and shaped appearance in the 1990s (e.g., Jennifer Lopez). If the past is any indication of the future, the ideal eyebrow shape will continue to evolve, and it is incumbent on the oculofacial plastic surgeon to maintain an awareness of these trends (▸ Fig. 7.2).

7.2.2 Volume and Facial Aging

A youthful eyebrow exhibits convexity and forward projection of the upper eyelid–brow complex on side profile (▸ Fig. 7.3). Loss of projection occurs with age, secondary to resorption of the frontal bone, soft tissue atrophy of the retro-orbicularis oculi fat, and tissue descent. Consideration to brow position and three-dimensional shape is critical to achieving optimal results in eyebrow rejuvenation. Replacement of volume with soft tissue fillers or autologous fat should be part of the modern surgeon's toolbox.

7.2.3 Eyebrow Height and Proportions

Like many concepts in facial aesthetics, there should be awareness of proportions and age appropriateness when thinking of optimal brow position. Although counterintuitive, a youthful brow position is relatively low set, an orientation that provides harmony with a relatively short, volume-rich lower eyelid–cheek transition. Facial rejuvenation surgical practices do, however, commonly perform vertical brow lifting techniques because the aging orbit accommodates a relatively higher brow position to maintain proportions with the longer length of the lower eyelid–cheek transition in age (▸ Fig. 7.4). In other words, to maintain harmony of the upper and lower eyelid aesthetic units, the aging face tolerates a relatively higher brow height to maintain similar proportions with the longer distance in the lower eyelid.[1] The aesthetic surgeon should keep proportions in

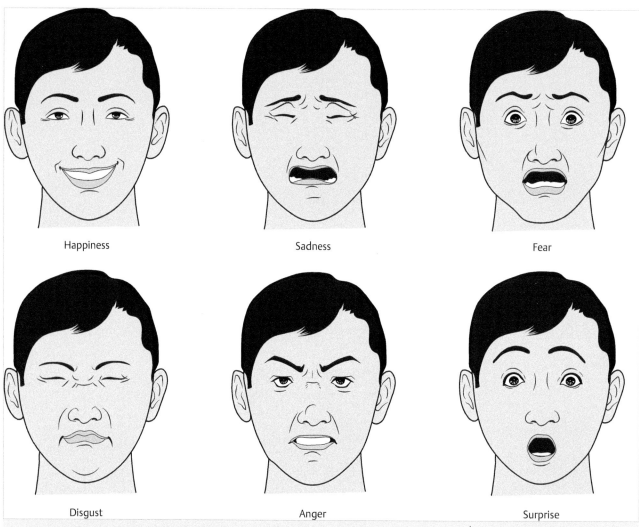

Fig. 7.1 Illustrations showing the power of eyebrow shape and appearance in conveying one's mood.

Below the figure, from left to right and top to bottom, the faces are labeled: Happiness, Sadness, Fear, Disgust, Anger, Surprise.

mind when assessing the potential for aesthetic improvement in the aging face. The surgeon should avoid overelevation of the youthful brow and consider the upper eyelid–eyebrow perceptual changes that may occur when shortening the lower eyelid–cheek transition with aesthetic lower eyelid blepharoplasty.

7.3 Patient Assessment

The first step to a successful surgery is gaining a realistic understanding of the patient's expectations. This should be married with the physical exam to determine whether one is a surgical candidate and which procedure to choose. There should be a discussion regarding the patient's desired eyebrow shape and position. It is always helpful to review photographs of youth to minimize the risk of choosing a procedure that may alter the patient's identity.

7.3.1 History

- Previous upper facial surgery, trauma, or facial paralysis?
- Current and previous use of facial neurotoxins and fillers.
- In females, it is useful to know whether the patient wears the hair up or down. This may influence the suitability for a scar along the hairline.
- Assessment of the patient's awareness of any preoperative asymmetry.
- If the surgeon suspects neurotoxin and/or injectable filler may be needed to optimize results after surgery, there should be an evaluation of the patient's willingness to have injectables postoperatively.
- If choosing a procedure with potential to affect sensory innervation, the surgeon should assess the patient's ability to tolerate scalp paresthesias postoperatively.

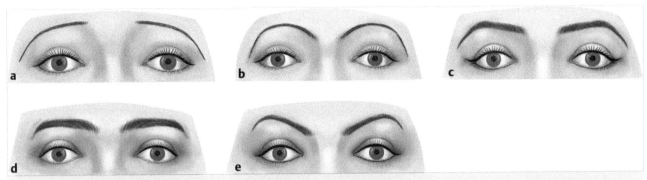

Fig. 7.2 Trends in eyebrow aesthetics. **(a)** 1920s: thin, downward slope. **(b)** 1930s: thin and rounded. **(c)** 1950s: thicker, filled in with make-up and exhibiting lateral arch. **(d)** 1980s: natural, less groomed. **(e)** 1990s: thin, lateral arch.

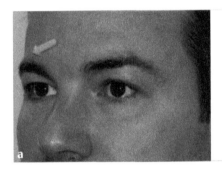
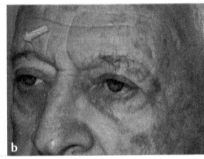

Fig. 7.3 A three-dimensional analysis of the youthful versus aging eyebrow. Oblique views of the eyebrow profile reveal the voluminous convexity of youth **(a)**. In contrast, the aging eyebrow profile exhibits loss of convexity secondary to soft tissue deflation, bony skeletal remodeling, and soft tissue descent (bottom) **(b)**.

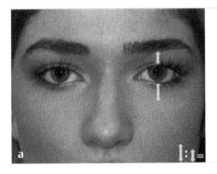
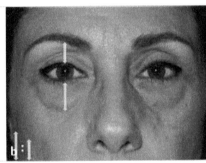

Fig. 7.4 Relative eyebrow position with age. **(a)** A youthful eyebrow position is set relatively low. The small distance from the eyelid–eyebrow transition matches the smaller lower eyelid–cheek transition length. **(b)** In contrast, the aging face tolerates a relatively higher vertical eyebrow height, to maintain aesthetic harmony with the longer lower eyelid–cheek transition length seen with age.

7.3.2 Physical Exam Checklist

- Preoperative eyebrow asymmetry?
- Brow height and shape (medial or lateral brow ptosis).
- Loss of brow convexity due to bony and soft tissue volume loss.
- Facial nerve weakness?
- Scalp and eyebrow hair density, thickness, and shape.
- Hairline: high or low?
- Quality of skin in brow and eyelid.
- Presence of blepharoptosis.

7.4 Risks of Surgery

- Patient dissatisfaction.
- Upper facial nerve damage.
- Loss of scalp sensation.
- Eyebrow asymmetry.
- Hematoma.
- Alopecia.
- Visible scar.

7.5 Choosing the Best Procedure/ Physician Decision-Making

Choosing the correct procedure is more important than steps of the actual procedure itself. An understanding of the capabilities and limitations of each approach allows the surgeon to educate the patient during the preoperative consultation, making them an informed partner in the decision process. The likelihood of an unhappy postsurgical patient may be minimized by understanding the strengths and weaknesses of each surgical approach and integrating these with a patient's individual desires and anatomy (▶ Fig. 7.5 and ▶ Table 7.1).

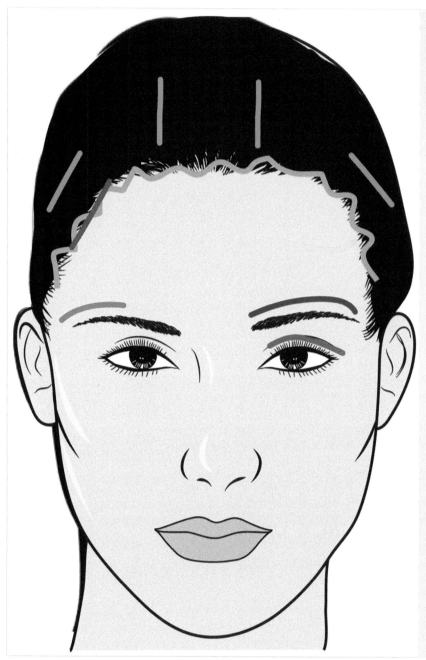

Fig. 7.5 Cutaneous incisions associated with eyebrow and forehead rejuvenation techniques. The incisions are color matched with their respective procedure names in Table 7.1.

7.6 Expert Tips/Pearls/Suggestions

7.6.1 Upper Eyelid Considerations

For optimal control of the upper eyelid–eyebrow complex, consider concurrently performing upper eyelid blepharoplasty with most eyebrow procedures. When present, also address coexisting blepharoptosis.

7.6.2 The Role of Nonsurgical Adjuncts

Patients unwilling to have postoperative injectables after surgical eyebrow rejuvenation must be warned about the possible limitation in the outcome and longevity of the procedure. Consider discounting or including postsurgical injectable treatment within the surgery fee to assist patients' understanding of the benefits of well-placed neurotoxin and filler.

7.6.3 Managing Asymmetry

Identify and photographically document any preoperative eyebrow asymmetry.
- Pay attention to any asymmetries that occur during facial animation and inform the patient that these dynamic facial asymmetries are usually not correctable with a static treatment such as surgery.
- Be aware of asymmetry that may be correctable when related to compensatory eyebrow elevation from ipsilateral blepharoptosis.

Table 7.1 Eyebrow contouring option summary

Procedure	Chapter	Optimal candidate	Gender	Risks	Addresses temporal ptosis?	Addresses medial ptosis?	Aesthetic patient-friendly?
Internal browlift	9	• Healthy soft tissue • Minimal lift needed	M/F	• Dimple • Tethering	✓	–	✓
Direct temporal	12	• Intact lateral brow cilia • Lateral brow ptosis	M	Scar (low)	✓	–	✓
Direct full	8	Facial nerve palsy	M/F	Scar (high)	✓	✓	–
Midforehead	10	• Deep forehead rhytids • High forehead	M/F	• Scar (high) • Paresthesia	✓	✓	–
Coronal pretrichial	11	• High forehead • Dense hair	M/F	• Scar • Paresthesia	✓	✓	✓
Coronal posttrichial	11	• Low forehead • Dense hair	M/F	• Alopecia • Paresthesia	✓	✓	✓
Temporal pretrichial	12	• Wears hair forward • Long temporal hairline	F	Scar (low)	✓	–	✓
Temporal posttrichial	12	Dense hair	M/F	• Alopecia • Facial nerve injury	✓	–	✓
Small incision temporal lift and fill	13	• Temporal brow ptosis • Volume loss	M/F	Facial nerve injury	✓	–	✓
Endoscopic browlift	14	• Dense hair • Low forehead	M/F	• Alopecia • Paresthesia • Frontal nerve injury	✓	✓	✓
Fat augmentation	16	Retro-orbicularis oculi and temporal fossa deflation	M/F	• Contour irregularity • Vision loss (rare)	✓	✓	✓
Neurotoxin	15	Periocular descent and rhytids	M/F	Temporary blepharoptosis	✓	✓	✓
Fillers	15	Retro-orbicularis oculi and temporal fossa deflation	M/F	• Contour irregularity • Vision loss (rare)	✓	✓	✓

• Review old photographs to assess whether asymmetry was present in youth.

7.6.4 Minimizing Hair Loss

Avoid direct cautery near the hair follicle base to minimize the risk of alopecia. Other methods to achieve hemostasis intraoperatively include chemical and mechanical vascular compression by injection of local anesthetic with epinephrine and use of external manual pressure, respectively.

Reference

[1] Gulbitti HA, Bouman TK, Marten TJ, van der Lei B. The orbital oval balance principle: a morphometric clinical analysis. Plast Reconstr Surg. 2018;142 (4):451e-461e

8 Direct Eyebrow Elevation

Nathan W. Blessing, Wendy W. Lee

Abstract

Direct brow elevation is an effective technique to elevate either the entire horizontal brow (full direct brow) or simply the tail or temporal aspect of the brow (temporal direct brow). Aesthetic and functional indications for direct brow elevation include improvement of the superior visual field, enhancement of the upper face by relieving falsely conveyed emotions (e.g., sadness with temporal brow ptosis, anger with medial brow ptosis, or tiredness/sleepiness with full brow ptosis), relief of eyelash ptosis from excess dermatochalasis, and a decrease in chronic frontalis overaction, which may lead to headaches. Direct brow elevation is functionally effective in all patients, and while this approach is not technically challenging, wound construction and closure is paramount to achieve an acceptable cosmetic outcome. The surgical scar is best camouflaged in those with thicker eyebrow hairs and may be visible postoperatively even with flawless technique. For these reasons, this procedure should be performed only after a careful discussion of the risks, benefits, and desired patient outcomes with a clear postoperative plan for possible visible scar management, including adjunctive therapies or planned makeup usage.

Keywords: eyebrow ptosis, direct brow elevation, temporal direct brow elevation

8.1 Introduction

Although there are many options for surgically elevating a droopy eyebrow, the aptly named "direct brow" technique addresses this sequela of the aging face or motor paralysis by directly excising and shortening the tissue immediately superior to the ptotic brow.[1] The incision may span the entire brow, such as in cases of seventh nerve paralysis, or simply the temporal portion in patients with isolated temporal brow ptosis, temporal hooding, and an irregular brow contour. This technique effectively and durably elevates the eyebrow to its natural resting position over the superior orbital rim. One of the main risks of this procedure is visible scarring; therefore, patient selection, preoperative counseling, and technically sound surgical technique are of the utmost importance to achieve a cosmetically acceptable outcome. Wound construction and meticulous closure are paramount. However, even with flawless surgical technique, the scar at the incision site is often still visible, especially when the medial brow is included, where the skin is thicker with more sebaceous units. Damage to the sensory branches of the supraorbital and supratrochlear neurovascular bundles is also a risk but can be avoided with a sound knowledge of the local anatomy and dissection in a more superficial plane when approaching that medial area.

8.2 Relevant Anatomy

The eyebrow is defined by the visible eyebrow hairs and their relationship to the nose, forehead, eyelids, and temples. The medial and central hair follicles are oriented in an obliquely superior plane, whereas the hair follicles in the temporal third of the brow are oriented more perpendicular to the skin edge[2,3] (▶ Fig. 8.1). Biologically, the eyebrow and brow hairs serve to protect the eyes from moisture, dust, and dander, which helps to maintain a clear visual axis.[4] The eyebrow is also a vital part of facial expression and can be voluntarily raised, lowered, or furrowed to convey a wide spectrum of emotions.[5] A ptotic brow can interfere with an individual's visual axis and unintentionally convey a sense of tiredness or sleepiness (▶ Fig. 8.2**a**, ▶ Fig. 8.3**a**). Additionally, ptosis of the medial head of the brow can convey anger, while ptosis of the lateral head of the brow may suggest sadness.[6]

The brow may be defined anatomically by several distinct changes from the nearby eyelids.[7] Dermatologically, there is a transition from the thin eyelid skin without subcutaneous fat to the thicker and more sebaceous brow skin that is contiguous with the skin of the forehead. There is an increasingly thick layer of subcutaneous fat separating the skin from the

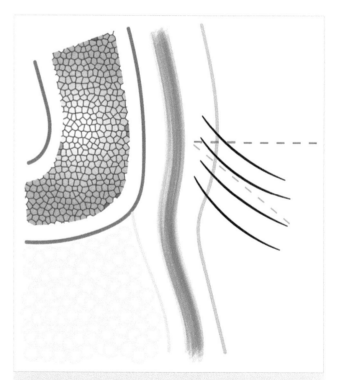

Fig. 8.1 Sagittal view of the normal relationship of the eyebrow to the adjacent anatomy. The medial and central hair follicles are oriented in an obliquely superior plane with respect to the skin edge. A skin incision perpendicular to the skin in the medial and central brow (*red dashed line*) will often transect hair follicles, resulting in brow hair loss inferior to the incision. A skin incision beveled superiorly in the plane of the follicles (*green dashed line*) minimizes unnecessary follicle transection. The upper incision should be similarly beveled to permit good wound closure. In temporal direct brow elevation, the hair follicles are oriented perpendicular to the skin (*red dashed line*) and no beveling is necessary.

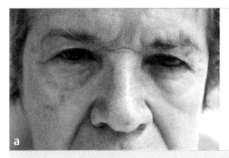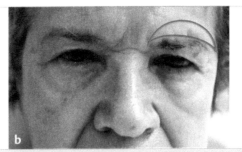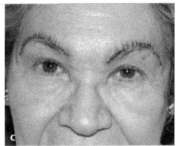

Fig. 8.2 An older female with age-related full horizontal eyebrow ptosis resting fully below the orbital rim. The brow has a flattened contour with secondary dermatochalasis **(a)**. An example of a full horizontal direct brow marking to elevate the entire eyebrow over the orbital rim and restore the normal female brow contour **(b)**. A 2-week postoperative photograph demonstrating a normal brow height and contour. No eyelid skin was removed. There is still residual crusting but the incision is healing nicely **(c)**.

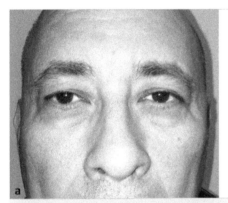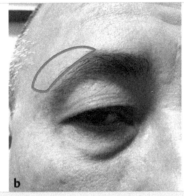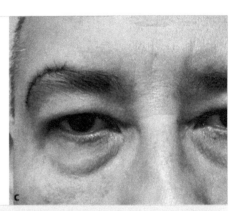

Fig. 8.3 A middle-aged male with age-related temporal brow ptosis. The downward temporal brow is causing secondary temporal dermatochalasis with hooding **(a)**. An example of a temporal direct brow marking to elevate the temporal eyebrow over the orbital rim and restore the normal flat male brow contour **(b)**. A 1-week postoperative photograph prior to suture removal. The brow has been restored to its normal height and contour and there is minimal postoperative edema or erythema **(c)**.

underlying muscular layer, which transitions from the circumferentially oriented orbicularis oculi, a brow depressor, to the vertically oriented frontalis muscle, a brow elevator. Above the arcus marginalis at the superior orbital rim but beneath the muscular layer, there is an additional fat pad overlying the periosteum labeled the brow fat pad or the retro-orbicularis oculi fat pad. This fat pad gives volume to the temporal aspect of the brow and is of particular aesthetic importance in women.[5]

The normal resting position of the youthful eyebrow is at or slightly above the superior orbital rim. The head, or most medial portion, of the eyebrow is also typically the thickest portion and begins at a line drawn vertically upward from the lateral nasal ala. The body, or central portion, of the brow continues laterally until arching and descending downward into the tail, the most lateral portion. The tail of the brow typically ends at an oblique line drawn from the lateral nasal ala intersecting with the lateral canthus.[8] The contour of a normal brow differs between men and women. Whereas the male brow is typically flatter with a small or absent peak (▶ Fig. 8.4**a**), the female brow arches upward over the lateral canthus to accent the underlying brow fat pad[9] (▶ Fig. 8.4**b**).

8.3 Goals of Intervention, Indications, and Benefits of the Procedure

The main goal of direct brow elevation is to meet the patient's postoperative expectations, which may be functional, cosmetic, or both.
- Improvement in the superior field of vision.
- Enhancement of the aesthetic of the face.
- Relief of brow skin hooding over the eyelashes.
- Decrease in chronic frontalis overaction to lift the brows away from the eyes, may also help alleviate frontal headaches.

8.4 Risks of the Procedure

- Infection.
- Bleeding.
- Pain.
- Visible scarring.
- Asymmetry.

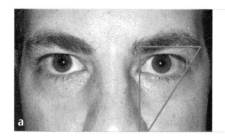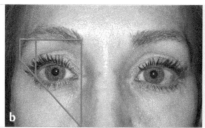

Fig. 8.4 The normal male brow contour is flat and rests just at or above the superior orbital rim (**a**), whereas the female brow contour is more arched temporally and rests above the temporal orbital rim (**b**).

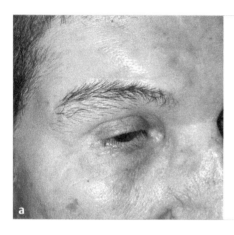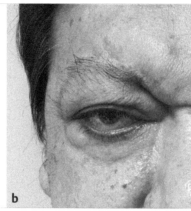

Fig. 8.5 A well-healed temporal direct brow incision (**a**) and full direct brow incision (**b**) are visible faintly above the superior brow hairs. Note that the medial portion of the full horizontal incision is more visible than the central and temporal portions (**b**).

- Feminization of the male brow.
- Overcorrection leading to a constant surprised look.
- Forehead numbness.
- Need for further procedures.

8.5 Preoperative Considerations and Patient Selection

Although effective in elevating the brow, the skin incision in direct brow elevation is only minimally camouflaged due to its placement just above the brow and the thickness of the skin being reapproximated with subsequent risk of scar contracture and depression (▶ Fig. 8.5**a**, **b**). This is in contrast to procedures such as the pretrichial temporal brow technique, internal brow-pexy, endoscopic browlift, and coronal browplasty, where the incisions are hidden among longer, fuller hair. The pretrichial technique also has risk of a visible scar, but this may be ameliorated by a trichophytic incision technique to encourage hair follicle growth through the incision site and/or the patient's hairstyle. The direct browlift technique is particularly suited to patients with thick, bushy eyebrows where superior brow hairs can mask the skin incision. It may also be a better surgical choice in patients where the skin incisions from alternative brow-elevating procedures may be more noticeable due to the patient's preferred hairstyle or a lack of hair. This often includes men with male-pattern hair loss and thick natural eyebrows. Some women may also be well suited for this procedure, particularly if they are willing to cover the resulting scar with makeup or permanent brow liner.

Preoperative patient discussion should include the risk of visible scarring and the proposed height and contour of brow elevation. Although the male brow is naturally flat, the full direct brow technique requires an arched incision to effect brow elevation and may result in a more arched brow contour. Even in women, in whom an arched brow is desirable, the contour may be unnatural in appearance and can result in a perpetually surprised look due to the amount of tissue that must be excised to achieve sufficient brow elevation.

The limited temporal direct brow technique has a decreased risk of scar contracture and depression because the temporal brow skin is often thinner and less sebaceous. Additionally, temporal brow ptosis is often more functionally limiting due to temporal hooding with blocking of the peripheral vision and aesthetically displeasing due to an unnatural brow contour. Whereas the full direct brow procedure creates an unnatural arched contour in both men and women, the temporal direct brow technique may restore a normal flat brow contour in men and a more arched lateral brow in women via excision of additional tissue.

8.6 Informed Consent

Informed consent should include a discussion of the risks, benefits, and expectations of the procedure as listed and explained above. The postoperative appearance may be roughly simulated for the patient using a few small pieces of plastic medical tape and a mirror.

8.7 Relative Contraindications

- Active local skin infection or inflammation.
- Recent history of skin cancer of the face.
- Systemic anticoagulation that cannot be suspended:
  - This is dependent on the surgeon's tolerance for intraoperative bleeding and the potential risk of postoperative hematoma formation. Excessive bleeding may

lead to an increase in cautery usage and loss of brow hairs inferior to the incision with a resultant increase in visible postoperative scarring.

- Recent upper face treatment with botulinum toxin (within 3–4 months).

8.8 Procedure

The procedure described may be done in an office-based setting or in an ambulatory surgery center.

8.8.1 Instrumentation

- Marking pen.
- Ruler and/or calipers.
- Local anesthesia: 2% lidocaine with 1:100,000 units of epinephrine (3–5 mL per side).
  - May augment with bupivacaine, ropivacaine, bicarbonate, and/or hyaluronidase.
- Castroviejo locking needle holder.
- Forceps (0.3 and 0.5 mm).
- Westcott and/or Stevens tenotomy scissors.
  - Monopolar cautery with a needle tip (optional).
- Sutures:
  - A 4–0 or 5–0 absorbable (e.g., polyglactin 910 [Vicryl] or chromic gut).
  - A 6–0 permanent suture (e.g., polypropylene [Prolene] or nylon).

8.8.2 Preoperative Checklist

- Informed consent.
- Instrumentation available.
- Patient demonstrates a clear understanding of the procedure to be performed and the desired outcome.
- Preoperative photographic documentation and visual field testing.
- Anticoagulation management (if necessary).

8.8.3 Operative Technique

Direct brow elevation may be quickly and effectively performed under local anesthesia with minimal instrumentation and minimal risk of bleeding. This may be advantageous in patients who are either unable or unwilling to undergo the general anesthesia required in other more extensive brow-elevating procedures. The most critical portions of the procedure include marking and wound construction/closure.

- Premedication with acetaminophen/codeine 300/30 mg or hydrocodone/acetaminophen 5/325 mg and diazepam 5 mg or lorazepam 1 mg may be given 30 minutes before the procedure.
- The incisions are marked in either the supine or sitting position.
  - Inferior marking is delineated within the first two to three rows of the superior brow hairs.
    1. Full direct brow marking starts starting at the medial head of the brow (▶ Fig. 8.2**b**).

2. Temporal direct brow marking starts at the temporal third of the brow where the brow descends laterally (▶ Fig. 8.3**b**).
  - Superior marking may be achieved with two methods. The highest point should be placed over the lateral canthus and each end tapered to form an ellipse.
    1. Manually raising the brow to the desired postoperative position: (a) the marking pen is rested over the inferior line; (b) the brow is dropped to its resting position; (c) The skin underneath the pen is marked.
    2. Estimation based on brow anatomy: upper marking is placed slightly larger than one brow width from the inferior marking.
- Local anesthesia is infiltrated into the marked areas and dispersed using compression with a 4 × 4 gauze, waiting 5 to 10 minutes for the full anesthetic and hemostatic effect.
- Skin incision:
  - The medial and central hair follicles are oriented in an obliquely superior plane. The lower incision should be beveled 45° superiorly to prevent follicle transection and subsequent hair loss as this may make the incision scar more visible. The upper incision should be beveled in parallel to permit good wound closure (▶ Fig. 8.1).
  - The temporal hair follicles are oriented perpendicular to the skin; for a temporal-only approach, the incision can be made perpendicular to the skin.
  - Cautery may be used but should be avoided in the superficial inferior wound margin to prevent hair follicle destruction.
  - The lower marking should be incised first from corner to corner in a smooth continuous fashion through the skin and subcutaneous fat. A second pass can then deepen the incision to at least the muscular layer or deeper to the periosteum. This can be performed with a blade or cutting cautery.
  - The superior incision is then incised using the same technique.
- Flap elevation:
  - May be performed with blunt-tipped surgical scissors such as Westcott or Stevens tenotomy scissors or monopolar cautery.
  - A flap is elevated at either the level of the superficial muscular plane or the preperiosteum.
  - Some practitioners excise full-thickness muscle to prevent bunching of the wound and enhance brow elevation, but this is not mandatory.
    1. Added risks include damage to the sensory fibers of V1 medially between the periosteum and muscular layer and bleeding from large caliber vessels.
    2. Medial flap dissection can be shallowed to a more superficial plane (superficial or lamellar muscle) to decrease the risk of forehead numbness or excessive bleeding.
- Wound closure is accomplished in layers.
  - Muscle or immediate premuscular tissue: interrupted 4–0 or 5–0 polyglactin 910 (Vicryl) or chromic gut.
  - Subcutaneous fat: buried interrupted 4–0 or 5–0 polyglactin 910 (Vicryl) or chromic gut.
  - Skin: Interrupted and running permanent sutures (6–0 polypropylene [Prolene] or nylon).

1. Excellent wound eversion is paramount to avoid a depressed scar: (a) vertical mattress sutures; (b) Running locking sutures; (c) Running horizontal mattress.

8.8.4 Expert Tips/Pearls/Suggestions

- The eyebrows should always be assessed as a functional subunit of the upper face; the presence of concomitant primary dermatochalasis and blepharoptosis should be identified and addressed.
- Patients receiving botulinum toxin treatments to the upper face should be assessed and treated when full muscular function is present for a predictable postoperative result.
- Care should be taken when elevating the full brow in men as extensive lifting with this technique imparts a feminine brow shape.
- Double-check all markings for symmetry and contour prior to cutting.
- The temporal portion of the marking may be flared outward in a lazy-S configuration lateral to the end of the temporal brow hairs to achieve additional temporal brow elevation.
- Marking in the sitting position allows for adequate compensation for the downward effects of gravity.
- For efficiency, the patient may be injected with local anesthetic following a quick prep with isopropyl alcohol pads prior to formal skin preparation and draping.
- The supratrochlear and supraorbital neurovascular bundles are approximately 17 and 27 mm from the midline at the orbital rim and the supraorbital notch is often palpable.
  - These can be marked as a reminder to stay more superficial above the muscular layer medially.

8.8.5 Postoperative Care

- Avoidance of heavy lifting, bending, and straining for 1 week.
- Showering from the neck down can be started the day after surgery; swimming or submerging the head should be avoided for 2 weeks after surgery.
- Ice should be applied for the first 48 hours postoperatively, 15 to 20 minutes on/off alternating while awake.
- Sleeping elevated on several pillows can help reduce postoperative edema.
- The wound should be kept clean and dry and dressed with antibiotic ophthalmic ointment (e.g., bacitracin, neomycin/dexamethasone, and erythromycin) three to four times daily.
- Pain management is typically achieved with ice and acetaminophen 500 to 1,000 mg every 6 hours.
- Prescription systemic anticoagulation can be resumed within 24 to 48 hours.
- Sutures are removed at postoperative week 1.
- Pigmented makeup should be avoided for at least 2 weeks to avoid permanent staining.
- Sun avoidance for 6 months.

8.9 Complications and Their Management

Most postoperative complications from this procedure are the result of poor communication between the patient and surgeon. Written instructions should be given to every patient and emphasized both preoperatively and postoperatively. A phone call the night or morning after surgery helps to reassure the patient and catch any misunderstandings before they become a problem. Residual brow ptosis is uncommon but can be revised after 4 to 6 weeks. Often, there is an unrecognized component of primary dermatochalasis that may be addressed via blepharoplasty. Visible scarring is the most common adverse outcome of this procedure, and management begins with a preoperative discussion of this risk. Almost all patients have a visible line (red, fading to pale white) present for 4 to 6 months after surgery. This line can be camouflaged with makeup after several weeks. Patients should be cautioned to avoid sun exposure for the first 6 months to prevent postinflammatory hyperpigmentation and scar thickening. There are topical creams and gels that can help the healing process (containing ingredients such as arnica, growth factors, antioxidants, and vitamin C), which can be applied 1 to 2 weeks after the surgery. Oral arnica may be started preoperatively and continued through the first several weeks after surgery, as long as bruising and swelling are present. Topical silicone may also help minimize visible scars. Laser therapy, both ablative and nonablative, can also be used to stimulate collagen and decrease the appearance of scars, if necessary. Rarely, an overtly visible scar may require direct excision and reconstruction.

References

[1] Booth AJ, Murray A, Tyers AG. The direct brow lift: efficacy, complications, and patient satisfaction. Br J Ophthalmol. 2004; 88(5):688–691
[2] Kersten RC, Kulwin DR. Direct, midforehead, and pretrichial browplasty. In: Tse DT, ed. Color Atlas of Oculoplastic Surgery. Philadelphia, PA: Wolters Kluwer Health/Lippincott Williams & Wilkins; 2011
[3] May M, Levine RE, Patel BC, Anderson RL. Eye reanimation techniques. In: May M, Schaitkin BM, eds. Facial Paralysis: Rehabilitation Techniques. New York, NY: Thieme; 2003
[4] Nguyen JV. The biology, structure, and function of eyebrow hair. J Drugs Dermatol. 2014; 13(1) Suppl:s12–s16
[5] Knize DM. Anatomic concepts for brow lift procedures. Plast Reconstr Surg. 2009; 124(6):2118–2126
[6] Knoll BI, Attkiss KJ, Persing JA. The influence of forehead, brow, and periorbital aesthetics on perceived expression in the youthful face. Plast Reconstr Surg. 2008; 121(5):1793–1802
[7] Lemke BN, Stasior OG. The anatomy of eyebrow ptosis. Arch Ophthalmol. 1982; 100(6):981–986
[8] Gunter JP, Antrobus SD. Aesthetic analysis of the eyebrows. Plast Reconstr Surg. 1997; 99(7):1808–1816
[9] Goldstein SM, Katowitz JA. The male eyebrow: a topographic anatomic analysis. Ophthal Plast Reconstr Surg. 2005; 21(4):285–291

9 Internal Eyebrow Lift

Ana F. Duarte, Alice V. Pereira, Juan A. Delgado, Martín H. Devoto

Abstract

The internal eyebrow lift has gained popularity since its first description in 1982. It allows brow stabilization and some elevation through an upper blepharoplasty incision. The procedure also minimizes temporal eyebrow descent that may occur due to eyelid skin and soft tissue removal after upper blepharoplasty. The procedure is safe, quick, and long-lasting and it does not require expensive equipment or additional incisions.

Keywords: brow ptosis, browpexy, upper blepharoplasty, browlift

9.1 Introduction

Aesthetic and functional assessment of the upper face requires a careful understanding of the upper face–eyebrow–eyelid continuum. The ideal eyebrow shape has been the subject of debate.[1] To optimize surgical lifting outcomes, each patient should be evaluated individually, taking into account the overall facial profile, age, gender, and ethnicity.[2-4] While patients may present with isolated eyelid or eyebrow complaints, a thorough upper facial rejuvenation requires assessment of both structures. The correction of dermatochalasis or eyelid ptosis in the presence of significant brow ptosis can reduce the compensatory frontalis contraction and aggravate brow descent if not concurrently addressed (▶ Fig. 9.1).[5]

Addressing brow ptosis with the internal browlift provides the advantages of a hidden scar, placed within a standard upper blepharoplasty incision, no additional incisions, no extended forehead dissection, and limited increased operative and recovery time.[6-12] The technique prevents lateral brow descent and may even achieve a mild-to-moderate eyebrow elevation (▶ Fig. 9.2). Medial brow lifting may also be attained through the same incision by weakening the eyebrow muscle depressors, allowing unopposed frontalis action.[9,10] Further benefits include minimal equipment cost, a shorter learning curve, and a lower risk of neurovascular damage because the procedure is performed under direct visualization.[7,8,13] The procedure may provide a cosmetic effect comparable to that produced by more aggressive techniques while minimizing complications.[8-12]

Internal browlift disadvantages include a limited amount of lift that can be achieved and questionable long-term results compared with brow lifting through direct, midforehead, coronal, and endoscopic approaches.[14,15] Damage to the neurovascular bundles (supraorbital and supratrochlear) remains a concern if the medial portion of the brow is accessed.[10] Here, we discuss our approach to internal eyebrow lifting.

9.2 Anatomic Considerations of the Upper Facial Continuum

The eyebrow and upper eyelid should be seen as a continuum.[1] In a patient presenting for upper blepharoplasty, the eyebrow position and shape should always be evaluated because its descent may be an important cause of postoperative eyelid skin redundancy and patient dissatisfaction.[16] It is important to recognize if brow ptosis has a lateral and/or medial component, as the causal forces and resultant corrective procedures are distinct. Further, it is important to maintain awareness of contemporary beauty ideals: the female eyebrow is arched laterally and positioned a few millimeters above the orbital rim,[3] while the male brow lies at the level of the orbital rim and is flat.[4] Brow volume should also be noted, in particular, the retro-orbicularis oculi fat (ROOF) pad position and volume. If a browlift is indicated and not performed, the possibility of postblepharoplasty brow ptosis from reduced compensatory frontalis contraction should be discussed with the patient. Older patient photographs assessing brow position in youth are a helpful guide on where to set the eyebrow position.

9.3 Goals of Intervention

- Brow stabilization.
- Treatment of mild-to-moderate temporal brow ptosis in patients who are undergoing upper blepharoplasty.

9.4 Risks

- Over- or undercorrection.
- Asymmetry.
- Brow ptosis recurrence.
- Bleeding.
- Infection.

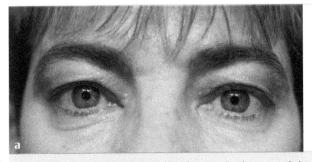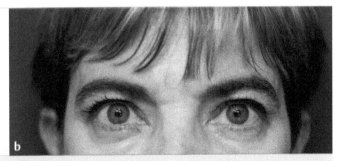

Fig. 9.1 Pre- **(a)** and postoperative **(b)** photographs showing a slight eyebrow ptosis induced after bilateral upper blepharoplasty alone.

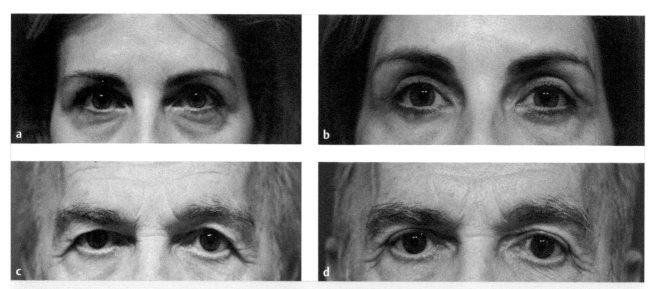

Fig. 9.2 Pre- **(a, c)** and postoperative **(b, d)** results of a female (superior) and a male (inferior) patient after upper blepharoplasty associated with a bilateral internal browlift.

- Transient edema.
- Eyelid, forehead, and scalp numbness.
- Temporary lagophthalmos.
- Eyebrow contour deformities.
- Skin dimpling.
- Prolonged forehead sensory loss from damage to the supraorbital and supratrochlear nerves.
- Consecutive eyebrow droop from damage to temporal branch of facial nerve.

9.5 Benefits

- Same incision as a standard upper blepharoplasty procedure.
- Limited tissue dissection.
- Quick procedure.
- Recovery time is the same as in upper blepharoplasty.
- Lower complication rate when compared to temporal or coronal lifts.
- The procedure may be used in thin-haired or bald patients.
- Minimal additional cost.

9.6 Informed Consent

The impact of browlift complications on the patient and the surgeon may be profound. It is easier to manage a dissatisfied patient when there has been a thorough preoperative discussion about the procedure, risks, benefits, and alternative approaches to manage the problem. The patient should be made aware of the possibility of additional surgery and financial responsibility.

9.7 Indications

- Mild-to-moderate temporal brow ptosis in patients who are undergoing upper blepharoplasty.[11]
- Mild-to-moderate temporal brow ptosis in patients with a high hairline or lengthened forehead.[11]

- Patient's general health makes a procedure under local anesthesia more suitable.[17]

9.8 Contraindications

- Severe brow ptosis requiring large eyebrow elevation.[10,14,18]
- Patient desire to address prominent horizontal wrinkles or redundant forehead skin.[18]
- Very thick-skinned patients where this minimally invasive technique is less effective.
- Very thin skin and ROOF, where the risk for dimpling is higher.

9.9 Patient Assessment

A good preoperative patient evaluation is essential to an excellent postoperative outcome. We focus on a patient's medical history, ophthalmic history, and external examination.

9.9.1 Medical History

Systemic conditions such as hypertension, diabetes, thyroid dysfunction, allergies, and autoimmune and hematologic disorders should be noted and managed preoperatively.
- Thyroid eye disease should be inactive for a period of at least 6 months.
- Antiplatelet drugs (such as aspirin, clopidogrel, and nonsteroidal anti-inflammatory agents), anticoagulants (heparin and warfarin), and supplemental medications should be recorded and withheld prior to surgery.

9.9.2 Ophthalmic History

A thorough ophthalmic history is important to avoid postoperative landmines in brow lifting surgery.

- History of previous facial surgical and nonsurgical treatments, with particular attention toward the use of neuromodulators and fillers.
  - A 3- to 6-month waiting period should be used in patients receiving these treatments to assess baseline eyebrow and eyelid positions.
- Previous refractive surgery or dry eye symptoms should be elicited because dry eye can complicate postoperative comfort and patient satisfaction.

9.9.3 Ophthalmic Examination

A complete ophthalmologic examination, including visual acuity, ocular motility, slit lamp examination, and tear film status, should be performed before every eyebrow and eyelid lift. Proceed with caution in patients with ocular surface staining, poor Bell's phenomenon, lagophthalmos, or decreased tear production.

9.9.4 Anatomic Evaluation: The Eyelid and Eyebrow Subunits

In assessing the upper facial continuum, careful attention must be given to each subunit separately.

The Eyelid

- Preoperative evaluation should include the upper margin–pupillary reflex distance (MRD1), margin crease distance, and margin fold distance with the brow in a neutral position to identify concurrent upper eyelid ptosis or any preexisting margin crease or fold asymmetries, respectively.
- The degree of eyelid hooding over the eyelid margin with and without digital brow suspension should be assessed.
- The prominence of the medial and central preaponeurotic fat pads should be noted.
- The presence of lacrimal gland prolapse should be identified.
- The presence of periorbital asymmetries should be documented.

The Eyebrow

- The presence, severity, and pattern of brow ptosis are determined with frontalis and glabellar muscles at rest, achieved by gentle downward pressure by the examiner's finger.
  - Notation of ptosis of the medial, central, and lateral brow should be made.
  - Inferior corneal limbus to inferior eyebrow hair (ILB) can be a useful measure to quantify the amount of eyebrow ptosis.
- The cause of an asymmetric brow position should be noted. Besides dermatochalasis or unilateral or asymmetric ptosis, mechanisms such as eyelid retraction, underlying bone asymmetry, previous trauma or surgery, facial nerve palsy, and ocular dominance should be identified.[19]
- If brow hair is plucked, it may be difficult to determine its actual inferior limit.
  - It is helpful to palpate brow fat and the transition between the brow and eyelid skin.
  - Brow ptosis is present when the brow is located below the superior orbital rim, or the ILB is less than 20 mm.[20]

9.10 Preoperative Checklist

- A full understanding of the patient's cosmetic concerns and expectations must be documented in the patient's chart.
- A complete preoperative evaluation should be documented.
- Preoperative photographs are important for surgical planning and to document pre- and postoperative findings. Standardized lighting conditions, the absence of makeup, and a fixed distance between the patient and photographer allow a more accurate retrospective comparison. Front full and close-up photographs in primary, downgaze, and upgaze as well as a lateral and/or oblique photographs allow a proper recording of the upper facial unit.
- OR checklist:
  - Signed informed consent documenting risks, benefits, and alternatives to the procedure.
  - Confirmation of the surgical indication.
  - Review anesthesia plan with the anesthesia provider. Anesthesia options should be discussed with the patient during the preoperative consultation.
    1. Upper blepharoplasty combined with internal browlift can be performed under local anesthesia and minimal oral sedation.
    2. If the patient is anxious or chooses not to be awake during the procedure, intravenous sedation or general anesthesia can be chosen.

9.11 The Procedure

The procedure may be performed in an office-based setting, outpatient surgical center, or hospital.

9.11.1 Instrumentation Needed

Instrumentation is similar to upper blepharoplasty.
- Curved spring scissors (Westcott).
- Forceps with and without teeth.
- Needle holder.
- Freer periosteum elevator.
- Catspaw and Desmarres retractors.
- Measuring caliper.
- Scalpel handle with a #15 blade.
- Unipolar cautery (with a Colorado or Colorado-like microdissection needle).

9.11.2 Sutures

- A 4–0 polyglactin 910 suture (Ethicon Vicryl) with a P-3 needle.
- A 6–0 polypropylene (Ethicon Prolene).

9.11.3 Operative Technique

With this technique, brow fixation is performed through an upper blepharoplasty incision.
- Preoperative surgical marking is made with the patient in the upright position.
  - The brow is suspended digitally and settled in its ideal location and a ruler is positioned at the peak level to

measure the amount of descent when the eyebrow is dropped. The same height is measured and marked cephalically to the brow.

○ Another mark may be placed laterally to raise the lateral third of the brow (► Fig. 9.3).

○ A third marking is placed to localize the medial supraorbital notch.

○ A standard blepharoplasty mark is finally performed, taking into account the final brow position.

• Topical proparacaine is instilled in both eyes prior to injection and before preparation of the face with povidone-iodine.

• Pain during anesthetic infiltration may be reduced by injecting a 1:5 mixture of anesthetic (lidocaine 2% with epinephrine:sterile saline) to the surgical area.

○ A higher concentration of local anesthetic (lidocaine 2% with epinephrine and/or bupivacaine 0.75%) may then be

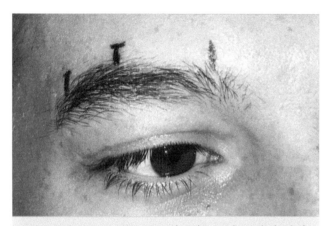

Fig. 9.3 Preoperative marking. Lateral markings indicate the level of desired eyebrow elevation at each point. Supraorbital notch location is marked medially.

painlessly infiltrated in each eyelid and brow area (► Fig. 9.4**a**).

• A bilateral standard upper eyelid blepharoplasty is performed.[21]

• Using blunt scissors or a monopolar cautery, dissection is carried out superiorly in the suborbicularis plane until the orbital rim is reached (► Fig. 9.4**b**).

• Stevens scissors are used for blunt dissection superficial to the ROOF, using a vertical and horizontal spreading motion (► Fig. 9.4**c**).

○ The goal is to create a pocket 1.5 to 2 cm above the superolateral orbital rim, being careful not to extend nasally to the previously marked supraorbital neurovascular bundle.

• Brow fat debulking has been described to thin lateral fullness.[22] We prefer not to do it as we believe this is important for the maintenance of a more natural and youthful volume and contour in this area.

• If there is significant medial brow ptosis, the medial depressor muscles (corrugator, depressor supercilii, and procerus) can be released/divided.[5,10]

○ The dissection proceeds medially in a suborbicularis plane using a scissor-spreading technique until the corrugator, depressor supercilii, and procerus are identified.

○ Care should be taken during dissection to minimize damage to supraorbital and supratrochlear neurovascular bundles to avoid sensory paresthesias.

○ The muscles are selectively divided using cautery and scissors to titrate protractor release.

Note: Too much muscle destruction may widen the intra-brow distance in an aesthetically displeasing way.

• A 4–0 polyglactin 910 suture is passed transcutaneously at the previously marked eyebrow location into the dissected plane. The suture is placed through the superior orbital rim ROOF, engaging periosteum at a level correlating with the

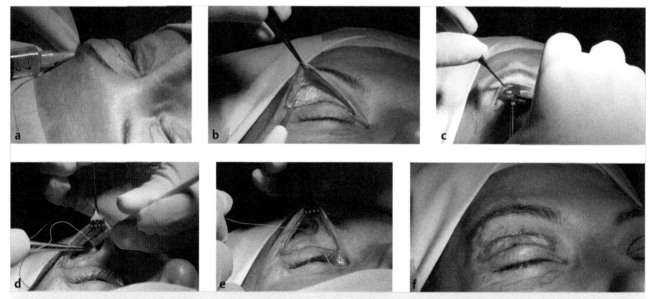

Fig. 9.4 Internal browlift technique. **(a)** Local anesthetic is infiltrated in the upper eyelid and brow area. **(b)** After upper blepharoplasty, dissection in the suborbicularis plane is performed to reach the orbital rim. **(c)** Blunt dissection is completed above the ROOF, using a spreading motion with Stevens scissors. **(d)** A 4–0 Vicryl suture is passed transcutaneously into the dissected pocket and placed through the superior orbital rim ROOF and periosteum and passed through the sub-brow tissue. **(e)** The suture is pulled from the skin into the dissected plane and tied. A second suture may be placed laterally. **(f)** Blepharoplasty incision is closed.

desired elevation (▶ Fig. 9.4**d**). The needle is passed through the orbicularis muscle and sub-brow tissue and the transcutaneous end of the suture is pulled into the dissected pocket. An optional second suture may be placed laterally in the same manner.

- Both purse-string sutures are tied (▶ Fig. 9.4**e**).
  - Care should be taken not to engage skin because it can cause visible puckering.
- A few variants of the transblepharoplasty browlift have been described. Burroughs's technique focused on weakening brow depressors achieving a natural, however limited, lift.[5] As an alternative to sutures, an absorbable anchoring device fixated to the frontal bone (Endotine, Coapt Systems, Palo Alto, CA) has also been described.[23]
- The blepharoplasty incision is ready for closure with a 6–0 Prolene suture (▶ Fig. 9.4**f**).
- Typical postoperative results are seen in ▶ Fig. 9.2.

9.12 Expert Tips/Pearls/Suggestions

- It is important to not overelevate the eyebrow, especially in patients with deep-set eyes because it may highlight the orbital rim and create a deep superior sulcus and a surprised, aesthetically unpleasant look.[24]
- Marked asymmetries in height should be avoided, as they may lead to a curious facial expression.[25]
- The final eyebrow shape is as important as its height. Always consider patient's sex, age, and facial features for optimal planning of which brow component (lateral, central, and medial) should be lifted.
  - An arched brow in a male patient is unnatural.
  - A medial brow peak creates a "surprised" look.
  - An exaggeratedly high lateral brow in comparison to the medial end creates an angry appearance.[24]

9.13 Postoperative Care Checklist

- Head of bed elevated 30°.
- Ice-cold compresses for 15 minutes every 2 hours during the first 48 hours.
- Regular ocular lubrication and antibiotic ointment for the upper blepharoplasty incision should be prescribed for 1 week.
- Use of sunglasses and sun avoidance to prevent squinting during the first postoperative month.
- Discuss possible outcomes during the initial postoperative period, including bruising and swelling, redness, or pain in the location of the browpexy suture.

9.14 Complications and Their Management

Complications are uncommon, can be avoided by meticulous technique, and may be treated with simple maneuvers.[10,13]

9.14.1 Bleeding

Significant bleeding may arise from the superficial temporal, supraorbital, and supratrochlear arteries. Hematomas are rare and, when small, resolve with time. A significant expanding hematoma should be treated with surgical drainage and vessel cauterization to achieve hemostasis.[13] Transient diplopia due to a hematoma in the vicinity of the trochlea has also been reported.[26] Adequate preoperative anesthetic injections with epinephrine, meticulous operative hemostasis, and postoperative care (head elevation, cold packs, and blood pressure control) decrease this risk.

9.14.2 Infection

Infections are rare and treated with topical antibiotics for superficial wound infections and combined topical and oral antibiotics for deeper infections. When infections do not resolve, culture and tissue biopsy are warranted to rule out atypical mycobacteria or organisms not susceptible to the initial treatment regimen.

9.14.3 Nerve Damage

Nerve damage may occur and is usually temporary, a result of anesthetic infiltration, direct injection into the nerve, blunt dissection, edema of the nerve sheath, aggressive traction during surgery, or cautery.[10,13,22]

Sensory Nerve Damage

With medial depressor muscle division, temporary neurapraxia of the supratrochlear and supraorbital nerve branches is expected, with sensory return typically within 2 to 3 weeks.

Motor Nerve Damage

Damage to the temporal branch of the facial nerve is the most worrisome local complication in browlift surgery.[13] Understanding seventh nerve anatomy and careful tissue retraction and dissection can minimize the risk of damage.[8]

- Should a paralysis develop, watchful waiting with patient reassurance and frequent follow-up is important.
- Contralateral neuromodulation with botulinum toxin may be used to improve symmetry until nerve function returns.
- If motor function does not return after a few weeks, nerve conduction studies are warranted.

9.14.4 Postoperative Lagophthalmos and Dry Eye

If lagophthalmos or poor orbicularis tone occurs, postoperative ocular lubrication is recommended until the eye discomfort resolves.

9.14.5 Residual Aesthetic Deformity

The most common reason for surgical revision is residual or recurrent aesthetic deformities.

Undercorrection

The majority of cases where a lower than desired effect is obtained are due to inappropriate browlift technique selection.[10,14,27] Effect attenuation over time may occur, and it can be prevented by simple measures such as botulinum toxin injections in the lateral orbital orbicularis muscle or the use of sunglasses and sun avoidance to prevent squinting in the first postoperative month.[10,13]

Overcorrection

Overresection of the medial brow depressors muscles may lead to widening and elevation of the medial brow, as well as glabellar contour defects. This will create an unfavorable brow shape, with a chronically surprised look.[24]

- In mild cases, botulinum toxin injections in the central frontal area may help.
- If pronounced, the medial brow can be surgically lowered. If this appearance results from insufficient lateral brow elevation compared to the medial area, an isolated lateral browlift may be repeated.

Brow Asymmetry

Some patients have brow asymmetry prior to surgery and many of them will still maintain it after surgery. If no asymmetry was present preoperatively, it is probably related to inappropriate suture placement and may require revision.

9.14.6 Skin Dimpling

It is important to place the browpexy sutures deep to provide long-lasting fixation and stability while allowing a good range of motion of the overlying soft tissues. Too superficial suture placement may cause skin dimpling or erosion. Massage may release skin dimpling. If it does not resolve, surgical revision may be necessary.

9.15 Summary

The internal eyebrow lift is a technically straightforward and quick approach to eyebrow stabilization and mild elevation. The approach is a nice adjunct to standard upper blepharoplasty where the same incision is used to achieve an improved upper facial aesthetic outcome.

References

[1] Lam VB, Czyz CN, Wulc AE. The brow-eyelid continuum: an anatomic perspective. Clin Plast Surg. 2013; 40(1):1–19

[2] Kunjur J, Sabesan T, Ilankovan V. Anthropometric analysis of eyebrows and eyelids: an inter-racial study. Br J Oral Maxillofac Surg. 2006; 44(2):89–93

[3] Codner MA, Kikkawa DO, Korn BS, Pacella SJ. Blepharoplasty and brow lift. Plast Reconstr Surg. 2010; 126(1):1e–17e

[4] Clevens RA. Rejuvenation of the male brow. Facial Plast Surg Clin North Am. 2008; 16(3):299–312, vi

[5] Burroughs JR, Bearden WH, Anderson RL, McCann JD. Internal brow elevation at blepharoplasty. Arch Facial Plast Surg. 2006; 8(1):36–41

[6] Zandi A, Ranjbar-Omidi B, Pourazizi M. Temporal brow lift vs internal browpexy in females undergoing upper blepharoplasty: Effects on lateral brow lifting. J Cosmet Dermatol. 2018; 17(5):855–861

[7] Cohen BD, Reiffel AJ, Spinelli HM. Browpexy through the upper lid (BUL): a new technique of lifting the brow with a standard blepharoplasty incision. Aesthet Surg J. 2011; 31(2):163–169

[8] Cintra HP, Basile FV. Transpalpebral brow lifting. Clin Plast Surg. 2008; 35(3):381–392, discussion 379

[9] Mokhtarzadeh A, Massry GG, Bitrian E, Harrison AR. Quantitative efficacy of external and internal browpexy performed in conjunction with blepharoplasty. Orbit. 2017; 36(2):102–109

[10] Georgescu D, Anderson RL, McCann JD. Brow ptosis correction: a comparison of five techniques. Facial Plast Surg. 2010; 26(3):186–192

[11] Nahai FR. The varied options in brow lifting. Clin Plast Surg. 2013; 40(1):101–104

[12] Ramirez OM. Transblepharoplasty forehead lift and upper face rejuvenation. Ann Plast Surg. 1996; 37(6):577–584

[13] Langsdon PR, Metzinger SE, Glickstein JS, Armstrong DL. Transblepharoplasty brow suspension: an expanded role. Ann Plast Surg. 2008; 60(1):2–5

[14] Pedroza F, dos Anjos GC, Bedoya M, Rivera M. Update on brow and forehead lifting. Curr Opin Otolaryngol Head Neck Surg. 2006; 14(4):283–288

[15] Slivinskis IB, Faiwichow L, Lemos Dias FC. Transpalpebral approach to the corrugator supercilii and procerus muscles. Plast Reconstr Surg. 2000; 105(2):803–804

[16] Lemke BN, Stasior OG. The anatomy of eyebrow ptosis. Arch Ophthalmol. 1982; 100(6):981–986

[17] Almousa R, Amrith S, Sundar G. Browlift—a South East Asian experience. Orbit. 2009; 28(6):347–353

[18] Leopizzi G. A transpalpebral approach to treatment of eyebrow ptosis. Aesthetic Plast Surg. 1999; 23(2):125–130

[19] Shah CT, Nguyen EV, Hassan AS. Asymmetric eyebrow elevation and its association with ocular dominance. Ophthal Plast Reconstr Surg. 2012; 28(1):50–53

[20] Putterman A. Evaluation of the cosmetic oculoplastic surgery patient. In: Cosmetic Oculoplastic Surgery. New York, NY: Grune & Stratton, Inc; 1982:11–26

[21] Zoumalan CI, Roostaeian J. Simplifying Blepharoplasty. Plast Reconstr Surg. 2016; 137(1):196e–213e

[22] McCord CD, Doxanas MT. Browplasty and browpexy: an adjunct to blepharoplasty. Plast Reconstr Surg. 1990; 86(2):248–254

[23] Evans GR, Kelishadi SS, Ho KU, Plastic Surgery Educational Foundation DATA Committee. "Heads up" on brow lift with Coapt Systems' Endotine Forehead technology. Plast Reconstr Surg. 2004; 113(5):1504–1505

[24] Yalçınkaya E, Cingi C, Söken H, Ulusoy S, Muluk NB. Aesthetic analysis of the ideal eyebrow shape and position. Eur Arch Otorhinolaryngol. 2016; 273(2):305–310

[25] Karacalar A, Korkmaz A, Kale A, Kopuz C. Compensatory brow asymmetry: anatomic study and clinical experience. Aesthetic Plast Surg. 2005; 29(2):119–123

[26] Mavrikakis I, DeSousa JL, Malhotra R. Periosteal fixation during subperiosteal brow lift surgery. Dermatol Surg. 2008; 34(11):1500–1506

[27] Presti P, Yalamanchili H, Honrado CP. Rejuvenation of the aging upper third of the face. Facial Plast Surg. 2006; 22(2):91–96

10 Midforehead Browlift Technique

Krishnapriya Kalyam, John B. Holds

Abstract

Brow ptosis cannot be ignored when evaluating a patient for rejuvenation of the upper third of the face. There are several techniques to address brow ptosis, and midforehead browlift has been performed for decades. It is a technically straightforward procedure and, with graded resection, can be used to lift any part of the brow and address the medial brow depressors. This technique has special utility in the treatment of brow ptosis associated with facial paralysis.

Keywords: browlift, midforehead browlift, facial paralysis

10.1 Introduction

Brow ptosis progresses with age causing functional and aesthetic complaints. The combination of loss of tissue volume and elasticity, effects of gravity, and contraction of the brow depressors results in forehead or brow ptosis with a tired, aged appearance and visual obstruction if severe. Significant unilateral eyebrow ptosis can also result from seventh nerve palsy following trauma, Bell's palsy, or other diseases. When evaluating options for rejuvenation of upper third of the face, brow ptosis is often found in conjunction with horizontal forehead rhytids and furrowing of glabella. Contraction of the frontalis muscle results in horizontal creases and the action of corrugator muscle results in vertical creases of the glabella. These creases deepen with age and become permanent.

There are several ways to perform a browlift depending on the amount of brow ptosis, tissue characteristics, hairline, forehead height, age, gender, and cosmetic expectations. Treatment options include nonsurgical treatments such as botulinum toxin denervation of the brow depressors, thread lifts and internal browpexy, direct browlift, midforehead browlift, pretrichial browlift, and coronal and endoscopic foreheadlift.[1]

The midforehead browlift approach described by Brennan and Rafaty in the 1980s takes advantage of the deep horizontal forehead furrows.[2] It can be useful in patients with broad or recessed hairline where a coronal or pretrichial approach may leave an unacceptable scar at the hairline. In addition, the midforehead approach allows ready access to the brow depressor muscles that may be resected and weakened. This technique is excellent in patients with facial palsy who have a significant brow ptosis and lack rhytids on the paralytic side.

In this procedure, appropriate amounts of midforehead skin and subcutaneous fat are removed with an incision generally based on a deep midforehead crease. It is performed bilaterally or unilaterally as needed with excellent functional and cosmetic outcomes.

10.2 Goals of Intervention/ Indications

- Elevate medial, central, and/or lateral eyebrow as needed.

- Camouflage scar in midforehead furrows.
- No hair loss or disturbance of the hairline or eyebrow.

10.3 Risks of the Procedure

- Bleeding.
- Infection—rare.
- Scarring.
- Forehead sensory or motor deficit.

10.4 Benefits of the Procedure

- Lift eyebrow bilaterally or unilaterally.
- Easy access to brow depressors if needed.
- Camouflage scar in forehead rhytids.
- Special utility in facial paralysis as a more natural contour can be achieved with elevation of the head (medial) brow to an optimal contour.

10.5 Informed Consent

- Include risks and benefits (as above).
- Emphasize incision location and months required for incision to mature and resolve incisional erythema.

10.6 Contraindications

- Very short forehead to hairline.
- Patient unwilling to accept incision location or time to heal.

10.7 Preoperative Assessment

- Preoperative assessment should be performed in an upright position with the face in repose.
- Redundant eyelid skin that extends beyond the lateral canthus provides clues for temporal brow ptosis.
- Relative position of brow to the orbital rim is noted.
  - A female brow typically rests above the orbital rim.
  - The male eyebrow generally rests at or near the orbital rim.
- Forehead and medial brow rhytids are noted.

10.8 The Procedure

This procedure can be done under local, monitored, or general anesthesia in an office-based procedure room, ambulatory operating room, or hospital-based setting. It can be performed unilaterally or bilaterally.

10.8.1 Instruments Needed

- Westcott and Kaye scissors.
- Needle drivers.
- The #15 Bard-Parker knife handle and blade.

- Paufique or heavier forceps.
- Knapp four-prong or similar size retractor.
- Sutures:
  - A 4–0 and/or 5–0 polyglactin 910 (Vicryl).
  - A 5–0 polypropylene P-13 (Covidien) or P-3 (Ethicon) needle.
- Local anesthetic:
  - Bupivacaine 0.5% with 1:100,000 epinephrine.
  - Lidocaine 2% with 1:100,000 epinephrine.

10.8.2 Operative Technique

- Patients are marked with the forehead relaxed in the upright position (▶ Fig. 10.1). Forehead incisions are marked so they

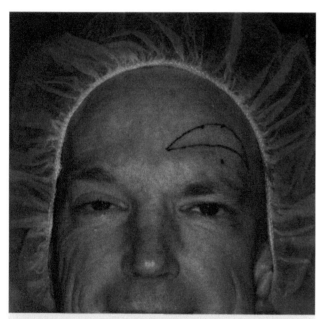

Fig. 10.1 Preoperative photograph showing markings of area of excision in a patient with unilateral brow ptosis from facial paralysis.

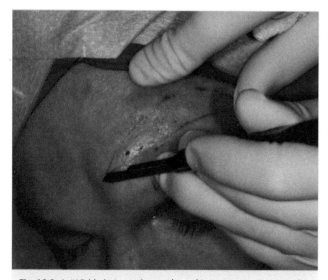

Fig. 10.3 A #15 blade is used to make a skin incision in an upwardly angling bevel of 45 to 75°.

are along one edge of a prominent horizontal forehead rhytid in the midforehead. Incisions can extend laterally to the temporal crest. The widest portion of skin excision should be at the point requiring the maximum brow elevation, usually over the lateral arch of the brow. The incisions can be staggered at different heights on each side, depending on the level of prominent furrows to further hide the scar.

- Anesthesia can vary from lightly sedated local to general anesthesia. Optionally, dilute anesthetic (0.2% lidocaine) is injected into the marked areas and under the area to be elevated. We first administer dilute anesthetic in all our cases. Either 2% lidocaine or 0.5% bupivacaine with 1:100,000 with epinephrine is reinjected for vasoconstriction and more prolonged anesthesia. Supraorbital and supratrochlear blocks are administered (▶ Fig. 10.2). A tumescent technique with dilute local anesthetic decreases later anesthetic requirements and decreases bleeding during the surgical dissection.
- A #15 blade is used to make a skin incision at the uppermost marked line perpendicular to the skin. An alternate technique is to incise with an upwardly angling bevel of 45 to 75°, opposite of how one might incise for a trichophytic forehead lift (▶ Fig. 10.3).
- Sharp dissection is carried down to the frontalis muscle and the skin and subcutaneous tissue is undermined (▶ Fig. 10.4). Undermining can be minimal or beneath the eyebrow.

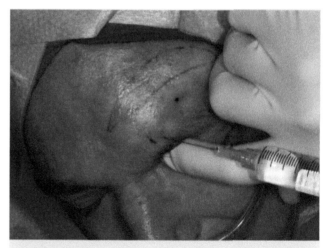

Fig. 10.2 Local anesthetic blocks are administered in area of excision and supraorbital block is given.

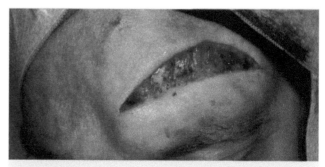

Fig. 10.4 Sharp dissection is carried down to frontalis muscle and the skin and subcutaneous tissue is excised.

Likewise, the undermined plane may be subcutaneous and superficial to all major neurovascular bundles or deep to the galea (▶ Fig. 10.5). Care is taken medially and laterally to avoid damage to nerves. After undermining and any galeal advancement, the undermined soft tissues and forehead skin are elevated and overlapped to determine if the proposed excision from the initial markings is appropriate and any adjustments made.

- Hemostasis is achieved with cautery.
- The skin is excised on each side (matching prior vertical or beveled incision).
- A two-layer closure is achieved using interrupted inverted, 4–0 or 5–0 polyglactin 910 (Vicryl) deep sutures (▶ Fig. 10.6). The skin is closed in a running vertical mattress fashion to

achieve optimal wound approximation and eversion of wound edges (▶ Fig. 10.7).
- Typical preoperative and postoperative results are shown in ▶ Fig. 10.8 and ▶ Fig. 10.9 for unilateral and bilateral cases, respectively.
  - In bilateral cases, the incisions are usually staggered vertically.
  - There is no need for a surgical drain.

10.9 Expert Tips/Pearls/Suggestions

- The beveled incision should be at a same angle at both inferior and superior skin incisions as with a trichophytic technique.
- Avoid deeper dissection to prevent injury to the neurovascular structures.
- A key to good cosmesis lies in good wound closure with appropriate tension and wound edge eversion.

10.10 Postoperative Care Checklist

- Ice is applied as tolerated to the operative sites for 48 hours.
- The patient is advised to sleep with the head of the bed elevated.
- Postoperative medications are given:
  - Antibiotic ointment (Neosporin or bacitracin) three times a day.
  - Oral pain medication, typically acetaminophen/hydrocodone, 5 mg/325 mg.
- Postoperative wound check at 7 to 10 days for suture removal.

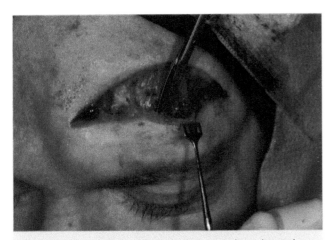

Fig. 10.5 Undermining is performed subcutaneously to elevate the brow. Care is taken to avoid injury to neurovascular bundles.

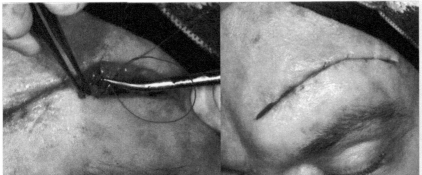

Fig. 10.6 Deep closure is performed using inverted interrupted 5–0 polyglactin sutures.

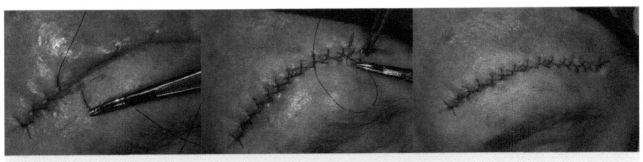

Fig. 10.7 Superficial skin is closed in a running vertical mattress fashion using 5–0 polypropylene suture.

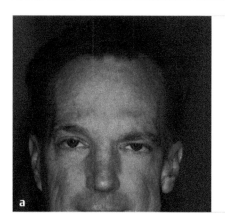
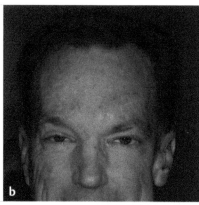

Fig. 10.8 Preoperative (a) and 1-month postoperative (b) after left midforehead direct browlift in a patient with left facial palsy and left brow ptosis.

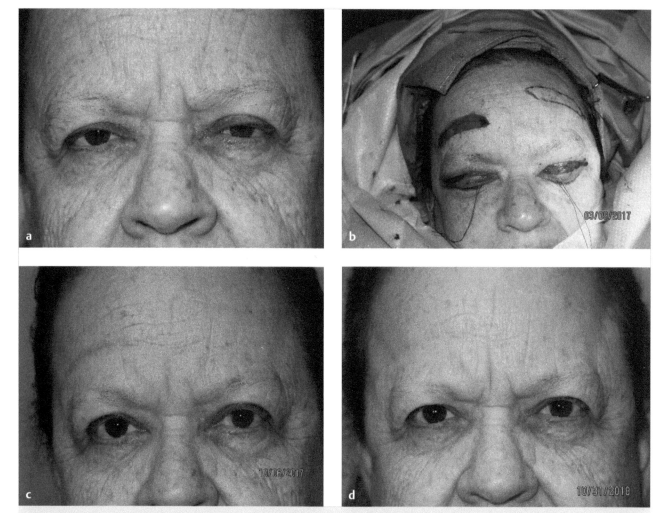

Fig. 10.9 Preoperative (a), intraoperative (b), 6-week postoperation (c), and 1-year postbilateral midforehead browlift (d), upper eyelid ptosis, and blepharoplasty. Note the staggered vertical heights of the incisions in this bilateral case, the erythema at the right side wound at 6 weeks, and resolution by 1 year. (These images are provided courtesy of Dr. Michael A. Burnstine.)

10.11 Complications and Their Management

- Bleeding—rare:
  - Pressure.
  - Open wound, cauterize, and close wound.
- Infection:
  - Oral antibiotics usually prevent wound infections.
- Undercorrection or contour abnormality:
  - The procedure may be repeated to address a contour abnormality or undercorrection through the same incision site.
  - Botox may be given to the frontalis of the opposite side to improve symmetry between the sides.
- Overcorrection
  - This rarely happens. Botox may be used to the frontalis on the ipsilateral side.
  - Galeal recession can be performed, if needed. However, with time, the brow will relax slightly.

- Scarring:
  - Combined steroids and 5-fluorouracil may be given into the scar in the early (first 2 months) postoperative period.
  - Carbon dioxide or erbium-doped yttrium aluminum garnet laser resurfacing may be utilized to level and obscure the incision 2 months or more postoperatively

10.12 Conclusion

Direct brow elevation through a midforehead approach is an excellent tool for brow elevation in facial paralysis patients and patients that do not mind a prolonged recovery period. It should be a tool in every oculofacial surgeon's armamentarium.

References

[1] Johnson CM, Jr, Waldman SR. Midforehead lift. Arch Otolaryngol. 1983; 109 (3):155–159

[2] Brennan HG, Rafaty FM. Midforehead incisions in treatment of the aging face. Arch Otolaryngol. 1982; 108(11):732–734

11 Open Coronal Pretrichial Browlift Surgery

Wesley L. Brundridge, Hans B. Heymann, Christopher M. DeBacker, David E. E. Holck

Abstract

Brow lifting is an integral part of facial rejuvenation. Forehead rejuvenation is able to restore a more youthful and aesthetically pleasing brow position and facial harmony. Currently, there are many well-described approaches available for forehead rejuvenation. Here, we describe the coronal pretrichial lift to elevate the eyebrow and enhance the upper face by addressing forehead rhytids and improving the brow to trichion distance.

Keywords: brow ptosis, glabella, forehead rejuvenation, browlift, coronal browlift, open browlift, pretrichial browlift

11.1 Introduction

The coronal open pretrichial browlift treats a descended brow line and addresses the aging forehead in a long-lasting way. It can be approached through either a pre- or posttrichial coronal incision.[1-10] Patients with a significant component of medial eyebrow ptosis, mechanical ptosis, vertical and horizontal glabellar rhytids, a high hairline, and a pronounced dorsal nasal root are well treated with this open technique because access and visualization for glabellar manipulation are excellent.[1-6] Coronal brow lifting incisions are less useful in male patients with male-pattern baldness due to a noticeable scar. Patients less concerned with forehead rhytids or cosmesis and who desire a procedure solely to expand their visual field may not require an open browlift.

11.2 Unique Anatomical Considerations in Coronal Brow Lifting

Age and genetics contribute to periorbital soft tissue descent and deflation. The subbrow fibrofatty soft tissue (the retro-orbicularis oculus fat pad or ROOF) descends over the orbital rim and into the eyelid, and may aggravate dermatochalasis and upper eyelid herniated orbital fat. These changes may alter the face and may emote a fatigued, angry, depressed, or sad appearance, as well as affect the superior field of vision. Altering the upper face through an open brow lifting approach requires a thorough understanding of brow anatomy to improve the facial aesthetic and to avoid complications.

11.2.1 The Eyebrow

Characteristics of the ideal brow have been described. The ideal height and contour vary by age and gender.

Eyebrow Position

The medial eyebrow should begin in the same vertical plane as the nasal ala and medial canthus. The temporal brow should end along the oblique line extending from the nasal ala through the lateral canthus. The eyebrow apex should lie directly over the lateral limbus.[11] For women, the brow begins at or slightly above the orbital rim prominence, arches upward as it sweeps laterally, and is at its maximal height at the two-thirds point. In men, the aesthetically pleasing brow should be flatter, straighter, and at or slightly below the orbital rim.[2]

Eyebrow Hair Orientation

The medial aspect of the brow has hairs that direct upward, the body of the brow has hairs that direct more horizontally, and the tail of the brow has hairs that may orient slightly downward. The tail of the brow often does not overlie the frontalis muscle because this muscle does not extend past the conjoint fascia separating the temporalis muscle laterally from the frontalis muscle centrally. This exacerbates temporal brow ptosis with age.

11.2.2 The Anatomic Layers

The scalp is composed of five layers: skin, subcutaneous tissue, aponeurosis, loose areolar tissue, and periosteum. The skin of the brow and forehead is thick and laden with sebaceous glands. The supraorbital ridge separates the midface from the forehead, and the hairline separates the forehead from the scalp. The galea aponeurosis connects anteriorly to the frontalis muscle, which serves as the primary brow elevator and posteriorly to the occipital muscle. The loose areolar tissue allows a safe, reliable dissection plane for the open browlift. It also allows easy access to the glabella with its corrugator and procerus muscles. The subcutaneous dissection also allows another dissection plane. Caution is necessary in the subcutaneous plane to avoid excess skin tension, which may cause overlying ischemia and necrosis.

11.2.3 The Muscles of Elevation and Depression

The muscles responsible for brow depression include the paired corrugator supercilii, procerus, and the orbicularis oculi muscles.[1,4] The temporoparietal fascia (TPF) is deep to the skin and subcutaneous tissue in the temporal region. It is contiguous with the superficial muscular aponeurotic system inferiorly and galea superiorly. Deep to the TPF is the deep temporal fascia. The deep temporal fascia divides at the supraorbital ridge into intermediate temporal fascia and deep temporal fascia, with an intermediate fat pad between the two layers. The dissection plane between the superficial and deep temporalis fascial plane is loose and often may be dissected digitally. The deep temporal fat pad lies below the deep temporal fascia. Traumatizing the deep temporal fat pad may cause atrophy and temporal wasting.[4]

11.2.4 The Sensory Supply

The sensory supply to the forehead and scalp includes the supratrochlear and supraorbital branches of the ophthalmic division of the trigeminal nerve. These may be easily identified in the subgaleal approach and preserved during dissection.[4] The supraorbital nerve can be seen exiting the supraorbital notch, or in 10% of cases from the supraorbital foramen.[5] There are multiple trunks to the supraorbital nerve as it exits the supraorbital notch or foramen. The zygomaticotemporal and auriculotemporal nerves, branches of the maxillary nerve and mandibular branches of the trigeminal nerve, supply the temple. The scalp is supplied by extensions of these nerves and also by branches of the dorsal rami of cervical spinal nerves and the cervical plexus.[1]

11.2.5 The Facial Nerve

The course of the temporal branch of the facial nerve must be appreciated during brow lifting. The temporal branch of the facial nerve emerges from the parotid gland approximately 2.5 cm anterior to the tragus and runs obliquely. It passes 1.5 cm lateral to the lateral orbital rim to innervate the frontalis muscle from its deep surface.[6] It is just superficial to the periosteum at the zygoma, and then it travels anterior to the superficial layers of the deep temporal fascia superiorly to ultimately reach the brow musculature from the undersurface. Fibers enter the underbelly of the frontalis muscle approximately 1 cm above the supraorbital rim. It is imperative to carefully dissect deep to the temporal fascia, staying anterior to the deep temporalis fascia to avoid functional and cosmetic complications from nerve injury (see "Upper Facial Danger Zones" in Chapter 2).[1]

11.2.6 The Vascular Supply

The vascular supply to this region is from branches of both the internal and external carotid arteries.[1,4] The supraorbital and supratrochlear arteries originate from the internal carotid system via the ophthalmic artery and supply the central anterior forehead and scalp. These arteries pierce the frontalis muscle a centimeter above the brow and lie more superficial. The remainder of the blood supply comes via the branches of the superficial temporal, zygomaticotemporal, posterior auricular, and occipital arteries, which all are branches of the external carotid.

11.3 Patient Evaluation

Preoperative evaluation of the browlift patient is a critical step. It is here that forehead length and contour, eyebrow shape and contour, forehead rhytids, and nasal root aging changes are addressed.

11.3.1 Forehead Length and Contour

The distance between the brow and hairline must always be considered in brow lifting. The typical youthful distances for forehead height are 4.5 to 5.5 cm.[3] The distance must be balanced with the upper and lower thirds of the face. Higher hairlines contribute to an aged face. A high hairline is better suited to the pretrichial open browlift incision to avoid unnaturally lengthening of the forehead. Hairline contour should also be

taken under consideration when planning the incision. The incision should be made in parallel to the shape of the hairline. Patients with a widow's peak should have the incision marked to avoid altering the central contour of the hairline.

11.3.2 Eyebrow Shape and Contour

Patients with nasal brow ptosis, mechanical ptosis from eyebrow descent, and lateral brow ptosis are ideal candidates for the pretrichial open-sky approach.

11.3.3 Forehead Rhytids

Prominent forehead rhytids are treated by elevation of the entire frontalis muscle, skin, and subcutaneous tissue as a unit. Scoring the underside of the frontalis muscle perpendicular to the frontalis muscle orientation can easily be performed with the open-sky approach and will weaken the horizontal lines.

11.3.4 Nasal Root

A prominent nasal root can be released through an open browlift. As needed for deep vertical and horizontal glabellar lines, release of the corrugator and procerus muscles, respectively, can offer long-lasting desirable reduction of these lines. Caution must be exercised to avoid overaggressive resection of the corrugator muscles to prevent splaying of the medial head of the brow as well as dimpling of the glabella postoperatively. An increased risk of hypesthesia may also be seen. The authors occasionally place soft tissue fillers in the area around the resected corrugator muscles to avoid these complications.

11.4 Goals of Intervention/ Indications

The main goal of the open browlift is to meet the patient's desires. The primary goal is to correct functionally limiting or aesthetically displeasing brow ptosis with associated forehead wrinkling by elevating the entire brow as a unit.[1]
- Improvement in the superior field of vision (functional brow ptosis with resultant mechanical upper eyelid ptosis).
- Improved eyebrow height.
- Improved eyebrow contour.
- Reduction of glabellar folds and the skin redundancy at the nasal root.
- Improved aesthetic treatment of forehead rhytids.
- Relief from nonsurgical applications to improve the eyebrow height and contour, specifically neurotoxins into the brow depressors and fillers to volumize.

11.5 Risks of the Procedure

- Bleeding (subflap hematoma formation).
- Infection (uncommon).
- Wound dehiscence (uncommon).
- Asymmetric brow position.
- Asymmetric hairline position.
- Overcorrection (aesthetically displeasing overelevation).

- Undercorrection.
- Damage to frontal (temporal) branch of the facial nerve, inducing brow ptosis.
- Sensory nerve deficit (prolonged anesthesia, paresthesia, and dysesthesia of the scalp and forehead).[9,10]
- Lagophthalmos from elevation of the eyebrow in conjunction with upper blepharoplasty.
- Skin necrosis.
- Prominent or irregular scar.
- Temporary or permanent eyebrow alopecia.
- Abnormal hair part (with posttrichial open browlift).
- Abnormal soft tissue contour.

11.6 Benefits of the Procedure

- Improvement of superior field of vision and mechanical ptosis.
- Aesthetic enhancement of the upper face, including the forehead, eyebrow, and upper eyelids.
- Improvement of glabella and nasal root.
- Improved eyebrow contour.
- Avoidance of nonsurgical preparations to create the desired brow height and contour (neuromodulation and filler volumization).
- Incision camouflage in posttrichial coronal browlift and relative incision camouflage in pretrichial coronal browlift.
- Low rate of serious complications.

11.7 Contraindications

- Lagophthalmos due to a deficiency of upper eyelid skin from prior blepharoplasty, other surgery, or trauma.
- Poor corneal protective mechanisms.
- A high hairline or male-pattern baldness is a relative contraindication to coronal incision brow lifting because the incision will be visible.

11.8 Informed Consent

- Include risks, benefits, and contraindications.
- Have the patients demonstrate their desired eyebrow position and contour with a mirror.
- Understand and convey what is a functional and what is an aesthetic outcome.
- Discuss the possible need for additional surgery to address upper eyelid ptosis, dermatochalasis and herniated orbital fat, crease reformation, and/or lacrimal gland prolapse, if present.
- Preoperative discussion of postoperative pain, swelling, and bruising that may persist for several weeks following surgery.
- Discuss temporary or prolonged numbness, paresthesias, and dysesthesias as possible sequelae of surgery: postoperative sensory disturbance such as itching or numbness can persist for months.
- Injury to the facial nerve is rare, but the consent should cover damage to the temporal branch of the facial nerve.
- Discuss possible early postoperative seroma or hematoma formation, which would require drainage (uncommon).

11.9 The Procedure

The procedure described can be done in an outpatient (ambulatory) surgery center, hospital, or in a well-equipped office-based setting. If cooperative ptosis surgery is planned, it should be performed prior to brow rejuvenation, which requires heavier anesthesia.

11.9.1 Instruments Needed (▶ Fig. 11.1)

- Sterile surgical marking pen.
- Ruler.
- Local (2% lidocaine with 1:100,000 U epinephrine mixed 1:1 ratio with 0.75% bupivacaine to inject incisions) and tumescent local anesthesia (mix 90 mL of normal saline, 60 mL of 1% lidocaine with 1:100,000 epinephrine, and 40 mL of 0.25% bupivacaine; 30–40 mL on 1.5-inch spinal needle).
- Adson (large-toothed) forceps.
- Facelift scissors.
- Bishop Harmon forceps.
- Bipolar cautery.
- Hemostat.
- Scalpel blades, #10 and #11.
- The 4 × 4 gauze and lap sponges.
- Freer periosteal elevator.
- Large two-prong skin hooks (two).
- Hemostat clamp.
- Monopolar (optional).
- Bipolar cautery.
- Westcott scissors.
- 0.5 or Bishop Harmon forceps.
- Headlight.
- Suction.
- Illuminated retractor.

11.9.2 Sutures Used

- A 5–0 chromic gut suture for everting the incision skin edges.
- Approximately 35 regular surgical skin staples with stapler.

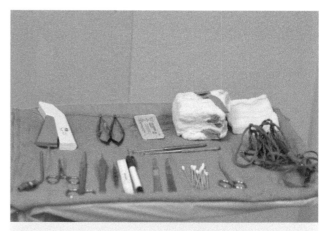

Fig. 11.1 Instruments used in coronal pretrichial brow lifting (see "Instruments Needed" for itemized description).

11.9.3 Preoperative Checklist

- Informed consent with documentation of desired patient preference for eyebrow height, contour, glabellar rejuvenation, and incision placement.
- Preoperative medical clearance, with stopping of all anticoagulants preoperatively (aspirin-containing medications 10 days preoperatively, nonsteroidals 4–5 days preoperatively, nutritional supplements, including garlic, ginkgo, ginseng, and ginger, and alcohol 4–5 days preoperatively).
- Instrumentation on hand.
- Preoperative photographic documentation (frontal view, lateral view [Frankfurt plane], oblique view, and demonstrating preoperative facial nerve function). This is essential for postoperative comparison.
- Give preoperative antibiotics within 1 hour of beginning surgery.
- Control blood pressure adequately before surgery.
- Encourage smoking cessation prior to surgery to facilitate better healing.

11.9.4 The Operative Technique

- Premedication with lorazepam 1 mg and acetaminophen/hydrocodone 5 mg/325 mg may be given 30 minutes before the procedure.
- The patient is marked in the preoperative area sitting up. Key anatomic landmarks are marked, including the supraorbital notch, supraorbital neurovascular bundle, and the course of the frontal branch of the facial nerve. The hairline incision is also marked (▶ Fig. 11.2).
  - Forehead incision:
    - Approximately 5 mm posterior to the trichion (the point where the normal hairline and middle line of the hairline intersect) for pretrichial incision.
    - Approximately 3 to 4 cm posterior to the hairline for posttrichial incision. The incision is extended further behind the temporal hairline. The higher the forehead, the greater the temporal extension.
    - An irregular incision is preferable to maximally camouflage the incision (▶ Fig. 11.3).
    - For a subcutaneous dissection, the incision is placed approximately 5 mm posterior to the trichion. It is typically extended to the temporal limbus. In patients with significant temporal hooding, the dissection is extended to the temporal crest. In these cases, we mark the temporal crest as the lateral extent of the dissection.
    - Widow's peak (if present): (1) Area of maximal brow elevation, approximately 5 cm on either side of the widow's peak. This typically corresponds to the temporal corneal limbus; (2) In general, the area of maximal elevation should be more lateral in a female to achieve a more feminine lateral arch.
  - Glabellar folds are marked, especially if the patient wishes these to be ameliorated.
  - Areas of caution.
    - Supraorbital neurovascular bundle.
    - Course of the frontal branch of the facial nerve (see "Upper Facial Danger Zones" in Chapter 2).
  - A preoperative decision is made with the patient on eyebrow shaping and amount of desired elevation.
- Local anesthesia is injected along the planned incision line, and the forehead is tumesced for hemostatic effect.
  - If a subgaleal dissection plane is anticipated, deeper tumescence is infiltrated.
  - If a subcutaneous dissection is planned, infiltration of tumescent anesthesia is placed in this superficial plane. Draping may be accomplished by wrapping surgical towels around the head to pull back the hair. They may be fixed using towel clamps or staples.
- An incision is made with a beveled #10 (subgaleal) or #11 (subcutaneous) blade (▶ Fig. 11.3).
  - A #10 blade is used to make the coronal or pretrichial incisions down to the subgaleal plane.
  - The shape of the forehead incision is generally 2.5 to 5.0 cm posterior to the frontal hairline in a coronal incision. The shape of the incision should parallel the shape of the hairline.
  - For pretrichial incisions, many surgeons advocate an irregular incision to aid in scar camouflage (▶ Fig. 11.3, ▶ Fig. 11.4).

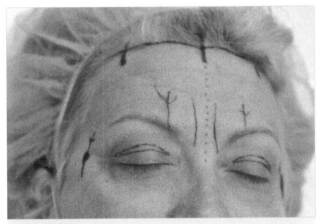

Fig. 11.2 Preoperative markings. The pretrichial incision is marked approximately 5 mm above the hairline. The central (widow's) peak is marked along with the planned maximal elevation corresponding to the temporal limbus (approximately 5 cm on either side of the widow's peak). The course of the frontal branch of the facial nerve and the supraorbital neurovascular bundle are marked. The glabellar folds are also marked.

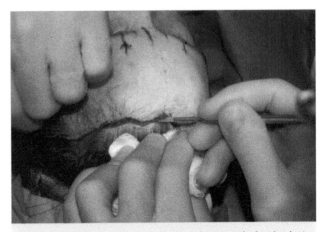

Fig. 11.3 A beveled incision is made along the premarked trichophytic incision. The incision follows the hairline contour in an irregular line.

- A subgaleal dissection plane is developed centrally. Frequently, this plane is loose and can be extended inferiorly using spreading technique with facelift scissors or digitally. Two-prong skin hooks are used to retract the flap for better visualization (▶ Fig. 11.4).
- In a subgaleal dissection, the temporal dissection plane is developed between the superficial and deep temporalis fascia. This is a loose areolar plane that is easily dissected digitally or with spreading motion of facelift scissors (▶ Fig. 11.5).
- Alternatively, a subcutaneous dissection may be developed using facelift scissors or digitally (▶ Fig. 11.6).
  - Tumescing in the subcutaneous plane makes this dissection easier.
  - Avoid cautery on the undersurface of the skin flap to avoid overlying skin necrosis. The subcutaneous dissection plane is not extended beyond the temporal crest.
- The temporal dissection plane is connected with the subgaleal dissection plane by dissecting the conjoint fascia overlying the temporal crest (▶ Fig. 11.7). This may be accomplished with facelift scissors face down along the bone of the crest to release the conjoint tendon (▶ Fig. 11.8). This maneuver creates a large released upper facial flap (▶ Fig. 11.9).
- Digital and/or blunt dissection is used when approaching the superior orbital rim to avoid injury to the supraorbital and supratrochlear neurovascular bundles until they are safely identified.
- Horizontal and vertical spreading with facelift scissors or alternatively a Freer periosteal elevator at the superior orbital rim from lateral canthus to lateral canthus is used to dissect into the ROOF to maximize forehead and brow mobilization.
- If the nasal root is an aesthetic concern, dissection is continued toward the radix of the nose to mobilize and elevate the soft tissue in this area.
- Hemostasis is maintained with bipolar cautery.
  - Avoid cautery on the undersurface of the forehead flap.
  - Use caution with cautery along the hair follicles at the incision site.
- The corrugator muscles are identified and dissected from surrounding neurovascular structures and subcutaneous soft tissue bluntly with a fine-tipped hemostat (▶ Fig. 11.10). If planned preoperatively:
  - The muscle is debulked/transected with bipolar cautery and Westcott scissors.
  - To avoid soft tissue depressions (dimpling), we occasionally take fibrofatty tissue dissected from the excised forehead flap and fixate this between the cut edges of the resected corrugator muscle using 5–0 fast-absorbing gut sutures (▶ Fig. 11.11).
- As desired, this same tissue may be placed along the superotemporal orbital rim to augment soft tissue deflation in this area (▶ Fig. 11.12, ▶ Fig. 11.13).

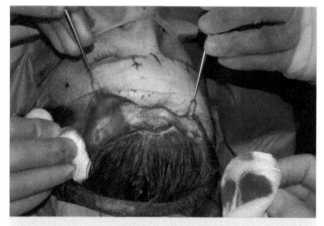

Fig. 11.4 A central subgaleal dissection plane is easily developed, and dissection in this loose plane may be extended manually or with spreading of facelift scissors. Caution is maintained as the surgeon approaches the superior orbital rim, and near the supraorbital neurovascular bundle.

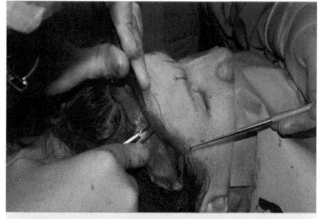

Fig. 11.5 The temporal dissection plane is developed between the superficial and deep temporal fascial planes. This is a loose areolar plane that may be expanded digitally or with spreading using facelift scissors. Caution is maintained inferiorly where the overlying frontal branch of the facial nerve resides.

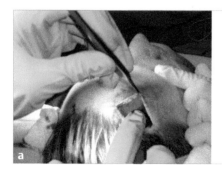
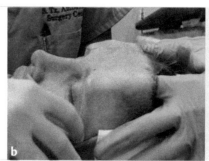

Fig. 11.6 A subcutaneous dissection plane may also be developed (a). Tumescence is carefully infiltrated in the subcutaneous plane to facilitate dissection. The incisional bevel is increased to better enter this plane. The undersurface of the dissection plane has a cobblestone appearance of the subcutaneous fat. Dissection may be accomplished with blunt spreading of facelift scissors and/or digitally. The lateral extent of the dissection is at the temporal crest. Dissection is continued to the superior orbital rim (b).

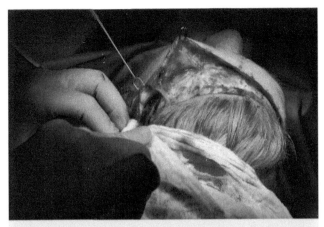

Fig. 11.7 Between the central subgaleal dissection plane and the temporal dissection plane, the adherent conjoined fascia is apparent.

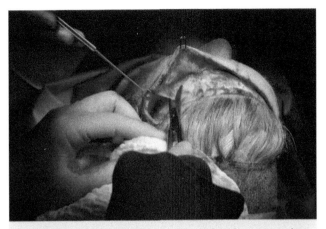

Fig. 11.8 The conjoined fascia is released with facelift scissors pushing against the periosteal plane.

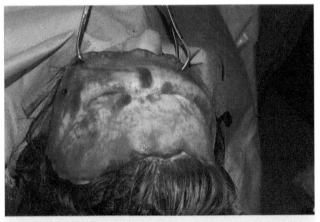

Fig. 11.9 The dissected subgaleal forehead flap is exposed and demonstrates the supraorbital neurovascular bundle and the glabella.

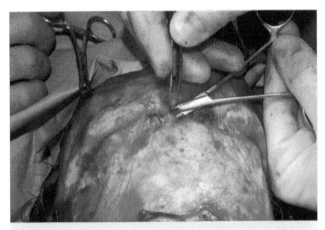

Fig. 11.10 If corrugator release is planned at preoperative evaluation, the corrugator muscle is dissected from the adjacent supraorbital neurovascular bundle, exposed, and managed by segmental weakening or transection.

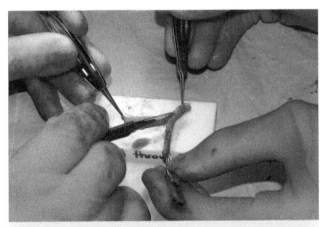

Fig. 11.11 If planned preoperatively, the fibrofatty subcutaneous tissue is dissected in the subdermal plane from the excised scalp segment.

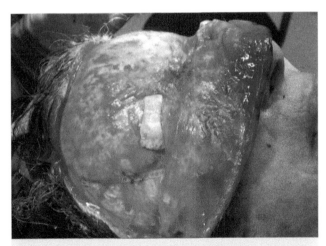

Fig. 11.12 The fibrofatty tissue may be fixated at the temporal brow to provide soft tissue augmentation to this area.

- If horizontal brow rhytids are to be addressed, scoring the frontalis muscle from the undersurface of the forehead flap to weaken the frontalis muscle may be performed at this step.
- A marking pen and ruler are used to mark the desired amount of skin and soft tissue to excise (▶ Fig. 11.14).
  - The amount of resection is determined preoperatively. In general, removing approximately 8 to 10 mm of tissue centrally and 12 to 15 mm temporally will result in an appropriate aesthetic result.
  - In a subcutaneous dissection, 10- to 15-mm central resection and 15- to 20-mm temporal resection will result in an optimal result.
- The incision is initially closed with 35 regular staples centrally and at the area of maximal elevation on both sides (▶ Fig. 11.15). The symmetry of the browlift is checked.
  - If further elevation is required, an additional tissue flap may be resected.
  - If one side or both eyebrows are overcorrected, posterior subgaleal dissection will lower the flap.

- A #10 or #11 blade and facelift scissors are used to remove the pretrichial skin (▶ Fig. 11.16).
- The incision is closed with approximately 35 regular stainless steel skin staples as well as sutures along the irregular incision line (▶ Fig. 11.17).

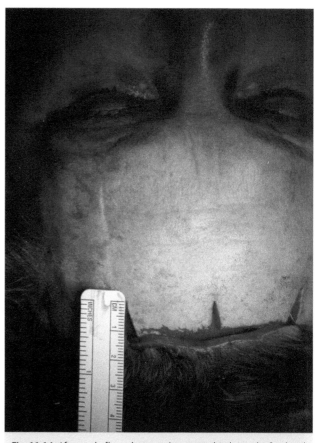

Fig. 11.14 After scalp flap release at the supraorbital rim, the forehead flap is advanced superiorly. The preoperatively planned amount of tissue to be excised is marked, and back cuts are made at the central (widow's peak) and area of maximal elevation (typically 5 cm on either side of the widow's peak).

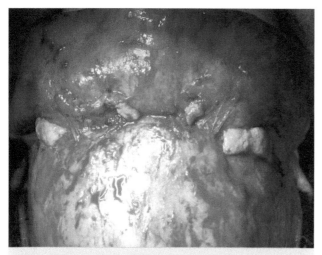

Fig. 11.13 The same fibrofatty tissue may be sutured to the free edges of the resected corrugator muscle centrally to avoid subcutaneous dimpling and maintain corrugator recession.

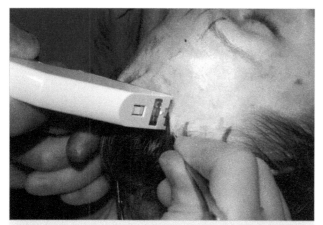

Fig. 11.15 Approximately 35 regular staples are used to fixate the advanced forehead flap. Symmetry is evaluated prior to excision of the scalp tissue.

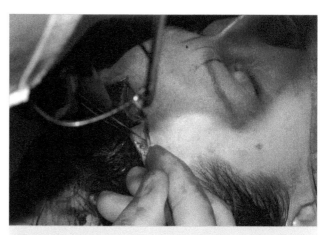

Fig. 11.16 Segmental excision of the scalp flap tissue. The excised tissue may be used for volume augmentation as seen in ▶ Fig. 11.11, ▶ Fig. 11.12, ▶ Fig. 11.13.

- In closing, the wound edges should be everted with Bishop Harmon forceps or Adson forceps.
  - Alternatively, simple interrupted and running sutures can be used to evert the wound edges. Caution is maintained to avoid wound tension, as this may cause hair follicle loss.
- Antibiotic ointment is placed on the incision site after the hair is washed. Use prewashed woven gauze bandage (e.g., Kerlix Bandage Rolls, Covidien Ltd, Dublin, Ireland) and wrap the head with moderate tightness. Bandaging with pressure should surround the brow incisions and also wrap under the

patient's chin for stabilization. The Kerlix dressing is covered with a Coban self-adherent bandage to apply further pressure to the flap. The surgeon should be mindful of the bandage tightness underneath the chin to minimize patient discomfort.
- Excellent, youthful results can be obtained with this upper facial surgery approach (▶ Fig. 11.18, ▶ Fig. 11.19, ▶ Fig. 11.20).

11.10 Expert Tips/Pearls/Suggestions

- Document other preexisting conditions such as preexisting facial nerve weakness, dermatochalasis, degree of steatoblepharon, lacrimal gland prolapse, or upper eyelid ptosis prior to performing the brow lifting surgery. Preexisting conditions may be corrected prior to brow lifting or concurrently.
  - Ptosis surgeries that require patient cooperation should be done prior to brow lifting.
  - Blepharoplasty surgery may be performed before or after the brow ptosis correction. Avoidance of excess tissue excision is paramount to avoid lagophthalmos.
  - Blepharoplasty incision geometry may change if performing both browlift and blepharoplasty concurrently. Elevation of the temporal eyebrow reduces the need for large lateral upper blepharoplasty incisions or lateral blepharoplasty incision flaring.

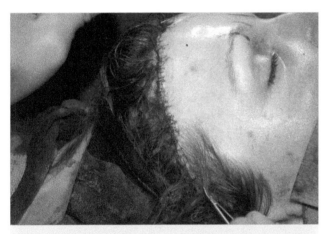

Fig. 11.17 The forehead flap is secured using 35 regular staples. The temporal soft tissue augmentation is preplaced.

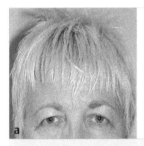 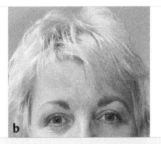 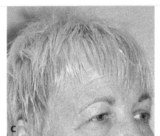 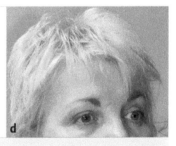

Fig. 11.18 (a–d) Pre- and postoperative view of open pretrichial browlift. The patient also underwent concurrent upper and lower eyelid blepharoplasty. Temporal view of pre- and postoperative open pretrichial browlift.

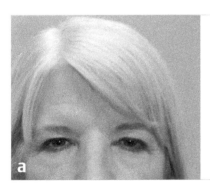 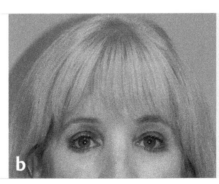

Fig. 11.19 (a,b) Pre- and postoperative view of open browlift with upper eyelid blepharoplasty.

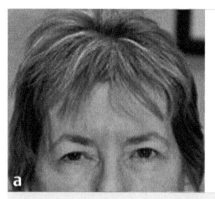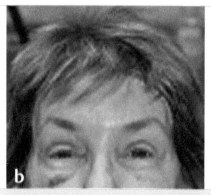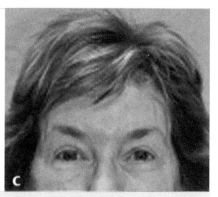

Fig. 11.20 (a–c) Pre- and postoperative views of open (pretrichial) browlift from a subcutaneous approach.

- While preparing for browlift surgery, emphasis should be placed on eye protection. The eye protective mechanisms should be evaluated, specifically amount of lagophthalmos, intactness of Bell's phenomenon, blink response, and presence of dry eye. If compromised, less tissue removal and brow elevation is recommended.
- The desired eyebrow height and contour and aesthetic differences between genders must be discussed before surgery.
  - The male brow tends to be straighter, thicker, and located at the superior orbital rim.
  - In females, the brow is often less prominent, higher, and has a lateral arch.
- Measure twice and cut once.
- Beveling the incision at the hairline allows hair to grow through the incision line.
- Over time, an irregular incision line provides better camouflage than a straight incision line.
- The extent of the lateral (temporal) dissection is determined by the forehead height as well as the amount of temporal elevation desired.
- Manual dissection is useful in the vicinity of frontal and facial nerves.
- Avoid aggressive dissection temporally overlying the temporal fat pad to avoid temporal hollowing.
- Dissect with caution around the supraorbital neurovascular bundle. The supraorbital nerve has multiple trunks and can be dissected from the surrounding tissue to allow maximal soft tissue release at the superior nasal orbital rim.
- Hemostasis is maintained with bipolar cautery.
  - Avoid cautery on the undersurface of the flap, especially along the frontal branch of the facial nerve.
  - Note: Cautery may be used on the undersurface of the flap to diminish horizontal forehead rhytids.
- Before closure, ensure symmetry between sides.
- Clean (shampoo) hair and wrap with a Kerlix headwrap.
- We do not typically use drains for forehead elevation.

11.11 Postoperative Care Checklist

- Cool compresses are applied to the operative sites for the first week postoperatively, 20 minutes on/20 minutes off while awake.
- The patient is advised to sleep with the head of the bed elevated.
- The patient may shower the next day. Wash hair with shampoo away from the fresh incisions.
- The wound should be kept clean and bacitracin antibiotic ointment applied three to four times daily.
- Postoperative medications are given:
  - Antibiotic eye ointment to the wounds on the eyelid, nonophthalmic topical antibiotic for scalp wounds.
  - Oral antibiotics.
  - Oral pain medication, typically acetaminophen/ hydrocodone, 5 mg/325 mg.
  - Antinausea medications as needed.
- Workouts and strenuous exercise should be avoided until the sutures/staples are removed at 10 to 14 days postoperation.
- Blood thinners like aspirin and nonsteroidals should be avoided for 1 week postoperatively.
- Encourage patient to keep Kerlix/Coban bandaging in place for 24 to 48 hours.
- Continue using medicated ointment to the incisions until staples are removed. Ointment can be tapered rapidly after removal.
- Blood pressure should be well controlled in the immediate postoperative period. Occasionally, two 0.1-mg clonidine pills are prescribed at home to maintain a lower resting blood pressure.

11.12 Complications and Their Management

In our experience, most suboptimal results in the coronal brow-lift stem from poor preoperative planning. Address any complications in an honest manner disclosing the nature of the complication, how it occurred, and what is the plan of action to resolve or mitigate it.

11.12.1 Expanding Hematoma

This complication is best prevented by stopping all anticoagulation in an appropriate time frame prior to the surgery, by maintaining careful hemostasis during surgery, and by controlling blood pressure after surgery. Select patients may benefit from anxiolytics. A pressure dressing with Kerlix and Coban is helpful for the first 24 hours postoperatively. A focal hematoma may be aspirated and pressure dressing placed. If more extensive, the flap must be lifted and the hematoma evacuated.

11.12.2 Scarring

The best defense against a noticeable scar is good surgical technique. If the trichophytic incision is formed anterior to the hairline, the incision may be visible. It is important to create the incision posterior to the anterior hairline wherein hair is thinner and less dense. This may be created 5 mm or more posterior to the hairline. Intraoperative beveling the incision allows for hair to regrow through the incision line. We also advocate creating an irregular jagged incision that makes the scar less visually significant. Postoperatively, the scar is best hidden if the patient wears the hair down until the wound has a chance to mature. If the scar is prominent, it can be injected with a steroid preparation. Resurfacing with dermabrasion or carbon dioxide laser may help for larger, more unsightly scars.

11.12.3 Postoperative Brow Asymmetry

Brow asymmetry may be minimized by preoperatively evaluating brow positioning and determining the amount of forehead flap to excise. Postoperatively, the surgeon must rule out asymmetric edema or frontal nerve weakness. If asymmetry following surgery persists and is cosmetically unacceptable, a return to the operating room may be necessary. Neurotoxin may be used in the postoperative period as a temporizing measure until a new surgical plan is developed.

11.12.4 Facial Nerve Damage

Damage to the facial nerve is uncommon, but can be seen if the frontal branch of the facial nerve is stretched intraoperatively. Most cases resolve over a period of weeks to months. Temporary weakening of the contralateral side with botulinum neuro-modulation may create better symmetry until the frontal weakness resolves.

11.12.5 Scalp and Forehead Numbness

Numbness, paresthesia, dysesthesia, and other sensory phenomenon (e.g., itching and pain) are commonly encountered postoperatively, sometimes lasting for months. This is best handled with reassurance that over time these sensations will resolve. Permanent numbness has been reported but is quite rare.[8] Medications for neuropathy such as gabapentin may be used to alleviate some of these symptoms.

11.12.6 Alopecia

Extensive alopecia is uncommon but can occur most commonly along the incision line. This complication may be avoided by beveling the incisions in the direction of the hair follicles at the beginning of the case and minimizing cautery at the wound edge with the incision created at least 5 mm posterior to the anterior hairline where the hair is thicker. Further, a beveled incision allows hair to grow through the incision site to make the scar less noticeable.

11.13 Alternative Approaches to the Open Browlift

Low to normal hairlines are the best candidates for a posttrichial coronal incision or subperiosteal approach with or without endoscopic guidance. In these patients, lengthening of the forehead has less impact to the final aesthetic outcome. The coronal posttrichial incision browlift has the advantage of immediate postoperative camouflage of the incision. The main disadvantages are elevation of the hairline, lengthening of the forehead, and the potential for alopecia along the incision.[6–10] In our practice, the subperiosteal approach, with or without endoscopic guidance, has supplanted the classic posttrichial browlift. The results are similar and the incisions are shorter.

Internal browlift, direct browlift, midforehead lift, temporal trichial, small incision lift and fill, endoscopic browlift, fat augmentation, and neurotoxin use are summarized in **Table 7.1**. Specific clinical indications for each procedure, gender preference, risks, and consequences of each approach are outlined in detail in fellow chapters.

References

[1] Fett DR, Sutcliffe RT, Baylis HI. The coronal brow lift. Am J Ophthalmol. 1983; 96(6):751–754

[2] Dayan SH, Perkins SW, Vartanian AJ, Wiesman IM. The forehead lift: endoscopic versus coronal approaches. Aesthetic Plast Surg. 2001; 25(1): 35–39

[3] Farkas LG, Eiben OG, Sivkov S, Tompson B, Katic MJ, Forrest CR. Anthropometric measurements of the facial framework in adulthood: age-related changes in eight age categories in 600 healthy white North Americans of European ancestry from 16 to 90 years of age. J Craniofac Surg. 2004; 15(2):288–298

[4] Puig CM, LaFerriere KA. A retrospective comparison of open and endoscopic brow-lifts. Arch Facial Plast Surg. 2002; 4(4):221–225

[5] Elkwood A, Matarasso A, Rankin M, Elkowitz M, Godek CP. National plastic surgery survey: brow lifting techniques and complications. Plast Reconstr Surg. 2001; 108(7):2143–2150, discussion 2151–2152

[6] Stuzin JM, Wagstrom L, Kawamoto HK, Wolfe SA. Anatomy of the frontal branch of the facial nerve: the significance of the temporal fat pad. Plast Reconstr Surg. 1989; 83(2):265–271

[7] Paul MD. The evolution of the brow lift in aesthetic plastic surgery. Plast Reconstr Surg. 2001; 108(5):1409–1424

[8] Cilento BW, Johnson CM, Jr. The case for open forehead rejuvenation: a review of 1004 procedures. Arch Facial Plast Surg. 2009; 11(1):13–17

[9] Lighthall JG, Wang TD. Complications of forehead lift. Facial Plast Surg Clin North Am. 2013; 21(4):619–624

[10] Riefkohl R, Kosanin R, Georgiade GS. Complications of the forehead-brow lift. Aesthetic Plast Surg. 1983; 7(3):135–138

[11] Westmore MG. Facial cosmetics in conjunction with surgery. Paper presented at: Aesthetic Plastic Surgical Society; May 7, 1974. Vancouver, BC, Canada

Bibliography

[1] Angelos PC, Stallworth CL, Wang TD. Forehead lifting: state of the art. Facial Plast Surg. 2011; 27(1):50–57

[2] Nahai FR. The varied options in brow lifting. Clin Plast Surg. 2013; 40(1):101–104

[3] Lee H, Quatela VC. Endoscopic browplasty. Facial Plast Surg. 2018; 34(2):139–144

[4] Isse NG. Endoscopic facial rejuvenation. Clin Plast Surg. 1997; 24(2):213–231

[5] Glogau RG. Aesthetic and anatomic analysis of the aging skin. Semin Cutan Med Surg. 1996; 15(3):134–138

[6] Fitzpatrick TB. The validity and practicality of sun-reactive skin types I through VI. Arch Dermatol. 1988; 124(6):869–871

[7] Walrath JD, McCord CD. The open brow lift. Clin Plast Surg. 2013; 40(1):117–124

[8] Hunt HL. Plastic Surgery of the Head, Face, and Neck. Philadelphia, PA: Lea and Febiger; 1926

[9] Javidnia H, Sykes J. Endoscopic brow lifts: have they replaced coronal lifts? Facial Plast Surg Clin North Am. 2013; 21(2):191–199

[10] Broadbent T, Mokhktarzadeh A, Harrison A. Minimally invasive brow lifting techniques. Curr Opin Ophthalmol. 2017; 28(5):539–543

[11] McCord CD, Doxanas MT. Browplasty and browpexy: an adjunct to blepharoplasty. Plast Reconstr Surg. 1990; 86(2):248–254

[12] Zarem HA. Browpexy. Aesthet Surg J. 2004; 24(4):368–372

[13] Massry GG. The external browpexy. Ophthal Plast Reconstr Surg. 2012; 28(2):90–95

[14] Graham DW, Heller J, Kurkjian TJ, Schaub TS, Rohrich RJ. Brow lift in facial rejuvenation: a systematic literature review of open versus endoscopic techniques. Plast Reconstr Surg. 2011; 128(4):335e–341e

[15] Vrcek I, Chou E, Somogyi M, Shore JW. Volumization of the brow at the time of blepharoplasty: treating of the eyebrow fat pad as an independent unit. Ophthalmic Plast Reconstr Surg. 2018; 34(3):209–212

[16] Flowers RS, Ceydeli A. The open coronal approach to forehead rejuvenation. Clin Plast Surg. 2008; 35(3):331–351

[17] Sundine MJ, Connell BF. The open browlift. Facial Plast Surg. 2018; 34(2):128–138

12 Pretrichial Temporal Browlift

John J. Martin, Jr.

Abstract

In many patients with aging, there can be a loss of volume in the lateral brow. This will cause the brow to descend, resulting in excess skin with hooding in the lateral portion of the upper lid. Failure to address a low brow position when doing an upper eyelid surgery can result in a heavy, undercorrected appearance postoperatively. There have been many procedures described for the elevation of the temporal brow. Many of them use an incision either at or behind the hairline in the lateral forehead. Dissection proceeds inferiorly to the orbital rim. The technique in this chapter uses an incision of an ellipse of skin and subcutaneous tissue in front of the temporal hairline. In contrast to other techniques previously reported, there is no dissection or undermining around the ellipse. Instead, the tissue is closed directly with deep and superficial sutures or staples. The procedure is quick with minimal bruising and swelling while consistently elevating the lateral eyebrow several millimeters.

Keywords: browlift, brow ptosis, blepharoplasty, ptosis

12.1 Introduction

When considering aesthetic surgery of the upper eyelid, it is important that the position of the eyebrow also be evaluated. In many patients with aging, there can be a loss of volume in the lateral brow causing brow descent and resulting in excess skin hooding in the lateral portion of the upper eyelid. Failure to address a low brow position when doing an upper eyelid surgery can result in a heavy, undercorrected appearance postoperatively.

There have been conflicting reports regarding the actual descent of the brow after upper eyelid surgery.[1-4] From personal experience, I have found several cases of brow descent after upper eyelid surgery. As the lateral brow is the area of major descent for most patients with secondary dermatochalasis, many surgeries have been described to elevate just this area.[5-10] While all of these surgical techniques demonstrated elevation of the lateral brow, they all incorporate dissection down to the orbital rim in either a subcutaneous plane or on top of the deep temporalis fascia. This dissection increases operative time, increases the risk of postoperative bruising and swelling, and can damage the temporal branch of the facial nerve. I describe an alternative approach here, which uses a pretrichial elliptical incision in the temporal forehead, removing skin and subcutaneous tissue with no inferior incision undermining.

12.2 Goals of Intervention/ Indications

- Improvement of superotemporal visual field.
- Elevation of ptotic brow to its proper anatomic position.
- Decreasing upper eyelid hooding and dermatochalasis.
- Decreasing need for neurotoxin to elevate brow.

12.3 Risks of Procedure

- Bleeding.
- Infection.
- Visible scar.
- Suture granuloma.
- Asymmetry of brows.
- Overcorrection.
- Undercorrection.
- Damage to temporal branch of facial nerve.

12.4 Benefits of Procedure

- Improvement of superolateral visual field.
- Elevation of the ptotic lateral eyebrow.
- Decreasing upper eyelid hooding and dermatochalasis.
- Decreasing the need for neurotoxins to elevate the lateral eyebrow.

12.5 Contraindications

- Low temporal hairline.
- Bald or severe recession of temporal hairline.

12.6 Informed Consent

- Include risks, benefits, and contraindications.
- Revision may be necessary if there is postoperative asymmetry.

12.7 Preoperative Evaluation

- For any patient interested in upper eyelid surgery, either blepharoplasty or ptosis, the eyelid will be evaluated for excess skin.
  - The brow should be elevated manually to determine the amount of laxity and the glide in the eyebrow tissues.
  - If the brow is below the orbital rim, it will need to be elevated to prevent persistent lateral hooding postoperatively.
  - It is helpful to demonstrate to the patient the different cosmetic appearance that will be obtained if the brow is elevated at the same time as upper eyelid surgery.
- A pretrichial temporal browlift can be done in any patient who has a good temporal hair tuft.
  - If a patient has an extremely low temporal hairline, this surgery may not be appropriate because it can move the brow too close to the hairline.
- Consider avoiding the pretrichial temporal browlift in patients with short hair or in patients who wear their hair away from their face hair as this does not provide the ability to conceal the small possibility of a visible scar.
- Preoperative full-face photographs are important.
  - Primary and lateral oblique views are important for pre- and postoperative comparisons.

12.8 The Procedure

The procedure can be performed in an outpatient surgery center or in an office-based setting. Local anesthesia or local with intravenous sedation may be employed.

12.8.1 Instrumentation

- Surgical marking pen.
- Local anesthesia:
  - Lidocaine 2% with 1:100,000 epinephrine—5 mL.
  - Marcaine 0.75% with epinephrine—4 mL.
  - Bicarbonate 8.4%—1 mL.
  - A 27-gauge 1.5-inch needle.
- A #15 Bard-Parker blade.
- Adson–Brown forceps.
- Plastics needle holder (Webster type).
- Monopolar cautery with Colorado tip.
- Sutures:
  - A 4–0 PDS.
  - A 4–0 Prolene or staples.

12.8.2 Preoperative Checklist

- Informed consent.
- Instrumentation.
- Preoperative photographs.

12.8.3 Surgical Technique

- Prior to surgery, an ellipse of tissue will be marked over the superotemporal brow. The brow will be manually elevated at the hairline to see which location will give the most natural appearance and best elevation to the temporal brow. The ellipse usually measures about 3 cm in length and 1 to 2 cm in width (▶ Fig. 12.1**a**). This can be estimated by manually elevating the brow to the desired level, measuring and marking this distance.

- Local anesthesia is injected into the area 10 minutes before incision.
- After cleansing the area, an incision is made along the previously drawn lines with a #15 Bard-Parker blade.
- A skin and subcutaneous tissue flap is excised preserving as much subcutaneous fat as possible using either scissors or the cutting Bovie (▶ Fig. 12.1**b**).
- Hemostasis is performed with monopolar or bipolar cautery.
  - Dissection should not be carried into a deeper plane to avoid injury to the temporal branch of the facial nerve.
  - Care is taken to avoid cautery at the base of hair follicles to minimize the risk of postoperative alopecia.
  - No undermining is done under the skin.
- The wound is closed in two layers.
  - The subcutaneous tissue is closed with interrupted 4–0 PDS suture (▶ Fig. 12.1**c**).
  - The surgical assistant can manually elevate the brow tissue to decrease tension on the wound during closure of the suture.
  - The skin can be closed with either staples or a running 4–0 Prolene suture (▶ Fig. 12.1**d**).
- Topical antibiotic ointment is applied to the wound.

12.9 Expert Tips/Pearls/Suggestions

- Make sure the ellipse is marked over the area of the brow that needs the elevation.
- You will usually need to take out more skin than you think to get a good elevation.
  - The lateral eyebrow should appear overcorrected on the table.
  - The patient should be informed that they will appear overcorrected for about 1 to 2 weeks postoperatively.
- Keep the dissection subcutaneous to avoid possible damage to the facial nerve.
- Bevel the incision to minimize the scar.
- The wound edges should be reapproximated after placement of the deep sutures.

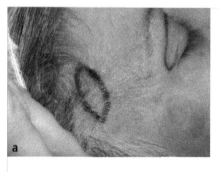
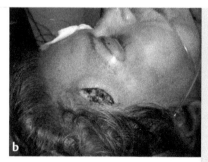
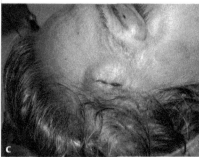
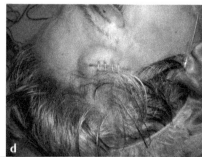

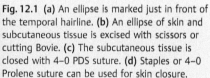

Fig. 12.1 (a) An ellipse is marked just in front of the temporal hairline. (b) An ellipse of skin and subcutaneous tissue is excised with scissors or cutting Bovie. (c) The subcutaneous tissue is closed with 4–0 PDS suture. (d) Staples or 4–0 Prolene suture can be used for skin closure.

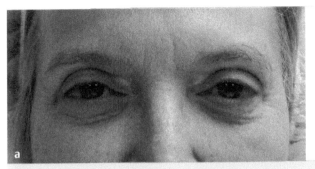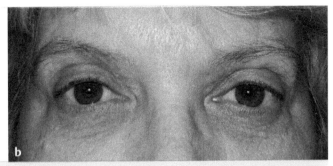

Fig. 12.2 **(a)** Preoperative photograph of the patient undergoing a pretrichial browlift only. **(b)** Postoperative photograph at 6 months after a pretrichial browlift.

- The staples/skin sutures may be removed in 10 days.
  - The closure is left in longer than upper eyelid sutures because of wound tension.
- If there is a noticeable scar, use silicone scar gel starting at 2 weeks postoperatively. Laser resurfacing may be helpful in the postoperative period.

12.10 Postoperative Care Checklist

- Ice for the first 48 hours, then warm compresses four times a day for 10 minutes.
- Keep wound clean with peroxide.
- Topical antibiotic cream two times a day.
- Shower and wash hair 1 day postoperatively.
- Minimal exercise for the first week.
- Suture/staple removal at 10 days.

▶ Fig. 12.2 illustrates a typical pre- and postoperative result. Note temporal eyebrow elevation and decreased lateral hooding.

12.11 Complications

There are a few complications with this procedure. They include scarring, granuloma formation, and over- and undercorrection. Alopecia should not be an issue because the incision is just in front of the hairline.

12.11.1 Scarring

The scar will usually remain red for a few weeks. Nonablative fractionated laser resurfacing and silicone scar cream can help improve the appearance of any scar that is irregular or slow to heal. It is rare to see any residual scar after a few months.

12.11.2 Suture Granuloma

If a suture granuloma occurs over the deep PDS suture, it is easily treated with a short course of antibiotics. If a suture extrudes through the wound, it should be removed.

12.11.3 Undercorrection

The pretrichial temporal browlift can be repeated after about 6 months if the brow remains low. If the brow height is adequate

but excess skin remains between the eyebrow and upper eyelid margin, a small lateral blepharoplasty may be performed.

12.11.4 Overcorrection

Overcorrection has never happened in the author's experience. The lift obtained is between 2 and 5 mm. If overcorrection does occur, a small amount of neurotoxin may be given to the frontalis muscle laterally. Massage may also help to lower the brow.

12.12 Conclusion

The pretrichial temporal browlift provides a quick and efficient option for the elevation of a low lateral eyebrow. The procedure does not require tissue undermining as the dissection involved is similar to a direct browlift, with the ellipse of excised skin placed at the hairline rather than directly above the brow. By moving the ellipse of excised tissue superiorly and further away from the brow, a larger amount of tissue needs to be removed to obtain a similar lift. The wound is closed in two layers. Limiting the dissection to just skin and subcutaneous tissue avoids the risk of damage to underlying nerves and provides 2 to 5 mm of lift. Patients are routinely happy with the results of the procedure.

References

[1] Prado RB, Silva-Junior DE, Padovani CR, Schellini SA. Assessment of eyebrow position before and after upper eyelid blepharoplasty. Orbit. 2012; 31(4): 222–226

[2] Lee JM, Lee TE, Lee H, Park M, Baek S. Change in brow position after upper blepharoplasty or levator advancement. J Craniofac Surg. 2012; 23(2):434–436

[3] Dar SA, Rubinstein TJ, Perry JD. Eyebrow position following upper blepharoplasty. Orbit. 2015; 34(6):327–330

[4] Hassanpour SE, Khajouei Kermani H. Brow ptosis after upper blepharoplasty. Findings in 70 patients. World J Plast Surg. 2016; 5(1):58–61

[5] Knize DM. Limited-incision forehead lift for eyebrow elevation to enhance upper blepharoplasty. Plast Reconstr Surg. 1996; 97(7):1334–1342

[6] McGuire CS, Gladstone HB. Novel pretrichial browlift technique and review of methods and complications. Dermatol Surg. 2009; 35(9):1390–1405

[7] Martin M, Shah CT, Attawala P, Neaman K, Meldrum M, Hassan AS. Objective brow height measurements following pretrichial brow lift and upper lid blepharoplasty. J Cutan Aesthet Surg. 2016; 9(2):93–96

[8] Nahai FR. The varied options in brow lifting. Clin Plast Surg. 2013; 40(1):101–104

[9] Broadbent T, Mokhktarzadeh A, Harrison A. Minimally invasive brow lifting techniques. Curr Opin Ophthalmol. 2017; 28(5):539–543

[10] Bidros RS, Salazar-Reyes H, Friedman JD. Subcutaneous temporal browlift under local anesthesia: a useful technique for periorbital rejuvenation. Aesthet Surg J. 2010; 30(6):783–788

13 Minimally Invasive Su-Por–Suture Temporal Brow Suspension: The Lift and Fill Technique

Michael A. Burnstine

Abstract

Temporal eyebrow ptosis is very common in the aging face. Understanding how to address the tissue descent and volume loss with Su-Por, high-density porous polyethylene, is described here. The procedure is minimally invasive and performed with small incisions, and the recovery time is rapid.

Keywords: browlift, small incision, minimally invasive, porous polyethylene, biointegration, Su-Por

13.1 Introduction

Many procedures have been developed to lift and fill the eyebrow tail for functional benefit and aesthetic enhancement. The lift and fill technique, too, was designed to elevate and provide fullness to the lateral eyebrow. The technique is quick and minimally invasive, and addresses the effects of aging: retro-orbicularis oculi fat (ROOF) atrophy and gravitational descent of the lateral eyebrow. The technique's novelty lies in its use of a thin profile Su-Por implant, which becomes biointegrated into the tissue.

Su-Por is a porous high-density polyethylene produced by Poriferous, LLC, and is described in the literature as safe and effective.[1-3] It is commonly used in surgeries that add more support for facial features.[4] Its pore size ranges between 100 and 250 µm, which is an optimal range for rapid fibrovascular ingrowth.[5] The pore size is sufficient to provoke an immune response, thus reducing the rate of infection and extrusion when compared to other porous implants. Incorporation of tissue into the Su-Por implant is rapid; soft tissue ingrowth has been shown at 1 week and bone ingrowth at 3 weeks after implantation.[1,6] In revision rhinoplasty, Romo et al found a complication rate of 2.6% after implantation of porous polyethylene into 187 patients.[7]

The advantages of the lift and fill technique over other suture suspension techniques and barbed suture techniques lie in its broad tissue integration. Elevating and suspending the ROOF with a porous scaffold along with deep anchoring of the tissue in the thick deep temporalis fascia plane prevents cheese wiring of the tissue. Most often, the lift and fill technique is combined with upper blepharoplasty, but it can be done in isolation. The procedure can be done in the office under local anesthesia or in an operating room setting with monitored or general anesthesia.

13.2 Goals of Intervention/Indications

- Elevate, stabilize, and add volume to the lateral eyebrow.
- Improve functional visual field when the lateral brow is ptotic preoperatively.

- Minimal incisions to the face, avoiding noticeable scars as seen in direct, midforehead, and coronal incisions.
- Minimal hair loss from small brow incision placement in the pre- or posttrichial space.

13.2.1 Risks of the Procedure

- Bleeding.
- Infection.
- Asymmetric eyebrow elevation.
- Palpable implant.
- Implant migration.

13.2.2 Benefits of the Procedure

- Aesthetic enhancement of the upper face.
- Lift of the lateral eyebrow tail.
- Youthful fullness of the eyebrow tail.

13.2.3 Informed Consent

- Include risks and benefits (as above).
- Mention implantation of a foreign material.
  - Though this use is novel, porous polyethylene has been used extensively in orbital and facial reconstruction for over 35 years.

13.3 Contraindications

- Active infection in the area of implant placement.

13.4 The Procedure

The procedure described is quick and easy to perform, and can be done in an outpatient surgery center or in an office-based setting.

13.4.1 Instruments Needed (▶ Fig. 13.1)

- Su-Por Airo brow implants (two):
  - Catalog number 4442: small, one per package.
  - Catalog number 4443: large, one per package.
  - Catalog number 4444: small, two per package.
  - Catalog number 4445: large, two per package.
- Ruler.
- Wright needle.
- Knapp lacrimal rake (two; B + L E4538).
- Tenzel-Cottle periosteal elevator (B + L E4595).
- Hemostat.
- Sutures.
  - A 4–0 Prolene, clear suture for fixation of implant.
  - A 6–0 Vicryl suture for wound closure.
  - A 6–0 Prolene suture for wound closure.

13.4.2 Preoperative Checklist

- Informed consent.
- Instrumentation on hand.
- Implants present.

13.4.3 Operative Technique

This procedure can be done under local, monitored, or general anesthesia in an office-based procedure room, ambulatory operating room, or hospital-based setting. Most often, it is performed in conjunction with an upper blepharoplasty.

- The blepharoplasty and eyebrow incisions are marked.
  - The hairline incision is typically 12 mm in length and in a pre- or posttrichial location. Its placement is determined by marking a direct line from lateral nasal ala through lateral canthus to the hairline (▶ Fig. 13.2).

- The blepharoplasty skin and fat (if needed) removal is completed.
- After the blepharoplasty is performed, the preperiosteal dissection is performed.
  - A lacrimal rake is used to pull the upper blepharoplasty incision toward the brow to facilitate this dissection (▶ Fig. 13.3).
- Dissection is performed in the preperiosteal plane. The tissue is elevated with a periosteal elevator. A large 2-cm tissue release is performed above the temporal superior orbital rim.
- Attention is then turned to incising the 12-mm hairline incision.
- Dissection is performed down through subcutaneous tissue and superficial temporalis fascia.
  - Blunt dissection is performed to the deep temporalis fascia with a hemostat while the lacrimal rakes are in place (▶ Fig. 13.4).

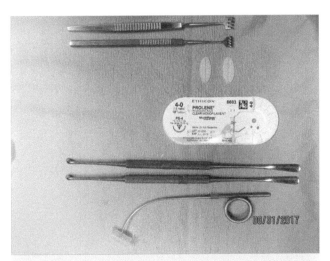

Fig. 13.1 The key instrumentation in the lift and fill technique includes two lacrimal rakes, two Su-Por Airo brow implants for bilateral cases, a clear 4–0 Prolene suture, a Tenzel-Cottle periosteal elevator, and a Wright needle.

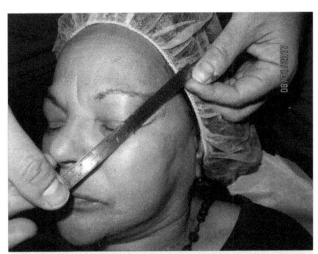

Fig. 13.2 The eyebrow incision is made in the desired vector of lateral eyebrow elevation. Typically, a line is drawn from the lateral nasal ala through the lateral canthus to the hairline. The hairline incision average size in 12 mm.

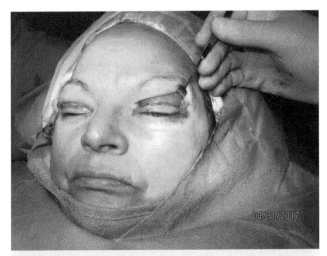

Fig. 13.3 A lacrimal rake is used to pull the upper eyelid incision to the lateral orbital rim prior to incising the tissue to the orbital rim.

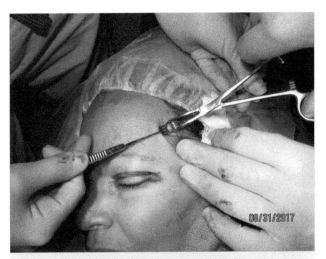

Fig. 13.4 Blunt dissection into the superficial temporalis fascia plane down to the deep temporalis fascia is performed with a hemostat to get to the desired plane.

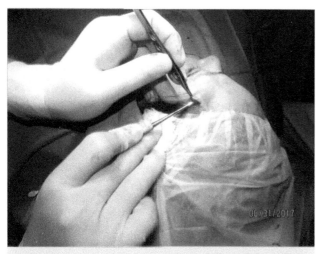

Fig. 13.5 A periosteal elevator may be used to release the conjoint tendon for greater elevation as needed.

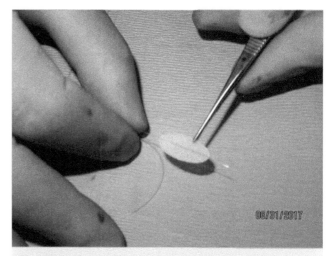

Fig. 13.6 A clear 4–0 Prolene suture is passed through the microchannel implant of the Su-Por Airo implant.

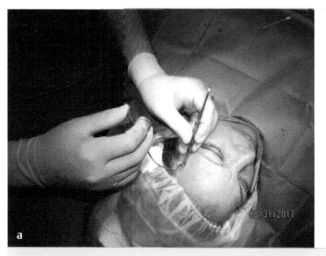

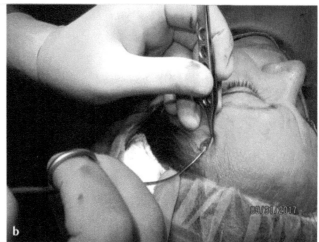

Fig. 13.7 The Wright needle is passed deep through the deep temporalis fascia (a), ensnaring a portion of the deep fascial plane (b).

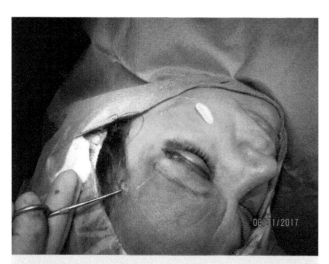

Fig. 13.8 Each arm of the clear 4–0 Prolene suture is passed through the eye of the Wright needle.

- A periosteal elevator may be used to release the conjoint tendon connecting the lateral subgaleal plane and the medial subperiosteal plane at the superior temporal fusion line (▶ Fig. 13.5). This is not needed in all cases.
- A clear 4–0 Prolene suture is threaded through the Su-Por implant microchannel (patent pending technology; ▶ Fig. 13.6).
- A Wright needle is passed through the hairline incision through the deep temporalis fascia (taking a small bite of it) to the lateral orbital rim in the preperiosteal plane (▶ Fig. 13.7a, b).
- Each arm of the Prolene suture threaded through the Su-Por Airo brow implant is passed through the eye of the Wright needle (▶ Fig. 13.8).
- The Wright needle is then brought back up through the hairline incision.
- The implant is brought into the desired location in the established plane after folding it slightly to buttress the ROOF tissue.

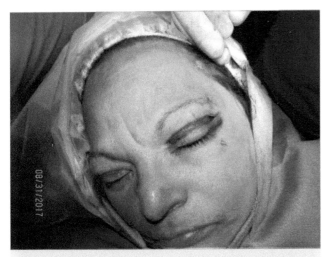

Fig. 13.9 The suture is tightened to the desired brow height and contour from the hairline incision.

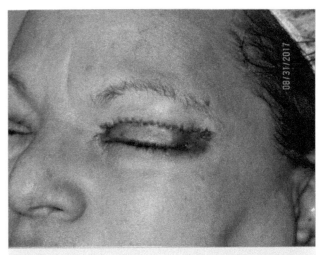

Fig. 13.10 The hairline incision is closed with 6–0 Vicryl followed by 6–0 Prolene, while the upper eyelid incision is closed with 6–0 Prolene alone.

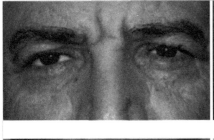
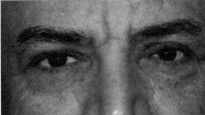
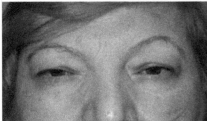
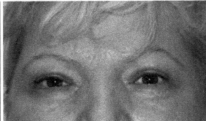

Fig. 13.11 Typical pre- (left-hand panels) and postoperative (right-hand panels) result. Each patient underwent bilateral upper eyelid ptosis repair, upper blepharoplasty, and the Su-Por temporal brow suspension: the lift and fill technique.

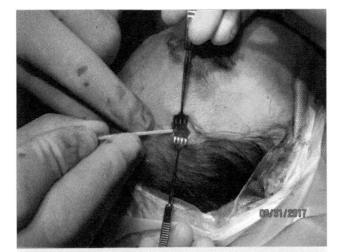

Fig. 13.12 Upon blunt dissection in the predeep superior temporal fascia plane, a tributary of the temporal artery may be encountered. It should be noted and avoided.

- The suture that has been passed through the deep temporalis fascia is then tightened, titrating the lateral eyebrow to the desired position (▶ Fig. 13.9).
- The wounds are closed with 6–0 Vicryl, followed by a running 6–0 Prolene sutures for the hairline incisions and a running 6–0 Prolene for the eyelid incision (▶ Fig. 13.10).
- Typical pre- and postoperative photographs are shown (▶ Fig. 13.11).

13.5 Expert Tips/Pearls/ Suggestions

- The 12-mm hairline incision is made in the vector of lift that the patient and surgeon desire. This should be demonstrated and discussed preoperatively.
- A wide preperiosteal release at the lateral eyebrow is required. However, the dissection should not be too wide. The success of the procedure depends on the "tissue drag" to elevate and suspend the ROOF fat.

- The surgeon must be mindful of the course of the superficial temporal artery and its tributaries within the superficial temporalis fascia on the deep temporalis fascia when dissecting the superior eyebrow incision (▶ Fig. 13.12).

13.6 Postoperative Care Checklist

- Ice is applied to the operative sites for 48 hours, 15 minutes on/15 minutes off while awake.
- The patient is advised to sleep with the head of the bed elevated.
- Postoperative medications are given:
  - Antibiotic eye ointment (bacitracin preferred) to the wounds.
  - An oral antibiotic because an implant is placed.
  - Oral pain medication, typically acetaminophen/ hydrocodone, 5 mg/325 mg.

13.7 Complications and Their Management

The implant suture suspension is a new technique with no reported complications to date. Theoretical complications include under- and overcorrection of the lateral eyebrow position, palpable implant, implant migration, hematoma, and infection. If the implant is palpable or otherwise bothersome, it can be explanted through the original blepharoplasty incision. If there is an under- or overcorrection, height can be modified through the hairline incision.

References

[1] Rah DK. Art of replacing craniofacial bone defects. Yonsei Med J. 2000; 41(6): 756–765

[2] Wellisz T. Clinical experience with the Medpor porous polyethylene implant. Aesthetic Plast Surg. 1993; 17(4):339–344

[3] Berghaus A, Stelter K. Alloplastic materials in rhinoplasty. Curr Opin Otolaryngol Head Neck Surg. 2006; 14(4):270–277

[4] Park HK, Dujovny M, Diaz FG, Guthikonda M. Biomechanical properties of high-density polyethylene for pterional prosthesis. Neurol Res. 2002; 24(7): 671–676

[5] Lin G, Lawson W. Complications using grafts and implants in rhinoplasty. Oper Tech Otolaryngol Head Neck Surg. 2007; 18(4):315–323

[6] Silver W, Dickson M, DeJoseph L. Implants and fillers for facial plastic surgery. In: Stucker F, de Souza C, Kenyon G, Lian T, Draf W, Schick B, eds. Rhinology and Facial Plastic Surgery. Berlin: Springer; 2009

[7] Romo T, III, Sclafani AP, Sabini P. Use of porous high-density polyethylene in revision rhinoplasty and in the platyrrhine nose. Aesthetic Plast Surg. 1998; 22(3):211–221

14 Endoscopic Upper Face and Eyebrow Lifting

Francesco P. Bernardini, Alessandro Gennai, David B. Samimi

Abstract

The authors describe the minimal incisions vertical endoscopic lifting (MIVEL) technique for periocular upper facial aesthetic rejuvenation. The technique emphasizes a scarless approach to address upper facial involutional changes by addressing the vertical vector of brow tissue descent with elevation and the three-dimensional volume loss with volume restoration.

Keywords: facial aging, minimally invasive surgery, endoscopic browlift, eyebrow rejuvenation, facial rejuvenation

14.1 Introduction

Scientific study supports the central role of the eyes in aesthetic facial rejuvenation. In a study by Nguyen et al, an eye-tracking system was used to show that age and fatigue judgments are based on preferred attention toward the eye region, and as a consequence, addressing the aesthetic of this area could be one of the most effective interventions to improve the appearance of an individual's face.[1] In a recent study of female aesthetic patients, the large majority (75%) reported the first signs of notable aging occurred around the eyes, and a similar majority described this region as the most desirable for rejuvenation.[2]

Attention to periocular signs of age is not a new phenomenon. Classic painters recognized and presented the signs of aging through the periocular area. In "The Old Man with a Gold Chain," Rembrandt (Art Museum, Chicago) was able to represent old age by focusing on the features of the periocular region in a subject with a hat and beard hiding much of his face (▶ Fig. 14.1). In the upper facial subunit, we notice forehead and brow descent (especially laterally), deepening of the upper sulcus, and dermatochalasis with lateral hooding. In 1645, Rembrandt similarly was able to represent the youthful upper periocular signs of beauty in a Dutch woman (▶ Fig. 14.2). The forehead shows no wrinkles, the brows are full, high, and arched, the sulcus is full, and the margin fold distance is low.

Surgeons dedicated to the periocular region should look at aging as being much wider and complicated than just the eyelids. Age-related changes of the eyelids are directly related to aging adjacent soft tissue. Schematically, we define the upper periocular aesthetic unit as being formed by: the superior complex (SC), including the forehead, the brow, and the upper eyelid; the lateral complex (LC), formed by the temple, the malar mound, and the lateral canthus; and the inferior complex composed of the lower eyelid and cheek (▶ Fig. 14.3). In the SC, descent plays a large role secondary to gravity forces and the continuous effect of the strong, synergistically acting depressor muscles: corrugator, depressor supercilii, procerus, and orbicularis oculi. Volume loss plays a relevant role, especially at the level of the brow fat, where it causes thinning of the brow, deepening of the sulcus, and loss of eyelid support with dermatochalasis. At the level of the LC, the temporalis fossa, located between the temporalis crest superiorly and the zygomatic arch inferiorly, has no room to descend, and its aging is determined

exclusively by volume loss. To achieve the most natural rejuvenation of the upper face, we aim to restore the position of the descended tissues and volume to the deflated tissue.[3] Here, we discuss the endoscopic browlift portion of our minimal invasive vertical endoscopic lift (MIVEL) technique for rejuvenation of the face. Specifically, we believe in tissue release, repositioning, and volume restoration[4-7] (▶ Fig. 14.4).

14.2 Goals of Intervention

- Natural-appearing rejuvenation of the upper facial aesthetic unit, most importantly the periocular region.
- Achieve three-dimensional rejuvenation with volume restoration (see Chapter 16 for fat grafting details).
- Maintain dynamic facial animation.
- Avoid traditional facelift approach of pulling skin along a horizontal plane in favor of vertical elevation.
- Avoid noticeable scars.

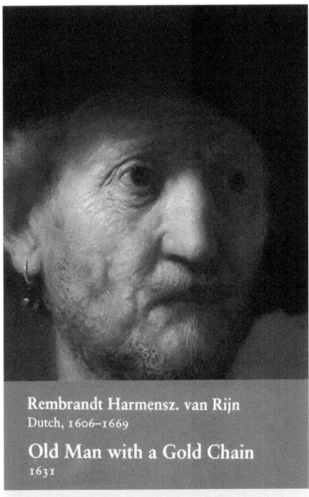

Rembrandt Harmensz. van Rijn
Dutch, 1606–1669

Old Man with a Gold Chain
1631

Fig. 14.1 Artists have understood the central role of the periocular area in conveying the aging face for centuries.

14.3 Risks

- Scalp paresthesia.
- Alopecia along incision site.
- Frontal branch facial nerve damage.
- Hematoma.
- Undercorrection.

14.4 Informed Consent

All patients should be aware of the high likelihood for transient forehead and scalp paresthesias after surgery. Patients should be made aware of nonsurgical alternatives such as neurotoxin and injectable fat or hyaluronic acid filler and the possible need for adjuvant filler or neurotoxin to maintain results. Although rare, the risk of alopecia and frontal nerve damage should be listed in the consent and understood by the patient.

14.5 Indications

- Age-related changes, including descent and deflation of the upper face.

14.6 Contraindications

- Unrealistic patient expectations.
- Overvolumization or overelevation from previous surgery.
- Thinning hair with preoperative alopecia.
- Significant hairline recession with preoperative forehead elongation.

14.7 The Procedure

The procedure is most commonly performed in an outpatient surgery center under general or intravenous monitored sedation.

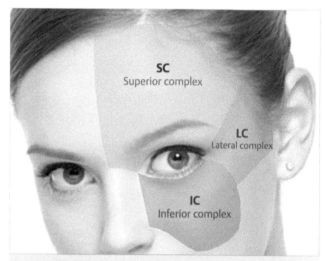

Fig. 14.3 Defining the periocular aesthetic units.

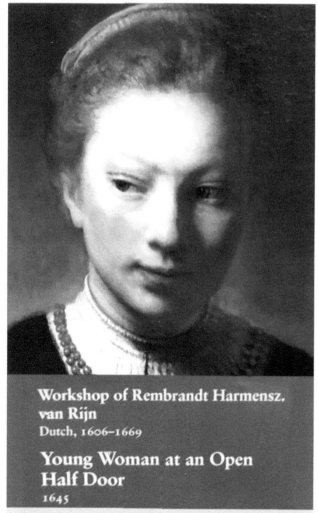

Fig. 14.2 Representative periocular area of the youthful face: a smooth lower eyelid–cheek transition, almond-shaped eyelid fissure, robust surrounding volume, and tight skin.

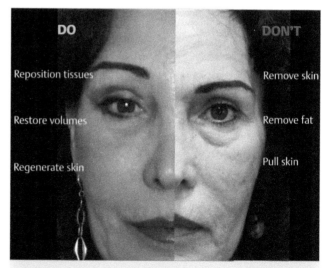

Fig. 14.4 Modern concepts in facial rejuvenation. The "Do Not" section describes what have been done in the past, with our modern version based on physiologically updated concepts.

14.7.1 Preoperative Checklist

- Signed consent in chart.
- Blood thinners have been stopped at an appropriate interval before surgery.
- Sterile instrumentation on hand.
- Full-face preoperative photographs available for review during surgery.

14.7.2 Instruments Needed (▶ Fig. 14.5)

- A 30° fiberoptic scope with endoscopic elevator that allows the surgeon to elevate tissue while viewing with one hand.
- Notable dedicated endoscopic instruments from left to right.
  - Long and regular periosteal elevators (Karl Storz #58210 FGA and UKA).
  - Midface dissector (Karl Storz, Model #50205 ZL).
  - Fine dissectors (Anthony Products Inc #67–20–53E).
  - Farabeuf retractors (Hayden Medical Inc #105–112).
  - Reverdin needle (seen centrally just to the right of the large hemostats, an instrument similar to a Wright needle, only longer, straighter, and finer, typically used by orthopedic surgery) (KLS Martin #20–721–19–07).
    - A Wright needle can be used as an alternative to the Reverdin needle (FCI Ophthalmics #WF-1000u).

14.7.3 Closure

- Temporal and paramedian fixation: a 3–0 Vicryl, tapered needle tip preferred (SH needle).
- Scalp staples for the closure of skin incisions behind hairline.

14.7.4 Local Anesthetic

- Tumescent solution for frontal, temporal, and malar regions: approximately 40 mL of 0.25% carbocaine or lidocaine with 1:400,000 epinephrine.
- Concentrated solution (20 mL of 1% carbocaine or lidocaine with 1:100,000 epinephrine) for upper periorbita, lateral canthus, glabella, and incision sites.

14.7.5 Fat Grafting

- Lipofilling of the face was performed in a manner consistent with the technique described by Dr. Coleman.[8]
- Recently, microfat grafting techniques have been introduced and performed by the senior authors, utilizing superficial injection of finer fat for concurrent rejuvenation of facial skin[4] (▶ Fig. 14.6).

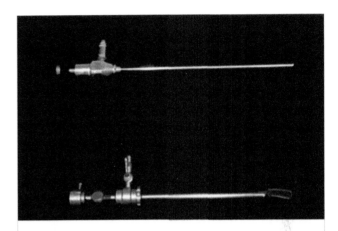

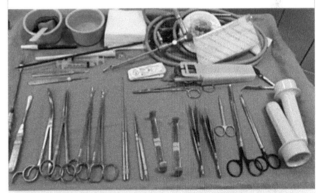

Fig. 14.5 Surgical instrumentation. The 30° fiberoptic scope with endoscopic elevator shown above is the most important component, allowing the surgeon to elevate tissue while viewing with one hand.

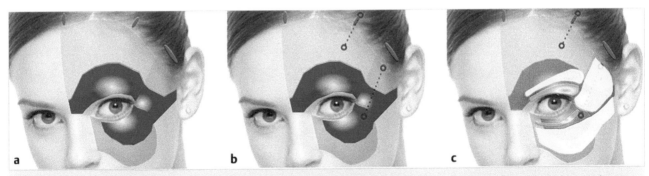

Fig. 14.6 (a) The *solid red lines* show the central, paramedian, and temporal incisions. The blue area shows the extension of the endoscopic dissection across the periocular unit. (b) The *dotted lines* show the vertical vectors of paramedian and lateral fixation. A vector similar to the temporal is used for malar fixation when necessary. (c) The fat is implanted in the dermal layer in the areas in *yellow* and in the suborbicularis plane in the areas in *orange*.

- Fat harvesting and injection are generally performed before incision to minimize the time from harvesting to injection and to place fat in undisrupted tissue planes.
- Details on fat grafting to the brow are described in Chapter 16.

14.7.6 Incision Placement (▶ Fig. 14.6)

- Vertical incisions: three total, all 1.5 cm in length, just behind hairline.
  - Single central: at midline.
  - Two paramedian: typically 5 cm on either side of central incision in females and 4 cm in males. The distance of the paramedial incision from midline dictates the location of the highest arch, thus being more lateral in the female patient.
- Temporal incisions: one on each side, 3-cm long, 1 cm behind and parallel to hairline. Incision should not extend above the superior extent of the temporalis muscle to ensure the presence of deep temporalis fascia for fixation. Superior extent of the temporalis can be determined with palpation while the patient bites down in the preoperative area.

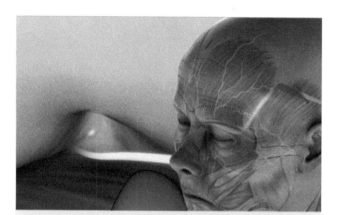

Fig. 14.7 Lysing of the conjoint tendon from lateral to medial ensures the creation of a single optical pocket in the correct planes: just above the deep temporalis fascia laterally and subperiosteal medially.

14.7.7 Operative Technique

The surgical technique has four general components: initial blind dissection without the endoscope, temporal endoscopic dissection, frontal endoscopic dissection, and fixation.

Areas of Blind Dissection

- Following intravenous sedation, local anesthetic injection, and sterile prepping and draping, incisions are made through marked sites with a #15 blade.
- In the frontal region, blind dissection may be performed quickly in a subperiosteal plane, trying to maintain an intact periosteum. This maneuver creates an optical pocket up to the "safety area," located 2 cm above the superior orbital rim. The frontal dissection extent will be up to the temporal fusion line, also known as conjoint tendon, laterally and 2 to 3 cm posterior to the hairline.
- In the temporal area, an optical pocket is created above the deep temporalis fascia. From the temporal dissection, the conjoint tendon (temporal fusion line) can be released to join the frontal and lateral pockets. Lysing the conjoint tendon from lateral to medial ensures that the procedure proceeds in safe planes: subperiosteal over the frontal region and just anterior to the deep temporalis fascia in the temporal region (▶ Fig. 14.7).

Temporal Endoscopic Dissection

- Once blind dissection is complete, the endoscope is entered through the temporal incision and directed toward the lateral canthus in a plane just above the deep temporalis fascia. The first landmark encountered is the sentinel vein, which should be left undisturbed.
- Lateral to the sentinel vein, blunt dissection reveals a neurovascular bundle, the zygomaticofacial nerve and vein. Lateral to this bundle is the zygomaticotemporal vein and nerve. These three structures act like electric posts above which runs the frontal branch of the facial nerve (▶ Fig. 14.8). Once the landmarks are visible, one can elect where to dissect.

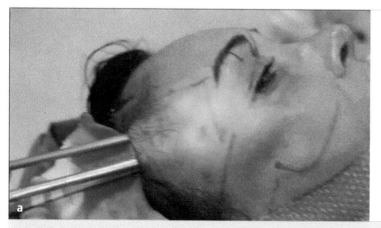
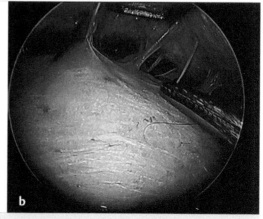

Fig. 14.8 Anatomic landmarks seen with external view of the dissection **(top)** and the endoscope view **(bottom)**. In the endoscopic view, the lateral orbit is on the left. The dissection is lateral to the sentinel vein and it shows the zygomaticotemporal (*blue arrow*) and the zygomaticofacial (*yellow arrow*) neurovascular bundles. Around and in front of the zygomaticotemporal bundle, the zygomatic cutaneous ligament (*orange arrow*) is exposed and starts to be bluntly elevated. The tunnel dissection will allow a safe dissection of the zygomatic arch and the prezygomatic space above the zygomatic muscles, which protect the zygomatic branch of the seventh nerve, which runs below them. (These images are provided courtesy of Dr. Francesco P. Bernardini.)

○ Lateral dissection between the sentinel vein and the zygomaticofacial bundle leads to the fat of the suborbicularis oculi fat (SOOF).

○ Dissection between the zygomaticofacial and zygomaticotemporal bundles provides access to the midface.

○ Medial to the sentinel vein is the lateral retinaculum and the lateral canthal tendon.

○ For a complete lateral dissection, it is necessary to free the tissue across the entire length of the zygomatic arch, elevate the SOOF, and release the lateral retinaculum.

Frontal Endoscopic Dissection

• The endoscope enters the paramedian incision and once the orbital rim is reached, blunt dissection elevates the periosteum from lateral to medial, and the supraorbital neurovascular bundle is encountered. All strands of periosteum need to be elevated around the bundle. The periosteum is very strong, and even small residual bands will prevent easy forehead flap mobilization.

• Medial to the supraorbital nerve, dissection will be aimed toward the glabella to elevate and release the corrugator and procerus muscles. The supratrochlear nerve resides between the fibers of the corrugator muscles.

Fixation

Fixation is performed in the paramedian and deep temporal regions.

Paramedian Fixation

The *Gennai stitch* is utilized for paramedian fixation, which determines the highest point of the brow (▶ Fig. 14.9, ▶ Fig. 14.10).

• Two small horizontal stab wound incisions are made in the forehead at the same level, one on each side, 1 to 2 cm below the paramedian incisions.

○ A greater paramedian to stab incision distance will provide a more robust forehead lift; however, there is more tissue bunching seen in the postoperative period.

– A Reverdin needle (an instrument analogous and replaceable with a Wright fascia needle) is passed in a subperiosteal plane from the forehead stab incision to the paramedian incision. The Reverdin needle is loaded with the suture thread and brought back out of the forehead stab incision, leaving the suture tail and needle outside of the paramedian incision. With the suture thread still loaded, the Reverdin needle is then passed superiorly from the stab incision to the paramedian incision in a subcutaneous plane superficial to the frontalis but deep to skin. The suture thread is then freed from the Reverdin needle, pulling the tail from the paramedian incision, through the wound and back out of the paramedian site: this maneuver lassos the frontalis and galeal tissue to elevate the forehead.

• The suture needle grasps the tissues deep to the skin at the posterior edge of the paramedian incision.

• All the deep tissues between the two incisions are brought together by tightening the suture, creating a temporary fold of redundant skin between the forehead and scalp incisions.

○ The amount of brow elevation is titrated by how tightly the suture is tied and how far the paramedian stab incision is placed. The longer the distance, the greater the elevation.

Deep Temporal Fixation

• Temporal fixation of the deep subcutaneous tissues of the elevated flap to the deep temporal fascia is performed with a 3–0 Vicryl suture. A tapered needle tip minimizes trauma and potential for cheese-wiring through the deep temporalis fascia. This fixation elevates and lateralizes the tail of the brow, the temporozygomatic area, and the corner of the eyelids, thereby elongating the eyelid fissure.

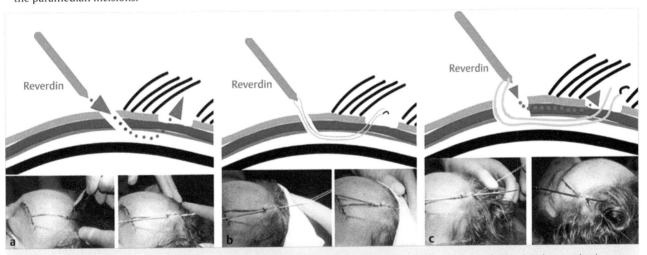

Fig. 14.9 The Gennai stitch for paramedian fixation. **(a)** Two small horizontal stab wound incisions are made in the forehead at the same level, one on each side, below the paramedian incisions. The Reverdin needle (a separate autoclavable instrument similar and replaceable with a Wright fascia needle) is passed from the forehead stab incision in a subperiosteal plane out of the paramedian incision. **(b)** The Reverdin needle is loaded with the suture and brought back out of the forehead incision, leaving the suture needle tip and tail outside the paramedian incision. **(c)** The tip of the Reverdin needle is passed superiorly in a plane deep to skin but superficial to frontalis out of the paramedian incision. The suture thread is freed from the Reverdin needle and the suture tail is pulled through the wound and back out of the paramedian incision.

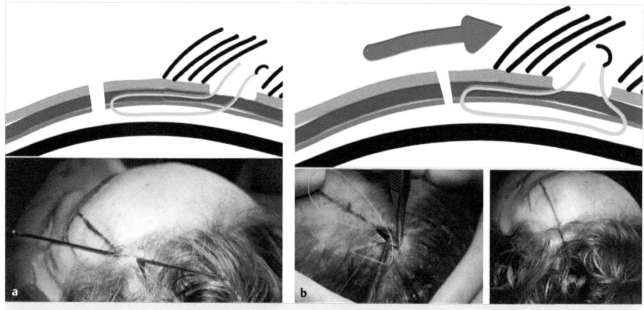

Fig. 14.10 Gennai stitch for paramedian fixation. (a) The suture is positioned anterior and posterior to the frontalis muscle in preparation to lift the forehead. (b) The suture needle grasps deep galeal tissue at the posterior edge of the paramedian incision. All the deep tissues between the two incisions are brought together by tightening the suture, creating a temporary fold of redundant tissue between the forehead and scalp incisions.

Results

Before and after images are shown in ▶ Fig. 14.11.

14.8 Postoperative Care Checklist

- With all sutures hidden behind the hairline, no topical medication is necessary.
- We recommend that patients do not pull on their hair and be extremely delicate when combing their hair for the first month.
- Prophylactic oral antibiotics are given for 1 week.
- Patients should avoid heavy lifting and strenuous activity for 10 days after surgery.
- Apply Botox at first postoperative visit and for the first few months after surgery to control the forces generated by the eyebrow depressors, specifically the orbital orbicularis laterally and corrugator muscles medially.

14.9 Expert Tips/Pearls/ Suggestions

- Fixation device: In the past, too much importance has been given to the strength of the fixation, with the idea that strong fixation with bone tunnels, endotines, and screws was necessary to support the tissues against gravity. The use of these fixations devices was associated with a limited dissection, especially of the temporal area, the lateral retinaculum, and the medial frontal periosteum. The authors believe that the most important factor for success is achieving a complete, tension-free flap that includes the forehead, temporal area, lateral retinaculum, SOOF, and zygomatic arch. Once soft tissue from the scalp to zygoma

is free, fixation can be achieved with simple, safe, and cost-effective sutures.
  - The role of fixation is to help maintain dissected tissues in optimal position until readherence into the new position during the healing process.
  - The time necessary to allow scar fixation is most likely less than the time of suture reabsorption.
  - Fixation with permanent devices is not necessary, nor do we recommend excision of scalp tissue, which can cause alopecia and visible scars, and does not add any value to the deep fixation. The authors have used fixation with the endotine device in more than 300 patients before switching to suture fixation, which has been now used in more than 200 patients.[3] The amount of elevation and the stability of the fixation have been compared with a lower complication rate.
  - In the suture fixation group, none of the patients experienced complications or referred any complaint other than a noticeable bulging of the skin folds of the forehead in the first 2 weeks, of which they were informed in advance.
- Fixation position: In planning the fixation position and ultimate natural shape of the brow, it is helpful to remember the different shape of the natural feminine eyebrow and carefully inspect each patient's old pictures.
  - The aim is to raise the tail of the brow and body until the final shape is naturally arched, ending with an elevated tail.
  - The more lateral to the midline of the forehead that the paramedian fixation is placed, the greater the effect on the tail. The closer the fixation is placed to the midline, the stronger the effect on the body or the head of the brow.
  - On average, the paramedian fixation is placed at 5 cm from the midline in a female patient and 4 cm in a male.
  - The lower the entry point on the forehead and the stronger the pull of the fixation, the larger the forehead skin fold

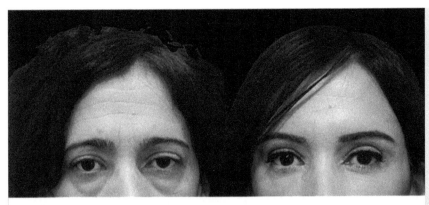

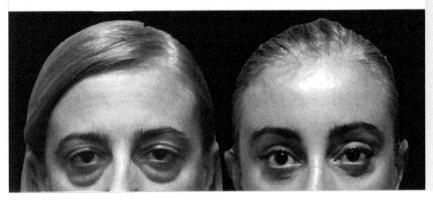

Fig. 14.11 Before and after patient examples. All patients underwent minimal invasive vertical endoscopic lift (MIVEL) of the upper face and lower eyelid blepharoplasty with concurrent upper and midfacial fat grafting. (These images are provided courtesy of Dr. Francesco P. Bernardini.)

results. Therefore, a heavier forehead, like a man's forehead, would require a stronger pull, resulting in a more visible skin fold.

- Surgical drain: A 10-French catheter and Jackson–Pratt-type bulb suction drain may be placed through one of the temporal wounds and positioned subperiosteally across the forehead just above the superior orbital rim before closing the wounds. With bulb suction, midfacial edema is minimized and the catheter can be used as a port to deliver 0.25% bupivacaine plain anesthetic solution for temporary postoperative pain management or in preparation for staple removal if needed. The drain is removed before or at the time of staple removal.

14.10 Complications and Their Management

- Facial nerve (VII) palsy: Proximity of the frontal branch of the facial nerve during surgical dissection leaves this branch susceptible to trauma. The risk for nerve damage is minimized by staying in the correct plane, using blunt dissection and avoiding cautery in the vicinity of the nerve, especially where the nerve crosses the zygomatic arch. When implementing these principles, nerve damage is rare and can be managed by injecting Botox on the contralateral side, minimizing the patient perception of dysfunction until recovery.
- Trigeminal nerve (V) damage: The supraorbital and supratrochlear branches of the trigeminal nerve (V1) can be

damaged at the time of frontal dissection where the nerve emerges from its foramen. With careful periosteal dissection under endoscopic visualization, the nerve can be freed from all periosteal attachments without damage. It is common that patients complain of hypesthesia in the scalp for up to 8 to 12 months. We have never encountered a case of permanent scalp anesthesia.

- Undercorrection: Surgical undercorrection can be managed with neurotoxin injection to relax brow depressor muscles and injectable filler to temples and brow when indicated.
- Overcorrection: An overarched or elevated brow may be noticed in the immediate postoperative period. The surgeon should offer reassurance that this resolves during recovery. Neurotoxin may be placed to selective portions of the frontalis if needed until resolution. The authors have never encountered a patient with complaint of overcorrection.

14.11 Conclusions

Rejuvenation of the upper face should address the specific aging changes that occur in each periocular region. Our approach to aesthetic improvement of the upper eyelid–eyebrow subunit emphasizes a minimally invasive, "scarless" technique, which addresses the vertical vector of tissue descent. We recommend concurrent volume restoration with fat grafting when indicated. Conservative removal of skin and/or fat in the eyelids may also be incorporated when needed.

References

[1] Nguyen HT, Isaacowitz DM, Rubin PA. Age- and fatigue-related markers of human faces: an eye-tracking study. Ophthalmology. 2009; 116(2): 355–360

[2] Sobanko JF, Taglienti AJ, Wilson AJ, et al. Motivations for seeking minimally invasive cosmetic procedures in an academic outpatient setting. Aesthet Surg J. 2015; 35(8):1014–1020

[3] Bernardini FP, Gennai A, Izzo L, Devoto MH. Minimal incisions vertical endoscopic lifting and fat grafting as a systematic approach to the rejuvenation of the periocular esthetic unit. Ophthal Plast Reconstr Surg. 2013; 29(4):308–315

[4] Bernard, ini FP, Gennai A, Izzo L, et al. Superficial enhanced fluid fat injection (SEFFI) to correct volume defects and skin aging of the face and periocular region. Aesthet Surg J. 2015; 35(5):504–515

[5] Ramirez OM. The central oval of the face: tridimensional endoscopic rejuvenation. Facial Plast Surg. 2000; 16(3):283–298

[6] Citarel, la ER, Sterodimas A, Condé-Green A. Endoscopically assisted limited-incision rhytidectomy: a 10-year prospective study. J Plast Reconstr Aesthet Surg. 2010; 63(11):1842–1848

[7] Bernardini FP, Skippen B, Gennai A, Zambelli A. Minimal incisions vertical endoscopic lifting (MIVEL) for the management of lateral canthal and lower eyelid malposition. Aesthet Surg J. 201 9; 39(5):472–480

[8] Coleman SR. Facial recontouring with lipostructure. Clin Plast Surg. 1997; 24 (2):347–367

15 Nonsurgical Management Techniques: Fillers and Neuromodulators

Jean Carruthers, Helen A. Merritt

Abstract

The brow and the periocular region form two-thirds of the "magic triangle," which explains the enormous social and psychological importance of this region. As a result, the brow is the most common facial site to receive aesthetic treatment, and the use of neuromodulators has become the most commonly performed aesthetic treatment worldwide. Age-related remodeling of the forehead and periorbita with loss of facial bone and soft tissue, descent of the brow with resultant glabellar and lateral canthal lines and folds, and temporal hollowing all contribute to a tired and aged appearance. Combination treatment of the upper face with neuromodulators and hyaluronic acid fillers has recently become a desired and popular treatment to address these changes. Neuromodulators can elevate the brows and reduce the persistent frown lines, crow's-feet lines, and horizontal forehead lines. Hyaluronic acid fillers smooth and recontour the medial glabellar complex and reflate the forehead, temple, and periorbital region.

Keywords: neuromodulator, filler, soft tissue augmentation, recontouring, combination therapy, maintenance therapy

15.1 Introduction

The clinical use of periocular neuromodulators and fillers has greatly expanded the treatment for periocular aging. Prior to these advances, individuals waited until they felt they needed surgical intervention such as blepharoplasty, facelift, and brow-lift and had these procedures performed in middle age. Now, younger patients often start with neuromodulators in the periocular region and add further treatment areas and combinations according to their developing aesthetic concerns.[1-3,4-7] With a developing global understanding of balancing physical health with emotional wholeness, patients often continue with these treatments into their 70s and 80s. Further, neuromodulators have been shown to reduce depression and to enhance self-esteem.[8,9] In short, these injection treatments have allowed patients to choose how they will traverse the inevitable aging process.

15.2 Properties of Botulinum Toxins and Periocular Fillers

It is important to understand the properties of what injectables a provider uses and the results that can be achieved. Physicians and surgeons who have a detailed understanding of the underlying anatomy and the subject's aesthetic goals will blend this knowledge with their own skill to produce a natural and enhanced appearance for their patients. Overcorrection is always to be avoided.

15.2.1 Botulinum Toxin Properties

Neuromodulator treatment of the periocular region is an important component of the modern aesthetic medical practice. Understanding the different toxins, their length of effect, and dilutions will deliver excellent outcomes and patient satisfaction.

Neurotoxin Mechanisms of Action

The strains of the anaerobic bacterium *Clostridium botulinum* produce eight distinct serotypes of botulinum neurotoxin (BoNT) designated A–H. All serotypes produce chemodenervation of skeletal muscles by blocking acetylcholine release from presynaptic motor neurons at the neuromuscular junction. There are differences in how they affect the intracellular "molecular machinery" and produce their clinical effect.

BoNT type A (BoNT-A) was the first serotype that Dr. Alan Scott, a pioneering San Francisco ophthalmologist, developed for use in humans to treat strabismus and blepharospasm.[10] Cosmetic use followed the use in blepharospasm.[11] Since the Food and Drug Administration (FDA) approval in 1990 of onabotulinumtoxinA (Botox/Botox Cosmetic), additional A formulations have been approved by the U.S. FDA and Health Canada: abobotulinumtoxinA (Dysport/Reloxin) and incobotulinumtoxinA (Xeomin). BoNT type B (BoNT-B) is also available in North America. RimabotulinumtoxinB (Myobloc/NeuroBloc) was FDA approved in 2000 for the treatment of cervical dystonia but has been used off-label to treat facial wrinkles.[12]

BoNT-A preparations have remained the preferred treatment for cosmetic applications, as BoNT-B has a shorter duration of effect, greater pain during injection, and other side effects compared to BoNT-A.[12] The onset of action is usually 24 to 48 hours after injection, with the full effect being noted at 5 to 7 days, peak effect at 30 days, and reduced effect over 3 to 6 months in most subjects. All approved neuromodulators differ in potency and clinical effect, and therefore, their units are not interchangeable. It is helpful to consult the product inserts and the peer-reviewed literature for further information.

Adverse Effects of Neurotoxin Treatment

The greatest complication of neurotoxin treatment is overcorrection or undercorrection. Overcorrection resolves over time, while further injection can address undercorrection.

15.2.2 Periocular Fillers Properties

Similar to neurotoxin usage, a detailed understanding of facial anatomy, proportions (volume), and periorbital fat distribution is critical to meet the patient's needs. Understanding how fillers work and how long they last given their molecular nature is important. Hyaluronic acid (HA) is the most abundant glycosaminoglycan in human tissue. It is a polymer that functions as a key structural component within the extracellular matrix, binding collagen and elastin fibers, stabilizing intercellular structures, and contributing to cell proliferation and migration. HA is composed of repeating subunits of *N*-acetylglucosamine and glucuronic acid, which in its natural, uncrosslinked state is catabolized in several days. The commercially produced injectable filler formulations are cross-linked and better able to resist degradation. Clinical effects of treatment typically persist for 4 to 12 months. While there are several manufacturing methods used to produce the various approved HA fillers, all are made by laboratory fermentation of *Streptococcus equi* with subsequent HA material modification. To have sustained tissue presence, they must be adequately cross-linked.

Because of the importance of vision, periocular injections should first and foremost be safe.[13,14] Reversibility with hyaluronidase is a desirable property of the HA group of fillers. In addition, the periocular skin is thinner and more delicate than that of the rest of the face and requires very careful injection technique with smooth and refined filler to give a positive aesthetic result both in contour and appearance of surface texture.[15]

Mechanism of Action: Space-Filling and Neocollagenesis

The efficacy of HA fillers has been initially attributed to their space-filling effect. More recent research suggests that HA may also induce neocollagenesis via changes in the structure and function of the cutaneous fibroblasts in the extracellular matrix.[16–18] Other non-HA fillers such as Radiesse and Sculptra are more commonly used in the mid- and lower face and other nonface areas such as chest and hands. The addition of 0.3% lidocaine to the HA fillers has become standard practice to improve patient comfort and tolerability.

- Gel hardness (G′): G′ is a measure of the amount of gel displaced based on the degree of stress applied to the gel. Hard gels (high G′) exhibit greater resistance to deformation, require greater injection pressure, and tend to provide a firmer feel under the skin. Soft gels may be beneficial for the treatment of areas with thin skin, such as the periorbital area or lips.
- Degree of cross-linking: The amount of uncross-linked (soluble) and cross-linked (insoluble) HA in a gel influences gel viscosity. Less cross-linked HA allows a smoother flow during injection but may contribute to a shorter duration of effect. Decreasing the amount of cross-linked HA also decreases the hardness of a gel.
- Particulate versus nonparticulate gels: Initial HA fillers were noncohesive biphasic fillers, characterized as cross-linked particles suspended in a noncross-linked HA matrix acting as a lubricant. These products (Restylane and Restylane Lyft [formerly Perlane]) have HA concentration of 20 mg/mL and are manufactured with nonanimal-stabilized HA technology where the gel is sized to a uniform particle volume and then mixed with uncomplexed HA to ensure that the material will flow on injection into tissue.[19]

Nonparticulate gels are characterized by a uniform, smooth consistency and so are monophasic. Juvéderm Ultra, Ultra Plus, Voluma, Volift, and Volbella are monophasic monodensified fillers, and in contrast to biphasic particulate gels, do not undergo sizing, a process that breaks down the gel. They contain a single phase of HA with a single density. Different families of monophasic monodensified fillers exist, depending on the manufacturing technology, such as the Hylacross technology (Juvéderm Ultra, HA concentration 24 mg/mL) or the Vycross technology (Juvéderm Voluma, HA concentration 20 mg/mL; Juvéderm Volift, HA concentration 17.5 mg/mL; and Juvéderm Volbella, HA concentration 15 mg/mL). Cohesive monophasic polydensified gels (Belotero range) were more recently introduced. In contrast to monodensified fillers, they are manufactured with the cohesive polydensified matrix (CPM) technology, resulting in a gel with nonuniform cross-linking and molecular weight and a viscosity that is lower than that of other fillers (comparing fillers targeting the same indication). These properties may allow for a more homogeneous intradermal distribution of the material.[20,21]

The cross-linking technology, the uniformity and size of the particles, and the gel formulation and the HA concentration of the filler determine its viscoelastic properties, and therefore its clinical effect. Fillers with high viscosity (G′) such as Restylane and Restylane Lyft are good solid support but do not spread as well for superficial filling. Belotero Balance has excellent spreadability and tissue integration due to having the lowest elasticity and viscosity. The Hylacross fillers (Juvéderm family) have intermediate viscosity and elasticity. Vycross fillers such as Juvéderm Voluma have low elasticity like Restylane and Restylane Lyft and are suitable for structural support, whereas the more elastic fillers such as Juvéderm Ultra and Belotero Basic are more elastic and spreadable and also helpful for more superficial application.[21]

Adverse Events and Hyaluronidase

The most frequent adverse effects associated with HA fillers are transient and mild, including pain, bruising, edema, and erythema at the injection site. Another common adverse event is the Tyndall effect in which blue light is reflected after a bolus of HA filler is placed superficially, particularly in the thin skin of the periocular region. Often a small dose of hyaluronidase is enough to reduce the nodule. Hyaluronidase can also be helpful for the restoration of symmetry.

Delayed inflammatory nodules may also occur. Our group conducted a retrospective chart review of our clinic patients who we treated with Juvéderm Voluma (HA-V) between February 1, 2009 and September 30, 2014 to evaluate for delayed onset nodules.[22] Of the 4,702 treatments using 11,460 mL of HA-V, 23 patients (0.5%) experienced delayed onset nodules. The median time from injection to reaction was 4 months, and median time to resolution was 6 weeks. Importantly, 9/23 (39%) had an identifiable immunologic trigger such as flu-like illness prior to the nodule onset. In our experience, effective treatments included oral prednisone, intralesional corticosteroids, and hyaluronidase. None of our nodules were of infectious etiology, and we feel they are largely immune-mediated responses to the short chains in HA-V. While delayed nodules are uncommon from HA-V (0.5%), it is important to be aware of this adverse effect and have a management protocol in place.

Inadvertent intravascular injection is also possible in superficial vasculature such as the supratrochlear vessels, but because they are arborizing with adjacent vasculature, the ischemic effects are much more limited. Intravascular injection can occur in a facial vessel where the flow is reversed, and the filler bolus canalized can block the central retinal artery. There is limited time to restore retinal circulation before the retinal tissue succumbs. There have been several cases now reported in the literature where periocular hyaluronidase in large doses has been injected in a retrobulbar, supratrochlear, and supraorbital approach where some or all vision was recovered.[23–25]

- Needle versus cannula: The theoretical risk of arterial wall perforation and emboli with cannulas is lower, but these complications can still occur with cannulas as with needles. Slow, small aliquot injection technique along with knowledge of the underlying vascular anatomy is essential. With both injection methods, the authors prefer to use an anterograde injection technique so that the soft bolus of filler rather than the tip of the needle or cannula pushes encountered vasculature gently aside. While both needles and cannulas are useful in practice and achieve excellent cosmetic results, cannula use in the deeper compartments among practitioners is encouraged to minimize complications.[26]
- Avoiding vascular complications: There are 98 reported cases of filler-induced blindness from 1906 to 2015.[27] There were over 3 million total reported aesthetic filler injections by the American Society of Aesthetic Plastic surgeons and the American Society for Dermatologic Surgery in 2016 and 2017.[28,29]

Although thankfully a rare event, physicians injecting in the periocular region and midface should be prepared with detailed knowledge of facial and vascular anatomy and have learned sophisticated injection techniques to prevent and if necessary treat inadvertent facial and periocular intravascular injection.[30]

15.3 Single Therapy and Combination Treatments in the Upper Face

In the past, neuromodulators were thought to be more appropriate for the upper face and fillers for the lower face. Now we feel that the refined clinical effect and longevity of response are best achieved with the use of combination therapy in the upper and lower face.[31] Below, we discuss the treatment of the different facial units.

15.3.1 Glabellar Frown Lines

The corrugator supercilii and orbicularis oculi muscles move the brow medially, and the procerus and depressor supercilii pull the brow inferiorly, thereby creating the frowning expression. The goal of neuromodulator treatment is to produce a weakening of these muscles but not to the extent that the upper face becomes immobile and (disturbingly) expressionless.

Individualization of the injection sites and doses to produce the desired aesthetic enhancement is a skill requiring a clear understanding of the underlying anatomy and the subject's desired treatment outcome. We currently use three to five injection sites when treating glabellar frown lines and vary the dosage, depending on the individual brow. The procedure effectively smooths the glabellar lines at rest and prevents their appearance when the patient attempts to frown for an average of 3 to 4 months[32,33] (▶ Fig. 15.1).

Glabellar folds may be present when the frown is activated but in more mature subjects may be present also at rest. In these subjects, we use combinations of neuromodulators and intradermal and subdermal forehead filler to achieve a

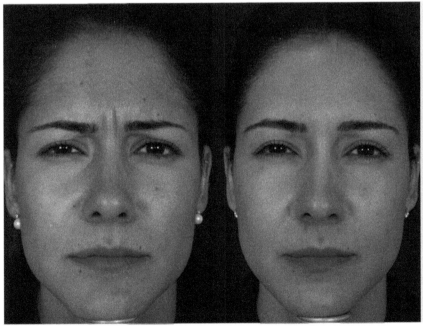

Fig. 15.1 Botulinum neurotoxin type A (BoNT-A) treatment of glabellar frown lines in a 32-year-old subject.

harmonious result in both the active and resting phases of expression[34] (▶ Fig. 15.2). In a comparative study, the aesthetic result lasted 30 weeks with the combination and 16 weeks with either neuromodulator or filler alone.[35]

15.3.2 Crow's-Feet

Crow's-feet lines radiate from the lateral canthus and are due to contraction of the lateral fibers of the orbicularis oculi muscle. Doses and sites vary according to the clinician; we evenly distribute injections among one to four injection sites, depending on the clinical effect desired. Results last approximately 3 months (▶ Fig. 15.3).

The elongated crow's-feet seen with maturity give the effect of tiredness and age. Sadly, using neuromodulator to chase the "long crows" is followed by an ipsilateral mouth droop due to weakening the zygomaticus muscles. The adjunctive use of fillers to gently lift the zygomatic area softens the etched appearance and improves the cheek contour for a more youthful appearance.

15.3.3 Horizontal Forehead Lines

Repeated contraction of the frontalis is the result of voluntarily lifting of the brows and is often seen when the subject has concurrent eyelid and/or eyebrow ptosis. The frontalis is a vertically oriented muscle and is the main brow elevator; it inserts superiorly into the galea aponeurotica and inferiorly into the skin of the brow. Weakening the frontalis muscle with the goal of eliminating horizontal forehead lines can result in undesired brow ptosis and an unattractive, "wooden" expression. Ideally, the individual will still be able to elevate the eyebrows (possibly to a lesser extent) after treatment (▶ Fig. 15.4). We believe that the brow depressors should *always* be treated at the same time as the frontalis, and this technique is described in the section "Brow Lifting and Shaping."

The use of dilute HA filler to the horizontal forehead lines softens etched lines and gives a mild browlift. After discussion, photography, and full informed consent, we mark the vessels to be avoided on the forehead supratrochlear, supraorbital, and temporal arteries. We use a diluted cross-linked HA product such as HA-V. The product comes in a 1-mL syringe, and we use a sterile fluid-dispensing connector (Braun Bethlehem, PA, FDC1000) plastic double Luer Lock to transfer 0.5 mL of HA-V into another sterile, Luer Lock 1-mL polycarbonate syringe. We now have two 0.5-mL syringes of HA-V to which we add 0.05 mL of 2% lidocaine with 1:200,000 epinephrine. The volume in each syringe is now 0.55 mL. We add a further 0.45 mL of preserved bacteriostatic saline, producing a final dilution of 50%. This mixture is then pushed back and forth 20 times

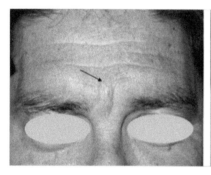
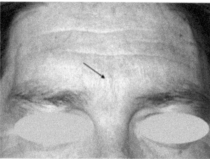

Fig. 15.2 Periocular BoNT-A with glabellar intradermal filler.

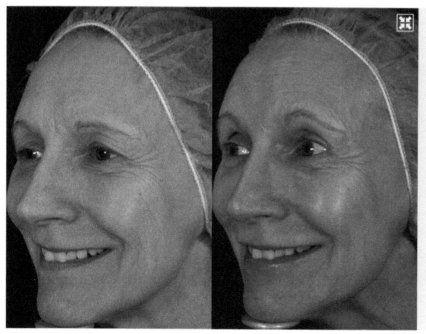

Fig. 15.3 BoNT-A treatment of lateral canthal rhytids ("crow's-feet").

through the fluid-dispensing connector to ensure even mixing. One half of this 50% mixture is then rediluted with 0.25 mL of bacteriostatic saline and mixed back and forth a further 20 times. This maneuver achieves the reduction in viscosity and the increase in moldability required. Each subject is photographed before and after the injection session, and the digital photographs are printed for the subject's chart and also kept electronically.

Three to five injection points are used in each area of the forehead: centrally between the supratrochlear vessels, more laterally between the supraorbital and supratrochlear vessels, and most laterally between the supraorbital vessels and the superficial temporal vessels.[36,37]

15.3.4 Brow Lifting and Shaping

Brow ptosis becomes obvious as we age, creating an angry, scowling expression. The shape and height of the eyebrow are determined by the opposing activity of the frontalis muscle, which elevates the brow, and the brow depressors. The medial brow depressors are the corrugator supercilii, the procerus, and the medial portion of the orbicularis oculi; the lateral depressor is the lateral portion of the orbicularis oculi lateral to the temporal fusion line. Previously, we believed that brow elevation was a result of the inactivation of the brow depressors. However, additional analysis of two dosing studies showed that central injections of 20 to 40 U of BoNT-A into the female glabella alone (with the most lateral injection at the midpupillary line) led to a dramatic lateral eyebrow elevation, followed by an entire browlift that peaked at 12 weeks post treatment.[32,33] Interestingly, too little BoNT-A (10 U) led to a brief *fall* in eyebrow position. We now believe that change in eyebrow position after glabella injection in women is due to diffusion of the BoNT-A into the lower frontalis muscle, which causes an increased resting tone in the remainder of the frontalis muscle and improvement in eyebrow position[38,39] (▶ Fig. 15.5).

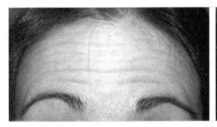 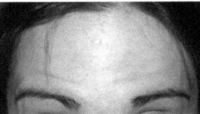

Fig. 15.4 BoNT-A treatment of horizontal forehead lines.

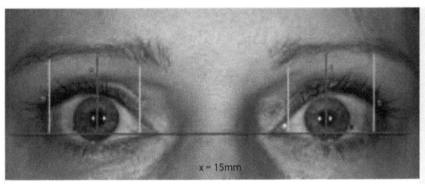

Fig. 15.5 BoNT-A treatment of glabellar frown lines causing elevation of the lateral brow where no neuromodulator was injected.

x = 15mm

Pre ● Right: Height$_a$ = 23.6mm   Left: Height$_a$ = 23.9mm
Height$_b$ = 22.4mm   Height$_b$ = 23.6mm
Height$_c$ = 20.1mm   Height$_c$ = 19.9mm

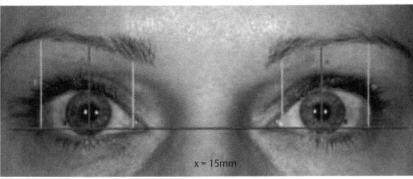

x = 15mm

Post ● Right: Height$_a$ = 24.8mm   Left: Height$_a$ = 24.5mm
Height$_b$ = 26.6mm   Height$_b$ = 25.3mm
Height$_c$ = 19.9mm   Height$_c$ = 20.2mm

15.3.5 Hypertrophic Orbicularis Oculi

We blink using the pretarsal portion of the orbicularis oculi muscle. Contraction of the pretarsal orbicularis during smiling decreases the height of the vertical palpebral aperture. When hypertrophied, the pretarsal orbicularis can give a "jelly roll" appearance to the lower eyelid, and some individuals may complain that they look overweight. We inject 2 U of BoNT-A into the lower pretarsal orbicularis, which gently opens the palpebral aperture both at rest and during smiling (▶ Fig. 15.6). Lateral orbital injections have a synergistic effect with these lower pretarsal eyelid injections and can be used as a safe way to enhance the lower eyelid effect.[40] This procedure is used only for patients with a normal preinjection snap test. Patients who have had previous lower eyelid ablative resurfacing or subciliary blepharoplasty without a coexisting canthopexy to support the normal position of the lower eyelid are not good candidates for this procedure.

15.3.6 Midface

Neuromodulator treatment weakens the upper nasalis and effectively softens the radial "bunny" lines. Bunny lines are typically treated in conjunction with the glabellar complex.

Particularly in subjects with a flatter nasal bridge, the use of diluted HA filler injected with a stepwise microbolus technique can restore a pleasing upper facial appearance. We use a 30-gauge mesotherapy needle while simultaneously tenting up with the nondominant hand the skin of the nasal dorsum away from the underlying periosteum with the dorsal nasal vessels below. We withdraw the plunger each time to be sure we are not intravascular. Very little filler volume is required.

Contraction of the lower nasalis muscle accentuates the nasal flare. Some individuals repeatedly and embarrassingly dilate their nostrils in social situations. The sides of the columella/septum become visible when the nostrils are prominently flared. In some individuals, this is a manifestation of oromandibular dystonia. Small doses (2–10 units) of BoNT-A have produced a satisfactory decrease in involuntary nostril flare in some patients for 3 to 4 months.

15.3.7 Temple

Volume loss in the temple is an early and subtle sign of aging that is more common in patients with low body fat and may lead to skeletonization of the bony lateral orbital rim.[41] Volumization of the temple with HA filler can improve the convexity between the brow and zygomatic arch, leading to a more youthful contour and overall appearance of the brow and face (▶ Fig. 15.7). HA fillers with higher G′ or viscosity are suitable for use in the temple to provide support of the more inferior structures and midface and can be administered with a needle or cannula.[42]

Excellent understanding of the complex vascular anatomy of this region is important for safe treatment. The optimal location for injection is between the superficial temporal vessels and middle temporal vein, approximately 1 cm posterior to the orbital rim along the temporal line of fusion and 1 cm inferior to this point[43] (▶ Fig. 15.8). An initial volume of 0.5 to 1 mL of HA can be placed on each side per treatment in a slow and controlled depot manner.[41,42] While subcutaneous or superficial injection techniques are described,[41] a preperiosteal depth of injection deep to the temporalis muscle is preferred to decrease the risk of vascular complications and blindness.[42,43]

15.4 Conclusion

The current use of neuromodulators and fillers has dramatically expanded the age range of subjects seeking aesthetic enhancement. Subjects also understand the marvelous synergy of facial recontouring with fillers and facial relaxation and elevation with neuromodulators. Most treatments require maintenance over the years. The neuromodulators and fillers are more successful when used together and also enhance the results of other treatments in our therapeutic armamentarium such as surgery and energy-based devices and lasers. These treatments

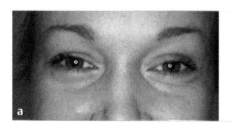
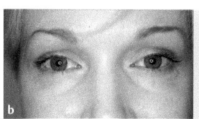

Fig. 15.6 BoNT-A treatment of hypertrophic orbicularis oculi. Eye widening effect is further enhanced with ipsilateral treatment of lateral canthal rhytids.

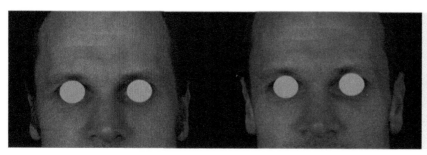

Fig. 15.7 Hyaluronic acid treatment of the temples.

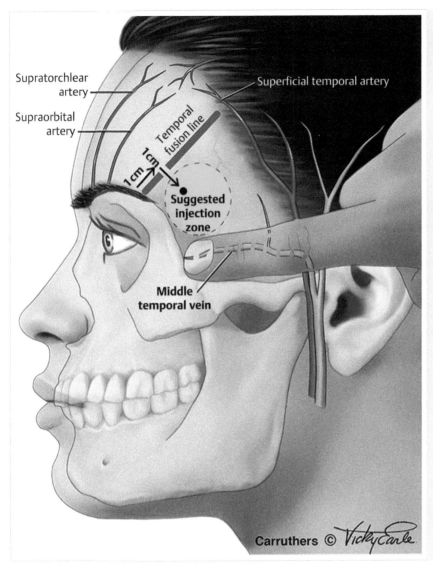

Supratorchlear artery

Supraorbital artery

Superficial temporal artery

Temporal fusion line

1 cm 1 cm 1 cm

Suggested injection zone

Middle temporal vein

Carruthers © VickyEarle

Fig. 15.8 The suggested safest injection zone for the temple is posterior to the superolateral bony orbital margin, 1 cm inferior to the temporal line of fusion and over 1 fingerbreadth above the superior border of the zygoma.

have been safe with the exception of the extremely rare filler-induced vascular occlusion.

References

[1] Morris D. Manwatching: A Field Guide to Human Behavior. New York, NY: H. N. Abrams; 1977

[2] Cather JC, Cather JC, Menter A. Update on botulinum toxin for facial aesthetics. Dermatol Clin. 2002; 20(4):749–761

[3] American Society of Plastic Surgeons. 2017 Plastic Surgery Statistics. 2017 Top Five Cosmetic Minimally-Invasive Procedures. 2017. Available at: https://www.plasticsurgery.com

[4] Richard MJ, Morris C, Deen BF, Gray L, Woodward JA. Analysis of the anatomic changes of the aging facial skeleton using computer-assisted tomography. Ophthal Plast Reconstr Surg. 2009; 25(5):382–386

[5] Rohrich RJ, Pessa JE. The fat compartments of the face: anatomy and clinical implications for cosmetic surgery. Plast Reconstr Surg. 2007; 119(7):2219–2227, discussion 2228–2231

[6] Carruthers J, Humphrey S, Beleznay K. Suggested safe injection zones for the temple. Dermatol Surg. 2017; 43:756–757

[7] Lambros V. Observations on periorbital and midface aging. Plast Reconstr Surg. 2007; 120(5):1367–1376, discussion 1377

[8] Hexsel D, Brum C, Siega C, et al. Evaluation of self-esteem and depression symptoms in depressed and nondepressed subjects treated with onabotulinumtoxinA for glabellar lines. Dermatol Surg. 2013; 39(7):1088–1096

[9] Kruger TH, Wollmer MA. Depression–An emerging indication for botulinum toxin treatment. Toxicon. 2015; 107 Pt A:154–157

[10] Scott AB. Botulinum toxin injection into extraocular muscles as an alternative to strabismus surgery. Ophthalmology. 1980; 87(10):1044–1049

[11] Carruthers JDA, Carruthers JA. Treatment of glabellar frown lines with C. botulinum-A exotoxin. J Dermatol Surg Oncol. 1992; 18(1):17–21

[12] Carruthers A, Carruthers J, Flynn TC, Leong MS. Dose-finding, safety, and tolerability study of botulinum toxin type B for the treatment of hyperfunctional glabellar lines. Dermatol Surg. 2007; 33(1 Spec No.):S60–S68

[13] Carruthers JD, Fagien S, Rohrich RJ, Weinkle S, Carruthers A. Blindness caused by cosmetic filler injection: a review of cause and therapy. Plast Reconstr Surg. 2014; 134(6):1197–1201

[14] Hong DK, Seo YJ, Lee JH, Im M. Sudden visual loss and multiple cerebral infarction after autologous fat injection into the glabella. Dermatol Surg. 2014; 40(4):485–487

[15] Carruthers J, Carruthers A, Humphrey S. Introduction to fillers. Plast Reconstr Surg. 2015; 136(5) Suppl:120S–131S

[16] Wang F, Garza LA, Kang S, et al. In vivo stimulation of de novo collagen production caused by cross-linked hyaluronic acid dermal filler injections in photodamaged human skin. Arch Dermatol. 2007; 143(2):155–163

[17] Turlier V, Delalleau A, Casas C, et al. Association between collagen production and mechanical stretching in dermal extracellular matrix: in vivo effect of

cross-linked hyaluronic acid filler. A randomised, placebo-controlled study. J Dermatol Sci. 2013; 69(3):187–194

[18] Quan T, Wang F, Shao Y, et al. Enhancing structural support of the dermal microenvironment activates fibroblasts, endothelial cells, and keratinocytes in aged human skin in vivo. J Invest Dermatol. 2013; 133(3):658–667

[19] Monheit GD, Narins RS, Mariwalla K. NASHA family. In: Carruthers J, Carruthers A, Dover JS, Alam M, eds. Procedures in Cosmetic Dermatology: Soft Tissue Augmentation. New York, NY: Elsevier; 2013:10–22

[20] Humphrey S, Fitzgerald R. Juvederm family. In Carruthers J, Carruthers, A, eds. Soft Tissue Augmentation. New York, NY: Elsevier; 2018:25–33

[21] Sundaram H, Cassuto D. Biophysical characteristics of hyaluronic acid soft-tissue fillers and their relevance to aesthetic applications. Plast Reconstr Surg. 2013; 132(4) Suppl 2:5S–21S

[22] Beleznay K, Carruthers JDA, Carruthers A, Mummert ME, Humphrey S. Delayed-onset nodules secondary to a smooth cohesive 20 mg/mL hyaluronic acid filler: cause and management. Dermatol Surg. 2015; 41(8):929–939

[23] Humphrey S, Weiss RA. Reversers. In: Carruthers J, Carruthers A, eds. Soft Tissue Augmentation. New York, NY: Elsevier; 2013:200–207

[24] Chesnut C. Restoration of visual loss with retrobulbar hyaluronidase injection after hyaluronic acid filler. Dermatol Surg. 2018; 44(3):435–437

[25] Goodman GJ, Clague MD. A rethink on hyaluronidase injection, intraarterial injection and blindness. Is there another option for treatment of retinal artery embolism caused by intraarterial injection of hyaluronic acid? Dermatol Surg. 2016; 42(4):547–549

[26] Chopra R, Graivier M, Fabi S, Nestor M, Meuse P, Mashburn J. A multi-center, open-label, prospective study of cannula injection of small-particle hyaluronic acid plus lidocaine (SPHAL) for lip augmentation. J Drugs Dermatol. 2018; 17(1):10–16

[27] Beleznay K, Carruthers JDA, Humphrey S, Jones D. Avoiding and treating blindness from fillers: a review of the world literature. Dermatol Surg. 2015; 41(10):1097–1117

[28] American Society of Aesthetic Plastic Surgery. 2016 Cosmetic Surgery National Database. 2016. Available at: https://www.surgery.org

[29] American Society for Dermatologic Surgery. ASDS Survey on Dermatologic Procedures. 2017. Available at: https://www.asds.net

[30] Fagien S, Carruthers J. Commentary on restoration of visual loss with retrobulbar hyaluronidase injection after hyaluronic acid filler. Dermatol Surg. 2018; 44(3):437–443

[31] Carruthers J, Burgess C, Day D, et al. Consensus recommendations for combined aesthetic interventions in the face using botulinum toxin, fillers, and energy-based devices. Dermatol Surg. 2016; 42(5):586–597

[32] Carruthers A, Carruthers J, Said S. Dose-ranging study of botulinum toxin type A in the treatment of glabellar rhytids in females. Dermatol Surg. 2005; 31(4):414–422, discussion 422

[33] Carruthers A, Carruthers J. Prospective, double-blind, randomized, parallel-group, dose-ranging study of botulinum toxin type A in men with glabellar rhytids. Dermatol Surg. 2005; 31(10):1297–1303

[34] Carruthers J, Carruthers A, Maberley D. Deep resting glabellar rhytides respond to BTX-A and Hylan B. Dermatol Surg. 2003; 29(5):539–544

[35] Carruthers J, Carruthers A. A prospective, randomized, parallel group study analyzing the effect of BTX-A (Botox) and nonanimal sourced hyaluronic acid (NASHA, Restylane) in combination compared with NASHA (Restylane) alone in severe glabellar rhytides in adult female subjects: treatment of severe glabellar rhytides with a hyaluronic acid derivative compared with the derivative and BTX-A. Dermatol Surg. 2003; 29(8):802–809

[36] Carruthers J, Carruthers A. Three-dimensional forehead reflation. Dermatol Surg. 2015; 41(1) Suppl 1:S321–S324

[37] Carruthers JDA, Carruthers Appreciation of the vascular anatomy of aesthetic forehead reflation. Dermatol Surg. 2018;44(Suppl 1):S2–S4

[38] Huilgol SC, Carruthers A, Carruthers JDA. Raising eyebrows with botulinum toxin. Dermatol Surg. 1999; 25(5):373–375, discussion 376

[39] Carruthers A, Carruthers J. Eyebrow height after botulinum toxin type A to the glabella. Dermatol Surg. 2007; 33(1 Spec No.):S26–S31

[40] Flynn TC, Carruthers JA, Carruthers JA. Botulinum-A toxin treatment of the lower eyelid improves infraorbital rhytides and widens the eye. Dermatol Surg. 2001; 27(8):703–708

[41] Buckingham ED, Glasgold R, Kontis T, et al. Volume rejuvenation of the facial upper third. Facial Plast Surg. 2015; 31(1):43–54

[42] Breithaupt AD, Jones DH, Braz A, Narins R, Weinkle S. Anatomical Basis for Safe and Effective Volumization of the Temple. Dermatol Surg. 2015; 41 Suppl 1:S278–S283

[43] Carruthers J, Humphrey S, Beleznay K, Carruthers A. Suggested Injection Zone for Soft Tissue Fillers in the Temple? Dermatol Surg. 2017; 43(5):756–757

16 Fat Augmentation of the Brow

Juliana Gildener-Leapman, Morris E. Hartstein

Abstract

A youthful upper lid–brow–temple complex is full and convex. With age, lipoatrophy and the associated volume loss contribute to lateral brow deflation and descent. Autologous fat is a biocompatible material that can be harvested and transferred to the brow alone or in conjunction with an upper blepharoplasty to restore the natural volume and convexities of the eyebrow region.

Keywords: autologous fat transfer, brow ptosis, brow contour, upper blepharoplasty, volume, negative vector, brow rejuvenation

16.1 Introduction

Understanding brow aesthetics and physiologic changes that occur to the brow with aging is key to determining appropriate surgical or nonsurgical management for any patient. There has been a significant evolution in brow aesthetic preferences as seen across cultures and fashion, suggesting that there is no single ideal brow shape and contour. Many studies[1-5] have attempted to find unifying principals for an objective brow aesthetic; however, no consensus has been reached. Ideal brow contour is an ever-evolving concept.

Nonetheless, a universally youthful upper lid–brow–temple complex is full with natural convexities. The aging process is associated with lipoatrophy and volume loss that contribute to lateral brow deflation and descent.[6,7] The recognition of volume loss in facial aging has found well-established treatments with autologous fat transfer and fillers, especially in the lower lid and cheek.[8,9] Until recently, however, the classic understanding of brow ptosis focused on gravitational descent, especially of the tail of the brow, with management mainly directed at surgical lifting.

Studies have revealed that there may be less brow descent with aging than previously thought.[10] In some cases, it has been shown that there is a paradoxical elevation of the medial brow with age associated with frontalis muscle tone compensating for blepharoptosis. The paradoxical elevation of the medial brow and the soft tissue deflation around the lateral brow together create a greater impression of lateral brow ptosis than may actually occur. Surgical brow lifting, which focuses solely on countering the gravitational forces that cause skin laxity and soft tissue descent, does not address the oftentimes more profound impact of volume loss. Volume loss with aging makes the bony orbit more visible and the lateral brow less visible as it dives posteriorly. A hollow between the bony orbit and the temporal fossa creates shadows and hides the tail of the brow, which is normally prominent in a youthful face. Surgical elevation alone may lead to further skeletonization of the orbital rim and an overelevated, unnatural appearing brow.[11] Lambros[10,12,13] and others[14,15-20] have discussed the important role of volume replacement in the upper lid and below the brow for periorbital rejuvenation. With this knowledge, the treatment paradigm for the aging brow is shifting toward volumization with hyaluronic acid fillers and autologous fat transfer.

Autologous fat is an abundant, biocompatible material that is relatively easy to harvest and long-lasting.[6,7,21,22] Patients already undergoing upper blepharoplasty are ideal candidates for intraoperative fat grafting to the brow and temporal fossa to provide an added rejuvenated effect. In our practice, autologous fat transfer has a noticeable synergistic effect with upper blepharoplasty to restore the natural convexities of the brow–temple complex (▶ Fig. 16.1, ▶ Fig. 16.2). It is a safe, rapid, and reliable procedure. It has the benefits of giving a natural restorative appearance, with fat biocompatibility potentially leading to greater longevity than alternative treatments. We have found this to be a useful enhancement for blepharoplasty patients who do not wish to undergo a browlift procedure or where a browlift would lead to an unnatural brow appearance. Here, we describe our experience with autologous fat transfer to the brow as a useful adjunct to the standard upper blepharoplasty.

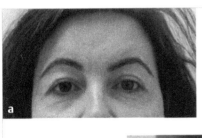
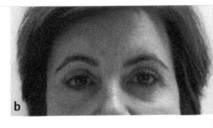
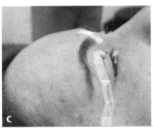

Fig. 16.1 (a) Preoperative frontal photograph of a patient with dermatochalasis and lateral brow ptosis and mild temporal fossa hollowing. **(b)** Postoperative frontal photograph of the same patient with autologous fat transfer to brow and temple with an improved anterior–posterior projection of the tail of the brow and fullness of the temporal fossa. **(c)** Immediate postoperative lateral photograph of the patient showing added volume and smooth contour to brow and temple after fat transfer procedure.

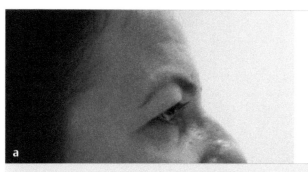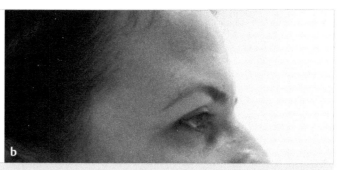

Fig. 16.2 **(a)** Preoperative photograph dermatochalasis with lateral hooding and lateral brow ptosis on a deflated superolateral orbital rim. **(b)** Postoperative photograph after upper blepharoplasty and autologous fat transfer demonstrating a subtle lift with a more youthful fullness and projection of the lateral brow.

16.2 Goals of Intervention

- To restore volume and the natural convexity to the eyebrow region using autologous fat.
- To enhance the upper blepharoplasty effect with autologous fat transfer.
- To minimize appearance of residual skin hooding after upper blepharoplasty.

16.3 Risks of Fat Grafting

- Contour irregularity.
- Eyebrow and eyelid asymmetry.
- Undercorrection/overcorrection.
- Infection.
- Fat migration.
- Fat necrosis.
- Fat embolism with stroke or blindness.

16.4 Benefits of Fat Grafting

- Restoration of a youthful brow contour with mild lift.
- Safe procedure with a low-risk profile.
- Autologous fat is biocompatible, integrates well into tissue, and is potentially permanent.

16.5 Informed Consent

Informed consent is obtained from all patients undergoing treatment. This includes an explanation of the aforementioned risks, benefits, and alternatives to these procedures.

16.6 Indications

A patient undergoing blepharoplasty with mild brow ptosis, loss of eyebrow convexity, and temporal fossa hollowing.

16.7 Contraindications

- Unmanageable patient expectations.
- Minimal fat to harvest.
- Medically unstable to have the procedure.

16.8 Preoperative Checklist

Prior to the procedure, it is important to have a clear informed consent, preoperative photographs, and instrumentation on hand. The procedure can be performed in a well-equipped office-based setting, surgery center, or hospital; it can be performed with local, monitored, or general anesthesia.

16.8.1 Instrumentation

- Standard blepharoplasty instruments.
- 18-gauge needle.
- Fat harvesting cannula (e.g., Tonnard).
- 10-mL Luer Lock syringe.
- Fat transfer device (Tulip or three-way stopcock).
- 1-mL Luer Lock syringes for fat grafting.
- Fat injection cannulas (0.9, 1.2 mm).
- Centrifuge (optional).
- 6–0 Prolene suture on PC-3 needle.

16.8.2 Operative Technique: Step by Step

Preparation

- Preoperative upper eyelid skin marking.
- Intravenous sedation.
- Topical anesthetizing eye drops.
- Local anesthesia to eyelid, periorbita, and fat harvest site.
- Sterile preparation and draping of operative sites.

Fat Harvest (▶ Fig. 16.3)

- Stab incision with a #15 blade in the upper outer thigh or in the umbilicus.
- Tumescence with dilute lidocaine (0.1% lidocaine and 1:1,000,000 epinephrine) using harvesting cannula for a volume of 20 mL. Wait at least 10 to 15 minutes before harvesting.
- Harvest fat with 10-mL Luer Lock syringe and harvesting cannula (e.g., Tonnard or Sorenson).
- Drain off supranate and infranate (filtration or centrifuge).
- Load fat into 1-mL Luer Lock syringes with transfer device (Tulip or three-way stopcock).
- Close wound site with 1 6–0 Prolene suture.

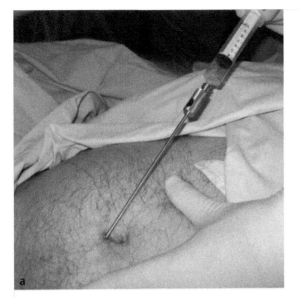
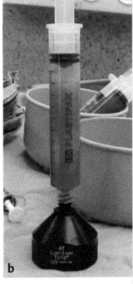

Fig. 16.3 (a) Fat harvest under low suction with 10-mL Luer Lock syringe. (b) Separation of fat from supranate and infranate on stand/transfer device (Tulip). (c) Load fat into 1-mL syringes for fat transfer.

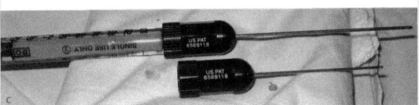

Upper Blepharoplasty

- Skin incision.
- Skin–muscle excision as needed.
- Cautery for hemostasis.
- Excise herniated fat pad(s), as needed.
- Close wound with a 6–0 Prolene suture in a running fashion.

Subbrow Fat Transfer (▶ Fig. 16.4)

- An 18-gauge needle stab incision temporal to the tail of the brow.
- Transfer fat in standard fashion (small aliquots, low pressure) using 0.9- or 1.2-mm cannulas.
- Transfer fat, cannula bevel down, in subdermal plane, posterior to brow and superior to brow in temporal region.
- Total fat transfer 1 to 2 mL per side.
- Massage fat.

16.9 Expert Tips/Pearls/ Suggestions

- The procedure is most useful in patients with moderate forehead skin laxity and a noticeable temporal hollow.
- Inject deep and massage the fat postinjection to ensure a smooth transition.
- Patients should be aware that they may have more postoperative upper lid swelling than with standard blepharoplasty alone.

16.10 Postoperative Care Checklist

- Antibiotic/steroid ointment (e.g., Maxitrol).
- Cold compresses for the first 24 to 48 hours.
- Follow-up in 1 week for suture removal.

16.11 Complications and Their Management

- Graft absorption:
  ○ Try a different filling agent like a hyaluronic acid filler.
- Undercorrection:
  ○ Supplement with hyaluronic acid or further fat harvesting and transfer.
- Overcorrection:
  ○ If still present after 6 months, consider surgical debulking or steroid injection.
- Contour irregularity:
  ○ Steroid injection and/or filler supplementation.
- Tissue necrosis or embolism:
  ○ Consider hyperbaric oxygen chamber.
- Infection:
  ○ Treat with oral antibiotics as needed.

16.12 Conclusion

Fat augmentation is a useful adjunct to the surgical enhancement of the upper eyelid–brow complex in restoring youthful volume and convexity to the aging brow.

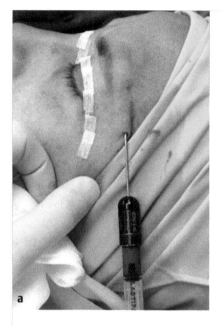
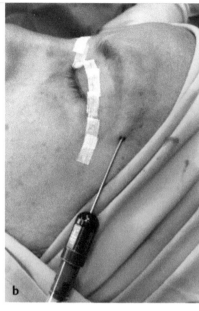
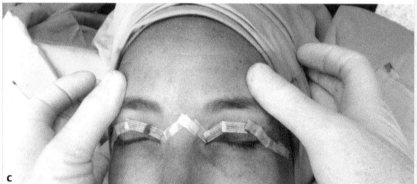

Fig. 16.4 Transfer fat with 0.9- or 1.2-mm cannula in small aliquots to brow (**a**) and superior brow in temporal region (**b**). Then massage of the fat for smooth contour (**c**).

References

[1] Hamamoto AA, Liu TW, Wong BJ. Identifying ideal brow vector position: empirical analysis of three brow archetypes. Facial Plast Surg. 2013; 29(1):76–82

[2] Freund RB, Nolan WB. Correlation between brow lift outcomes and aesthetic ideals for eyebrow height and shape in females. Plastic Reconstr Surg 1996;97(7):1343–1348

[3] Gunter JP, Antrobus SD. Aesthetic analysis of the eyebrows. Plastic Reconstr Surg 1997;99(7):1808–1816

[4] Griffin GR, Kim JC. Ideal female brow aesthetics. Clin Plast Surg. 2013; 40(1):147–155

[5] Baker SB, Dayan JH, Crane A, Kim S. The influence of brow shape on the perception of facial form and brow aesthetics. Plast Reconstr Surg. 2007; 119(7):2240–2247

[6] Collar RM, Boahene KD, Byrne PJ. Adjunctive fat grafting to the upper lid and brow. Clin Plast Surg. 2013; 40(1):191–199

[7] Ciuci PM, Obagi S. Rejuvenation of the periorbital complex with autologous fat transfer: current therapy. J Oral Maxillofac Surg. 2008; 66(8):1686–1693

[8] Coleman S, Saboeiro A, Sengelmann R. A comparison of lipoatrophy and aging: volume deficits in the face. Aesthetic Plast Surg. 2009; 33(1):14–21

[9] Pu LL, Coleman SR, Cui X, Ferguson RE, Jr, Vasconez HC. Autologous fat grafts harvested and refined by the Coleman technique: a comparative study. Plast Reconstr Surg. 2008; 122(3):932–937

[10] Lambros V. Observation on periorbital and midface aging. Plastic Reconstr Surg 2007;120(5):1367–1376; discussion 1377

[11] Chen HH, Williams EF. Lipotransfer in the upper third of the face. Curr Opin Otolaryngol. Head Neck Surg. 2011; 19:289–294

[12] Lambros V, Amos G. Three-dimensional facial averaging: a tool for understanding facial aging. Plast Reconstr Surg. 2016; 138(6):980e–982e

[13] Lambros V. Volumizing the brow with hyaluronic acid fillers. Aesthet Surg J. 2009; 29(3):174–179

[14] Rohrich RJ, Pessa JE. The fat compartments of the face: anatomy and clinical implications for cosmetic surgery. Plast Reconstr Surg. 2007;119(7):2219–2227

[15] Bucky LP, Kanchwala SK. The role of autologous fat and alternative fillers in the aging face. Plast Reconstr Surg. 2007; 120(6) Suppl:89S–97S

[16] Holck DE, Lopez MA. Periocular autologous fat transfer. Facial Plast Surg Clin North Am. 2008; 16(4):417–427, vi

[17] Sozer SO, Agullo FJ, Palladino H, Payne PE, Banerji S. Pedicled fat flap to increase lateral fullness in upper blepharoplasty. Aesthet Surg J. 2010; 30(2):161–165

[18] Massry GG. Nasal fat preservation in upper eyelid blepharoplasty. Ophthal Plast Reconstr Surg. 2011; 27(5):352–355

[19] Lam SM, Glasgold R, Glasgold M. Analysis of facial aesthetics as applied to injectables. Plast Reconstr Surg 2015;136(5, Suppl):11S–21S

[20] Sykes JM, Cotofana S, Trevidic P, et al. Upper face: clinical anatomy and regional approaches with injectable fillers. Plast Reconstr Surg. 2015; 136(5) Suppl:204S–218S

[21] Yaremchuk MJ, O'Sullivan N, Benslimane F. Reversing Brow Lifts. Aesth Surg J 2007;27(4):367–375

[22] Jatana KR, Smith SP, Jr. The scientific basis for lipotransfer: is it the ideal filler? Facial Plast Surg Clin North Am. 2008; 16(4):443–448, –vi–vii

Section III Involutional Ptosis

17 Involutional Ptosis: Etiology and Management

Farzad Pakdel, Helen A. Merritt

Abstract

Involutional upper eyelid ptosis is the most common type of blepharoptosis, most commonly due to disinsertion, attenuation, or related changes to the levator aponeurosis and muscle. A variety of etiologic and precipitating factors may lead to this type of acquired eyelid malposition. Classic presentation includes decreased palpebral fissure, decreased palpebral fissure on downgaze, decreased margin reflex distance 1, elevated eyelid crease and fold, and normal or near-normal levator function. Involutional ptosis has both functional and aesthetic impact. This type of eyelid ptosis should be differentiated from other types of acquired ptosis, as some of them may be secondary to serious or even life-threatening causes. Successful surgical management is guided by the severity of ptosis and the response to phenylephrine testing.

Keywords: involutional eyelid ptosis, aponeurotic ptosis, blepharoptosis

17.1 Introduction

Involutional ptosis describes the subset of acquired blepharoptosis most commonly due to stretching or disinsertion of the levator aponeurosis.[1] The appearance is classically characterized by a decrease in margin reflex distance 1 (MRD1), normal levator function, elevated upper eyelid crease and fold, and decreased palpebral fissure in downgaze.

Involutional ptosis is the most common etiology for ptosis encountered in an oculoplastic practice, found to make up greater than 60% of ptosis cases in large tertiary referral centers.[2] The prevalence of involutional ptosis increases with age, with average age of presentation in the seventh decade of life; however, younger patients can be affected.[2-4] Patients with this condition often present with consequent visual field complaints and concern about aesthetic appearance. Appropriate assessment to rule out other causes of acquired ptosis is essential. In this chapter, we provide information to understand and manage involutional blepharoptosis.

17.2 Etiology

Involutional ptosis is most commonly due to disinsertion or attenuation of the levator aponeurosis. Intraoperative anatomical findings may also include a lateral shift of the tarsal plate and dehiscence of the medial limb of Whitnall's ligament.[5] Intraoperative and histopathological observations of these patients have noted a small subset with fatty degeneration of levator muscle, which may point to a concurrent myopathic component in some cases.[5]

Classic associated risk factors for the development of involutional ptosis include habitual eyelid rubbing, contact lens use, and history of ocular procedures or surgery. Frequent lid rubbing in patients with irritation due to keratoconjunctivitis, blepharitis, or dry eye can contribute to microtrauma to the levator complex. Similarly, patients that wear hard or soft contact lenses may have chronic microtrauma to the levator muscle during lens placement, lens removal, and blink, contributing to levator dehiscence over time[6] (▶ Fig. 17.1). Chronic eyelid inflammation may also

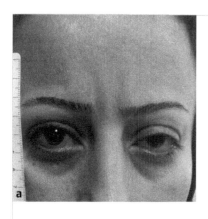
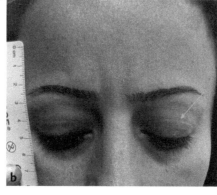
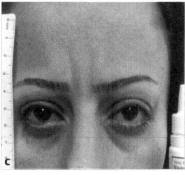
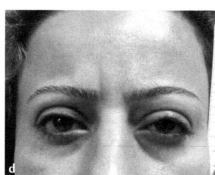

Fig. 17.1 Progressive aponeurotic ptosis in a 32-year-old woman after hard contact lens wear for keratoconus. **(a)** Left eyelid ptosis and elongated margin fold distance (MFD). **(b)** Downgaze view showing elevated left eyelid crease (*blue arrow*). **(c)** Correction of ptosis after application of topical phenylephrine. **(d)** One month after Müller's muscle–conjunctival resection. Ptosis is corrected, and MFD is symmetric.

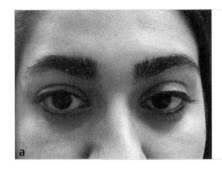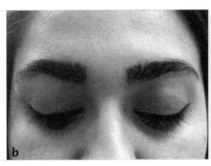

Fig. 17.2 Left involutional ptosis after bilateral adenoviral keratoconjunctivitis 1 year prior. Eyelid ptosis persisted long after resolution of the infection. Levator function was 16 and 14 in right and left side, respectively. **(a)** Asymmetric MRD1 and MFD. **(b)** High eyelid crease and decreased palpebral fissure in downgaze.

contribute to levator disinsertion[7] (▶ Fig. 17.2). Blepharochalasis syndrome, a condition characterized by recurrent, idiopathic episodes of upper eyelid edema, has an association with both primary and recurrent involutional ptosis.[8]

Blepharoptosis that develops after ocular surgery can involve disinsertion of the levator aponeurosis and thereby may be considered a subset of involutional ptosis. Postoperative ptosis may result less commonly from myogenic, neurogenic, or mixed mechanism changes.[9] Etiologic factors for postoperative ptosis may be multifactorial and include soft tissue inflammation, anesthetic myotoxicity, or iatrogenic trauma to the levator muscle (▶ Table 17.1). Ptosis has been reported after a wide spectrum of ocular surgeries, including cataract, glaucoma, vitreoretinal, pterygium, and refractive operations. The incidence of ptosis after intraocular and ocular surface surgeries averages 6% (range: 4–21%).[10,11] Usually, eyelid ptosis is transient and lasts less than 6 months.[12] Changing the technique of cataract surgery from extracapsular cataract extraction to phacoemulsification has significantly reduced the incidence of postcataract surgery ptosis.[13] Additionally, dehiscence of the levator aponeurosis has also been observed after sub-Tenon's injection of corticosteroids.[14,15]

17.3 Clinical Presentation

Patients with involutional ptosis typically present with unilateral or bilateral decreased palpebral fissure, decreased palpebral fissure on downgaze, decreased MRD1, elevated upper eyelid crease and fold, and normal levator excursion (LE)[16] (▶ Fig. 17.3). These patients may demonstrate chronic frontalis activation and eyebrow elevation to compensate eyelid ptosis. Thus, relaxation of the frontalis muscle by cosmetic botulinum toxin to the forehead may unmask or aggravate eyelid ptosis. In some patients with levator disinsertion and fair skin, the iris and pupil may be visible through the eyelid skin. Additionally, a subset of patients with involutional blepharoptosis may demonstrate eyelash ptosis.[17]

Presenting symptoms vary in severity and range from minor cosmetic concern to visual significance. Patients with visual field obstruction may complain of a superior or peripheral visual field deficit or difficulty reading, as the eyelid droops in downgaze.[18]

Cosmetic complaints are often related to anatomic changes in the aesthetic subunits of the eyelid–brow complex, including eyelid or brow height, margin fold asymmetry, or associated dermatochalasis (▶ Fig. 17.4). Additionally, some patients may complain of cephalgia or forehead fatigue as a result of chronic frontalis muscle contraction.

Table 17.1 Etiologic factors of blepharoptosis after ocular surgery

Eyelid edema

Hematoma

Blepharospasm secondary to irritation, pain, photophobia, and inflammation

Anesthesia myotoxicity

Levator damage by eyelid speculum

Levator damage by bridle suture

Horizontal stretching of the eyelid by speculum

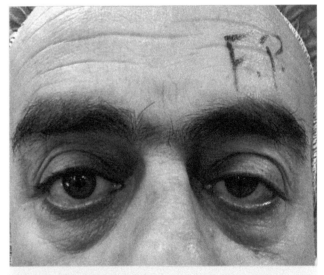

Fig. 17.3 Left aponeurotic ptosis after chalazion removal. Note asymmetric eyelid contour.

17.4 Evaluation

Careful evaluation of patients with upper eyelid ptosis is important to correctly identify the etiology, determine the functional and aesthetic impact, and guide management. A comprehensive history should include systemic conditions, medications with attention to anticoagulants and antiplatelets, and history of previous eye surgery or trauma. History should include the onset and progression of ptosis symptoms, alleviating and aggravating factors, and impact of ptosis on aesthetic concerns or activities of daily living. Review of past photographs may help clarify onset, progression, and associated conditions. Attention to concurrent involutional changes such as brow ptosis, dermatochalasis, lower eyelid malposition, and facial asymmetry is important. Additionally, a complete ophthalmic

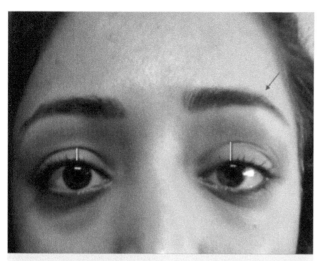

Fig. 17.4 Mild left involutional ptosis. Asymmetric MFD is the most important aesthetic issue in this patient. Note compensatory left brow elevation (*black arrow*).

Table 17.2 Red flags in patients with acquired eyelid ptosis

Clinical finding	Suggestive disease state
Abnormal extraocular movements	Third nerve palsy and hereditary or acquired myopathies or neuropathies
Asymmetric pupils	Horner's syndrome and third nerve palsy
Variable ptosis (change in eyelid height in different occasions or in fatigue state)	Myasthenia gravis, involutional ptosis, and myopathic conditions
Absence or decreased sweating in the ipsilateral face	Horner's syndrome
Episodic eyelid swelling	Blepharochalasis and orbital inflammatory disease
Fullness in upper eyelid	Orbital inflammatory disease and orbital tumor
Family history of myopathic disorders	Chronic progressive ophthalmoplegia, myotonic dystrophy, and oculopharyngeal muscular dystrophy
Hypoglobus	Mucocele, orbital tumor, and congenital or acquired orbital deformity

examination should be performed with attention to vision and health of the ocular surface.

The upper facial surgeon must differentiate involutional ptosis from acquired neurogenic etiologies such as myasthenia gravis, third nerve palsy, and Horner's syndrome. A comprehensive work-up is mandatory before therapeutic intervention when any atypical features are discovered (▶ Table 17.2). The patient should, therefore, be assessed carefully for signs and symptoms of concurrent diplopia, limitation of extraocular movements, anisocoria, and variability/fatigability, as these are not features of involutional ptosis.

External photographs and visual field testing are important to document preoperative findings and confirm visual significance of involutional ptosis.

17.4.1 Evaluation of Eyelid

Quantitative eyelid evaluation in patients with involutional ptosis is essential to confirm correct diagnosis and guide management. The following measurements should be noted.

Palpebral Fissure (PF)

The palpebral fissure is measured vertically from the margin of the upper eyelid to the margin of the lower eyelid with the patient's eyebrow relaxed in primary gaze and the contralateral eyelid elevated.

Palpebral Fissure on Downgaze (dPF)

The vertical palpebral fissure height should again be measured with the patient in downgaze. Involutional ptosis is associated with a smaller palpebral fissure measurement in downgaze than primary gaze.[18] The contralateral eyelid is elevated.

Margin Reflex Distance 1 (MRD1)

MRD1 is the distance between the pupillary light reflex and the upper lid margin with the patient's eyebrow relaxed in primary gaze and the contralateral eyelid elevated. The severity of ptosis is defined according to the MRD1 measurement. In cases of asymmetric ptosis, the MRD1 of each eye should be evaluated with the contralateral eyelid lifted to unmask latent ptosis due to Hering's law.

Eyelid Crease (MCD)

The shape, number, and position of the eyelid crease should be assessed. The main prominent crease should be identified and measured in millimeters. Crease height is measured when the patient looks down with the brow slightly elevated. Eyelid crease height may vary with age, sex, and race, and may be higher in women and Caucasians. Normally, crease position in Caucasian women is 8 to 10 mm and in Caucasian men is 6 to 8 mm. In involutional ptosis, the crease may be elevated, duplicated, or absent.

Levator Excursion (LE)

LE or function is determined by the distance of the upper eyelid excursion from downgaze to upgaze with the brow stabilized. Levator function below 12 mm is considered abnormal. Levator function is typically normal in patients with aponeurotic ptosis, although a subset of patients with involutional ptosis may have a borderline or decreased measurement.[16]

Margin Fold Distance (MFD)

MFD is the measurement between the upper eyelid margin and fold with the patient in primary gaze and is equivalent to tarsal platform show.[19] MFD is an important eyelid aesthetic measurement and may be asymmetric or increased in patients with involutional ptosis (▶ Fig. 17.4). Consideration of this measurement is critical to achieve postoperative symmetry and patient satisfaction.

Phenylephrine Test

Topical phenylephrine (2.5 or 10%) is applied to the ptotic eye, and MRD1 is measured after a period of 3 and 5 minutes. About 60% of patients with involutional eyelid ptosis may demonstrate > 1.5-mm response after this preoperative phenylephrine test.[20] This is a critical test to guide management, as patients with a good response to phenylephrine and good LE may have the best results after Müller's muscle–conjunctival resection (MMCR) surgery.[21]

17.5 Management

The main treatment for correction of involutional ptosis is surgery to reposition or advance the levator aponeurosis. Goals of ptosis surgery include symmetric improvement of palpebral fissure, MRD1, MCD, and MFD. Surgical management may be guided by the severity of ptosis and the response to phenylephrine. While the decision to repair ptosis from an anterior versus posterior approach is a subject of controversy among some oculoplastic surgeons, this section aims to briefly present each technique in a fair and evidence-based manner. Details regarding surgical techniques for the correction of involutional blepharoptosis, including anterior levator surgery, MMCR, and the Fasanella–Servat procedure, are covered in detail in other parts of this book.

The surgeon must decide which approach is most appropriate for each patient. In patients with mild to moderate ptosis (1–3 mm) and good response to phenylephrine testing, posterior ptosis repair with MMCR may be performed.[22,23] Advantages of this technique include a faster surgery, more rapid recovery, minimal postoperative eyelid swelling, and lower probability for eyelid contour deformity.[23] Additionally, there is no need for patient cooperation with a posterior approach. In patients with incomplete or poor response to phenylephrine or more severe involutional ptosis, a superior tarsectomy may be added to the MMCR or a Fasanella–Servat tarsectomy may be considered.[24,25]

In patients with moderate to severe ptosis, poor response to phenylephrine testing, or decreased levator function, an anterior approach to the levator and aponeurosis muscle may be necessary. Anterior levator surgery techniques include levator tuck, levator advancement, and levator resection. Generally, levator advancement is more effective when the patient has a pure levator aponeurosis dehiscence and good levator function.[26,27] Levator tuck may be considered in patients with mild ptosis and good levator function. Levator resection may provide the ability to correct more severe ptosis, especially in those with decreased levator function.[26,27] These techniques are illustrated in other chapters.

Patients with involutional eyelid ptosis frequently have concurrent dermatochalasis. Conversely, those seeking upper eyelid blepharoplasty may have some degrees of involutional ptosis. Concurrent upper eyelid blepharoplasty may be performed simultaneously with either posterior or anterior ptosis surgical approach. The ultimate goal of involutional ptosis repair is a happy patient with improved visual field who has symmetric eyelid height, contour, and crease and fold distances.

References

[1] Dortzbach RK, Sutula FC. Involutional blepharoptosis. A histopathological study. Arch Ophthalmol. 1980; 98(11):2045–2049

[2] Lim JM, Hou JH, Singa RM, Aakalu VK, Setabutr P. Relative incidence of blepharoptosis subtypes in an oculoplastics practice at a tertiary care center. Orbit. 2013; 32(4):231–234

[3] Hashemi H, Khabazkhoob M, Emamian MH, et al. The prevalence of ptosis in an Iranian adult population. J Curr Ophthalmol. 2016; 28(3):142–145

[4] Gonzalez-Esnaurrizar G. The epidemiology and etiology of ptosis in a ophthalmic center. Invest Ophthalmol Vis Sci. 2008; 49(13):640

[5] Shore JW, McCord CD, Jr. Anatomic changes in involutional blepharoptosis. Am J Ophthalmol. 1984; 98(1):21–27

[6] Hwang K, Kim JH. The risk of blepharoptosis in contact lens wearers. J Craniofac Surg. 2015; 26(5):e373–e374

[7] Fujiwara T, Matsuo K, Kondoh S, Yuzuriha S. Etiology and pathogenesis of aponeurotic blepharoptosis. Ann Plast Surg. 2001; 46(1):29–35

[8] Collin JR. Blepharochalasis. A review of 30 cases. Ophthal Plast Reconstr Surg. 1991; 7(3):153–157

[9] Baggio E, Ruban JM. [Postoperative ptosis: etiopathogenesis, clinical analysis, and therapeutic management. Apropos of a series of 43 cases]. J Fr Ophtalmol. 1998; 21(5):361–373

[10] Mehat MS, Sood V, Madge S. Blepharoptosis following anterior segment surgery: a new theory for an old problem. Orbit. 2012; 31(4):274–278

[11] Altieri M, Truscott E, Kingston AE, Bertagno R, Altieri G. Ptosis secondary to anterior segment surgery and its repair in a two-year follow-up study. Ophthalmologica. 2005; 219(3):129–135

[12] Bernardino CR, Rubin PA. Ptosis after cataract surgery. Semin Ophthalmol. 2002; 17(3–4):144–148

[13] Puvanachandra N, Hustler A, Seah LL, Tyers AG. The incidence of ptosis following extracapsular and phacoemulsification surgery: comparison of two prospective studies and review of the literature. Orbit. 2010; 29(6):321–323

[14] Song A, Carter KD, Nerad JA, Boldt C, Folk J. Steroid-induced ptosis: case studies and histopathologic analysis. Eye (Lond). 2008; 22(4):491–495

[15] Ideta S, Noda M, Kawamura R, et al. Dehiscence of levator aponeurosis in ptosis after sub-Tenon injection of triamcinolone acetonide. Can J Ophthalmol. 2009; 44(6):668–672

[16] Frueh BR. The mechanistic classification of ptosis. Ophthalmology. 1980; 87 (10):1019–1021

[17] Malik KJ, Lee MS, Park DJ, Harrison AR. Lash ptosis in congenital and acquired blepharoptosis. Arch Ophthalmol. 2007; 125(12):1613–1615

[18] Olson JJ, Putterman A. Loss of vertical palpebral fissure height on downgaze in acquired blepharoptosis. Arch Ophthalmol. 1995; 113(10):1293–1297

[19] Goldberg RA, Lew H. Cosmetic outcome of posterior approach ptosis surgery (an American Ophthalmological Society thesis). Trans Am Ophthalmol Soc. 2011; 109:157–167

[20] Grace Lee N, Lin LW, Mehta S, Freitag SK. Response to phenylephrine testing in upper eyelids with ptosis. Digit J Ophthalmol. 2015; 21(3):1–12

[21] Maheshwari R, Maheshwari S. Muller's muscle resection for ptosis and relationship with levator and Muller's muscle function. Orbit. 2011; 30(3):150–153

[22] Putterman AM, Urist MJ. Müller's muscle-conjunctival resection ptosis procedure. Ophthalmic Surg. 1978; 9(3):27–32

[23] Dresner SC. Further modifications of the Müller's muscle-conjunctival resection procedure for blepharoptosis. Ophthal Plast Reconstr Surg. 1991; 7(2):114–122

[24] Patel RM, Aakalu VK, Setabutr P, Putterman AM. Efficacy of Muller's muscle and conjunctiva resection with or without tarsectomy for the treatment of severe involutional blepharoptosis. Ophthal Plast Reconstr Surg. 2017; 33(4):273–278

[25] Samimi DB, Erb MH, Lane CJ, Dresner SC. The modified Fasanella-Servat procedure: description and quantified analysis. Ophthal Plast Reconstr Surg. 2013; 29(1):30–34

[26] Thomas GN, Chan J, Sundar G, Amrith S. Outcomes of levator advancement and Müller muscle-conjunctiva resection for the repair of upper eyelid ptosis. Orbit. 2017; 36(1):39–42

[27] Ben Simon GJ, Lee S, Schwarcz RM, McCann JD, Goldberg RA. External levator advancement vs Müller's muscle-conjunctival resection for correction of upper eyelid involutional ptosis. Am J Ophthalmol. 2005; 140(3):426–432

18 External Levator Advancement with Orbicularis-Sparing Technique

Magdalene Y. L. Ting, Jessica R. Chang, Sandy Zhang-Nunes

Abstract

External levator advancement is an optimal procedure for moderate to severe aponeurotic ptosis. This technique has the advantage of addressing both dermatochalasis and ptosis simultaneously through a single incision. With practice and a precise awareness of anatomy, this procedure allows the surgeon a high degree of control over eyelid contour, height, and symmetry. This chapter describes external levator advancement using an orbicularis muscle–sparing technique to maintain blink and minimize exposure keratopathy and lagophthalmos.

Keywords: aponeurotic ptosis, involutional ptosis, external levator advancement

18.1 Introduction/Goals of Intervention

External levator advancement (ELA) is a workhorse procedure for aponeurotic/involutional ptosis, which arises from attenuation of the levator aponeurosis resulting in its elongation or dehiscence from the tarsus.[1–3] Aponeurotic ptosis is characterized by decreased palpebral fissure (PF) in primary and downgaze, decreased margin reflex distance 1 (MRD1), increased margin crease and margin fold distances (MFD), normal Bell's phenomenon, and normal levator excursion (> 10 mm; ▶ Fig. 18.1).[2,3] Evaluation for concurrent dermatochalasis, brow ptosis, lagophthalmos, and dry eye should be performed prior to surgery.

The main goals of ELA include elevating the eyelid height (MRD1) to improve the superior visual field in primary gaze, improve PF on downgaze for reading, improve aesthetic eyelid contour and symmetry, and avoid lagophthalmos. To achieve the best results, reversible sedation should be used with local anesthetic so that the patient may cooperate with instructions from the surgeon to allow for intraoperative adjustment of eyelid height, contour, and symmetry. In experienced hands, this approach is very effective in establishing good eyelid position, with reported success rates ranging from 77 to 95%.[4,5] Primary external levator surgery is less complex than reoperation.[6] With practice, ELA can be a very predictable and successful technique alone or combined with blepharoplasty for patients who need simultaneous dermatochalasis and ptosis management.

18.2 Risks

Ptosis repair is an elective surgery and it is vital for the surgeon to have a thorough preoperative discussion with the patient. Main surgical risks include:
- Prolonged bruising and swelling of the eyelids (including lower eyelids).
- Exacerbation or new development of dry eye symptoms from exposure keratopathy.
- Contour abnormalities.
- Undercorrection.
- Overcorrection.
- Scarring.
- Lagophthalmos (incomplete eyelid closure).
- Orbital hemorrhage.
  - The risk may be slightly higher with an external levator surgery than blepharoplasty or posterior approach surgery that does not violate the orbital septum.
  - A disastrous orbital hemorrhage could lead to vision loss.
  - Less severe hematomas may cause delayed wound healing and/or recurrent ptosis.
- Damage to adjacent structures, including:
  - Trochlea medially, causing double vision.[7]
  - Lacrimal gland injury laterally.
- Wound infection or dehiscence.

18.3 Benefits
- Improvement in MRD1, PF, and superior visual field.
- Improved aesthetic appearance of face.

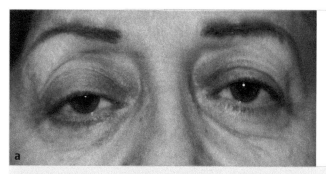
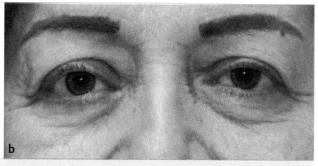

Fig. 18.1 (a) Before photograph of patient who underwent right upper eyelid external levator advancement ptosis repair. Note the elevated eyelid crease and compensatory brow elevation for the patient to see. (b) Six-month postoperative photograph, showing the right upper eyelid ptosis correction, with ensuing bilateral relaxation of the brows, decreased MFD, and now apparent residual dermatochalasis, which the patient did not want addressed at the time.

- May be performed with blepharoplasty without an additional incision.
- Allows for creation or adjustment of eyelid crease.
- Allows for intraoperative adjustment of eyelid contour and treatment of concurrent lacrimal gland prolapse (see Chapter 26).

18.4 Informed Consent

- What is ptosis?
- Surgical steps for ptosis repair.
- How will ptosis surgery benefit vision and appearance?
- Major risks and complications of the procedure.
- Alternatives to surgical repair:
  ○ No surgery.
  ○ Blepharoplasty only.
  ○ Posterior approach ptosis surgery.
- Anesthesia risks.

18.5 Indications

- Ability for patient to cooperate intraoperatively.
- Desire for improved facial aesthetics with an improved MRD1 and PF.
- Normal levator excursion (> 10 mm).
- Compromise of superior visual field leading to decreased quality of life and function, such as difficulty reading, peripheral vision obstruction affecting driving or ambulating, or difficulty with work requirements.

18.6 Relative Contraindications

- Severely decreased blink reflex (such as in Parkinson's disease patients).
- Loss of corneal sensitivity.
- Significant keratoconjunctivitis sicca and resultant exposure keratopathy.
- Paralysis or weakness of orbicularis oculi muscle.
- Absent Bell's phenomenon (involuntary upward excursion of eye with attempted lid closure).
- Abnormal levator excursion (< 10 mm).
  ○ External levator *resection* is an option for some patients with 5- to 10-mm levator function (See Chapter 30).
  ○ Frontalis suspension is the option for patients with levator excursion less than 4 mm (See Chapter 29).

18.7 The Procedure

The procedure can be performed under local or monitored anesthesia in an office-based setting, outpatient surgical center, or hospital.

18.7.1 Preoperative Checklist

- Review chart to confirm patient, informed consent signed, and past surgical, medical, and ocular histories.
- Confirmation of aponeurotic ptosis with decreased PF in primary and downgaze, decreased MRD1, increased margin crease distance, and MFD with normal levator excursion.

- Confirm ptosis is not variable to rule out myogenic (or neurogenic) ptosis.
- Confirm no severe dry eye or lagophthalmos and normal Bell's phenomenon.
- Discuss upper eyelid crease and fold distances with patient to determine whether simultaneous blepharoplasty is warranted (See Chapter 6).
  ○ Set the crease at 8 to 10 mm in Europeans.
  ○ Set the crease at 6 to 8 mm in East Asians who desire a double eyelid.
- Preoperative photographs, documenting the ptosis (primary and oblique views).
- Anticoagulation status.

18.7.2 Instruments Needed

- Castroviejo calipers.
- #15 Bard-Parker blade.
- Westcott scissors (both sharp and blunt-tipped).
- 0.3-mm Castroviejo forceps.
- Curved Castroviejo needle driver.
- Small two-prong skin retractor.
- 22-gauge needle.

18.7.3 Sutures Used

- The 5–0 Vicryl on a spatulated needle (or 6–0 nylon or Prolene for nondissolving suture, frequently used in reoperations).
- The 6–0 Prolene or 6–0 fast-absorbing or plain gut for skin closure.

18.7.4 The Operative Technique: Step by Step

- The patient is marked along the desired upper eyelid crease (8–10 mm from margin) in the upright position.
  ○ If any skin needs to be excised, a modified ellipse is marked for a simultaneous blepharoplasty.
- The patient is positioned supine in the operating room.
- The eyelids and face are prepared with 5% Betadine and draped in the usual sterile fashion for ophthalmic plastic surgery—the entire face is exposed, with nasal cannula for supplemental oxygen as needed.
- After Betadine cleansing, both upper eyelids are infiltrated with an equal amount of 1:1 mixture of lidocaine 2% with 1:100,000 epinephrine mixed with 0.5% bupivacaine (+/– about 0.2 mL of hyaluronidase per 10 mL).
  ○ No more than 1.5 mL per eyelid is injected to minimize the effect of the epinephrine on Müller's muscle.
- The preoperative skin markings are checked in the supine position by remeasurement and confirmation with the pinch test.
- An incision is made with a #15 Bard-Parker blade along the markings. Any marked excess skin is removed using Westcott scissors and 0.3-mm forceps, preserving underlying orbicularis to maximize postoperative eyelid closure. Hemostasis can be achieved with minimal bipolar or monopolar cautery.

- The patient's baseline eyelid position is assessed. The epinephrine in the block and the supine patient position usually partially corrects the patient's ptosis. Knowing the baseline position in this state helps assess how much intraoperative overcorrection should be targeted.
- Holding the inferior skin edge with forceps, Westcott scissors are used to cut straight down to the tarsus at the lower edge of the incision. The incision is extended medially to just before the punctum and laterally to approximately 3 mm nasal from the lateral canthus.
- A Colorado needle tip cautery and a "Q-tip roll technique," can be used for focal cautery to achieve hemostasis.
- A two-prong skin retractor is placed at the level of the pupil on the lower edge of the incision for inferior retraction by an assistant.
- The orbicularis is tented superiorly with forceps, and the dissection is made down to the orbital septum, angling the Westcott scissors superiorly to peel the orbicularis muscle away from orbital septum. Care must be taken to avoid injury to the levator aponeurosis during dissection. Because the dissection is started inferiorly at the level of the tarsus, it is important to recognize that the levator has been disinserted and to carefully search for the inferior edge of the aponeurosis.
- The septum is opened, and orbital (preaponeurotic) fat is exposed superiorly.
  - Anatomically, the levator is just posterior to this fat pad and is further exposed with blunt dissection (▶ Fig. 18.2).
  - To aid in exposing the levator aponeurosis, the patient can be asked to look up and down to visualize the levator muscle action.
  - Forced generation of the levator muscle can be tested by grasping the levator with toothed forceps and asking the patient to look up while pulling the levator aponeurosis down.
    – If no force is felt, the surgeon is most likely grasping the orbital septum.
- Müller's muscle is carefully peeled off the underside of the levator aponeurosis with sharp Westcott scissors to allow for

easy advancement. If Müller's muscle is violated, a significant amount of bleeding can occur.
- The patient is asked to open the eyes, and the eyelid position is reexamined to check the new baseline eyelid position before advancement because exposure of the levator aponeurosis may make the ptosis appear to be improved.
- A horizontal mattress suture between the levator and tarsus is begun with a 5–0 polyglactin suture with spatulated needle (or 6–0 Prolene or nylon) placed in a backhanded fashion through the levator at the desired height.
- Before passing the suture through the tarsus, the eyelid is lifted off of the globe to avoid ocular penetration. A protective corneal shield may also be used to prevent ocular injury. The needle is passed partial thickness through the tarsal plate approximately 8 mm above the lid margin (▶ Fig. 18.3a). One should be able to feel the firmness of the tarsus when making the tarsal bite. The lid is everted to ensure the needle does

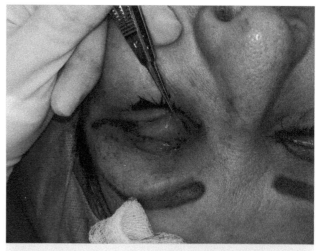

Fig. 18.2 The levator muscle is pulled forward for visualization after dissection from the orbital septum and preaponeurotic fat.

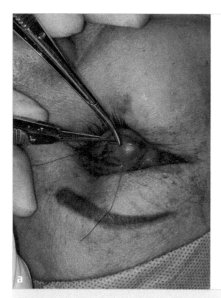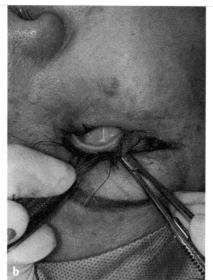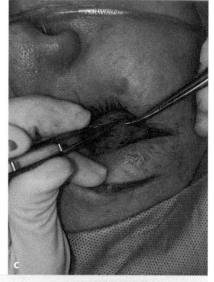

Fig. 18.3 After passing the 5–0 Vicryl suture through the levator aponeurosis at the desired height for advancement, the needle is passed through the tarsal plate at the level of the lower edge of the incision, approximately 8 mm above the lid margin (a). The lid is everted to ensure the needle does not travel full thickness through the eyelid (b). The needle will then be passed back through the levator to complete the horizontal mattress suture (c).

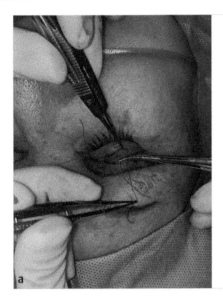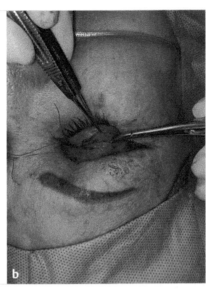

Fig. 18.4 The suture is tied temporarily to allow for intraoperative assessment of the eyelid position **(a)** with a slip knot **(b)**.

not travel full thickness through the eyelid tarsus (▶ Fig. 18.3**b**).

- The suture is passed through the levator again in the opposite direction to complete the horizontal mattress suture (▶ Fig. 18.3**c**). The suture is tied temporarily to allow for intraoperative assessment of the eyelid position (▶ Fig. 18.4).
- Eyelid position is reassessed by asking the patient to look up, down, and straight. The surgeon has to be mindful of the local anesthetic epinephrine effect on both the orbicularis oculi and levator muscles.
- Additional horizontal mattress sutures may be placed medially and laterally to support the central suture or adjust contour. Both the central and medial sutures are tied down temporarily, and the patient's eyelid position is re-evaluated (▶ Fig. 18.5).
- If the contour or height of the eyelid requires adjustment, the temporarily tied sutures can be released by pulling on the shorter end.
  - If the suture needs to be relaxed, it is temporarily retied in a hang-back fashion.
  - If it needs to be advanced, the placement on the levator can be adjusted (▶ Fig. 18.6) or the suture can be removed entirely and replaced.
- Once the ideal contour and height are achieved (▶ Fig. 18.7), the sutures are permanently tied down, being careful to not adjust the levator aponeurosis position from the desired temporarily tied location (▶ Fig. 18.8).
  - Overtightening may cause the suture to cheese-wire through the tarsus, advance the levator aponeurosis, or crimp the levator aponeurosis.
- The orbicularis muscle is redraped over the advanced levator aponeurosis. The lid can now be reinjected with more local anesthetic for comfort during closure or excess skin removal. The skin is closed using a suture of choice, such as a running 6–0 Prolene or plain gut. The goal is to achieve excellent eyelid height, contour, and eyelid crease and fold symmetry (▶ Fig. 18.9).

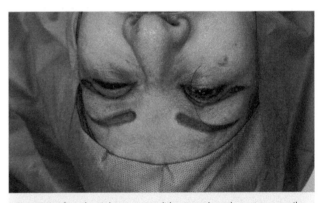

Fig. 18.5 After the right upper eyelid sutures have been temporarily tied down, then the patient's eyelid position is re-evaluated. The right upper eyelid has been advanced, the left side has not.

18.8 Postoperative Care Checklist

- Apply combination antibiotic and steroid ointment to the eye and the eyelid sutures twice daily for 1 to 2 weeks.
- Use ice packs to reduce lid swelling and pain (20 minutes on/20 minutes off while awake for the first few days). This is started in the recovery room.
- The patient can shower the next day and pat dry. Avoid rubbing, submerging face in water, bending over, heavy lifting, and vigorous activity for the first few days.
- If the patient sleeps in prone position, consider sending the patient home with eye shields and medical tape to use while sleeping. The patient should sleep with head elevated above heart level for first few days to minimize swelling.
- Patients may restart all usual home medications immediately after surgery, except anticoagulants, which may sometimes be held until the next day.
- Follow-up appointment is made in 1 to 2 weeks to assess operative outcome.

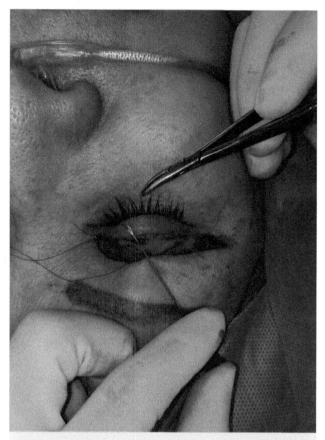

Fig. 18.6 To avoid having to remove the whole suture or use multiple double-armed sutures, a 22-gauge needle can be used to pass through the new desired position on the levator.

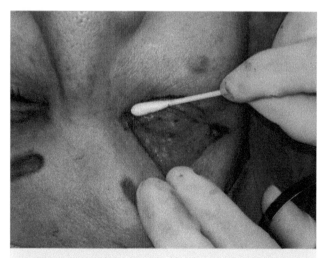

Fig. 18.8 Once the ideal contour and height are achieved, the sutures are permanently tied down one by one, being careful to not adjust the levator aponeurosis position from the desired temporarily tied location. One should not overtighten the suture.

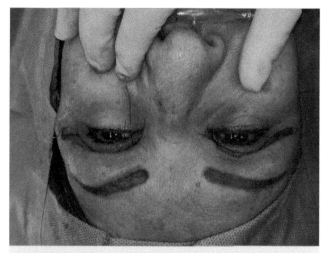

Fig. 18.7 After both levator aponeuroses have been temporarily advanced, the lids are assessed for symmetry, height, and contour.

18.9 Expert Tips/Pearls/ Suggestions

- Other periocular concerns must be addressed when present.
  - Severe dermatochalasis can cause mechanical eyelid ptosis and blepharoplasty may augment the surgical result.
  - Brow ptosis may contribute to mechanical eyelid ptosis. At times, concurrent eyebrow ptosis repair may need to be performed to adequately improve the superior visual field, especially laterally.
  - Lacrimal gland prolapse should be noted and addressed (See Chapter 26).
- Crease formation:
  - Set the crease at 8 to 10 mm in Europeans.
  - Set the crease at 6 to 8 mm in East Asians who desire a double eyelid.
- Excising too much eyelid skin can cause lagophthalmos.
- Measure twice and cut once.
- If simultaneous blepharoplasty is planned, check the preoperative markings in the supine position by remeasuring the patient using Castroviejo calipers to ensure at least 20 mm of skin remains for adequate lid closure. For example, if the upper eyelid crease is set at 8 mm from the margin, one leaves at least 12 mm superiorly between the superior skin incision and inferior edge of the eyebrow. The amount of skin to be excised should be confirmed with the pinch test to prevent postoperative lagophthalmos.
  - Many patients remove some of their brow hairs (cilia); therefore, measure from the transition from thin eyelid skin to thicker eyebrow skin rather than where the brow cilia begin.
  - Slightly less than 20 mm of skin remaining can be acceptable if there will be uncorrected brow ptosis and the pinch test demonstrates additional skin may be removed.

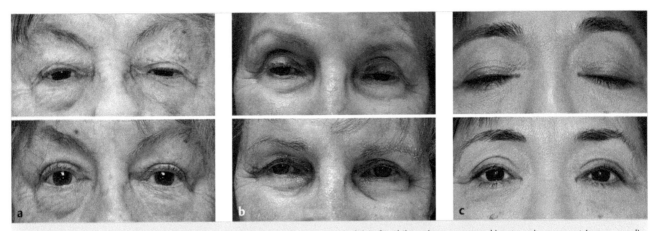

Fig. 18.9 (a–c) Representative pre- and postexternal levator aponeurosis repair. **(a)** Before bilateral upper external levator advancement (upper panel) and after bilateral upper eyelid ptosis repair (1 year) (lower panel). **(b)** Before bilateral external levator advancement (upper panel) and after 1 week (lower panel). **(c)** Before (upper panel) and 9 months after (lower panel) bilateral upper eyelid external levator advancement with lid crease external modification.

- Because levator advancement can be graded, undercorrection can be purposely targeted to reduce the severity of exposure keratopathy related to weak orbicularis, preexisting dry eye, and/or absent Bell's phenomenon.
- Infiltrate the same amount of local anesthetic on each side, with or without hyaluronidase (about 0.2 mL in a 10-mL preparation). Whichever technique you use, be consistent to develop predictable surgical outcomes.
- Care must be taken when passing the partial-thickness tarsal bite. The eyelid should always be everted to rule out full-thickness suture passage, which can cause postoperative eye pain from the suture abrading the cornea. If the suture pass is full thickness, remove the suture and repass it.
- Passing the tarsal suture lower than 8 mm above the lash line can help if lash eversion is needed; however, there is a greater risk of causing a peak in the eyelid contour, especially with floppy eyelids.
- Intraoperative adjustment of the eyelid position and contour.
  - To avoid removing the whole suture or using multiple double-armed sutures, one can use a 22-gauge needle to pass the suture ends through the new desired position on the levator (▶ Fig. 18.6).
  - A 22-gauge needle can be passed through the new desired position on the levator.
  - One arm of the 5–0 Vicryl suture is pulled back out of the levator and passed through the lumen of the 22-gauge needle to allow it to be retrieved into its new location through the levator.
  - The same is done with both arms of the suture, unless one arm still has the needle on, then this is simply backed out, and replaced at the desired higher location on the levator aponeurosis.
  - This method avoids repassing the tarsal bite, minimizing trauma to the tarsus and meibomian glands.
- Aim for slight overcorrection due to the patient's ptosis being corrected by supine position and epinephrine effect on Müller's muscle.
- If unsure whether the patient's eyelid is elevated sufficiently to desired level and appropriate eyelid contour attained, sit the patient upright intraoperatively to evaluate.
- For patients who need crease formation, a few supratarsal fixation sutures can be placed with 6-0 or 7-0 Vicryl.
  - The orbicularis muscle is secured beneath the skin at the lower edge of the crease incision to the levator aponeurosis at that level of the incision. Three to four sutures can be placed across the eyelid.
  - If only minimal crease support is needed, the skin closure can be modified by grasping a small wisp of levator at the lower edge of the incision and incorporating that into the closure with every other suture bite.

18.10 Complications and Their Management

The most difficult aspect of ptosis surgery is creating and sustaining symmetry between both eyelids.[1-5]

18.10.1 Undercorrection

Undercorrection is the most common complication.
- If mild, reassess after 3 months to ensure residual ptosis is not from postoperative edema.
- If severe, the surgeon can consider early reoperation within 1 week.
- The patient should be reminded no surgical correction is permanent, and their ptosis can recur with the passage of time. Ptosis recurrence may present sooner if they sleep on one particular side/eyelid (restretching the levator), wear contact lenses, or undergo procedures utilizing an ocular speculum.

18.10.2 Overcorrection

- If mild, lid pulls/massage may be helpful to stretch the levator (pulling down on lashes and/or eyelid to keep retracted eyelid down, while patient looks up). The authors do this fairly aggressively in the office first, then instruct the patient to do the same at least for 5 minutes five times a day.

- If severe, early reopening of wound and releasing the levator back to desired location may be required.

18.10.3 Lagophthalmos

Lagophthalmos, which is inadequate eyelid closure, is often temporary and requires lubricating ophthalmic ointment as a temporizing measure. If this does not resolve and worsens pre-existing dry eye and exposure keratopathy, early retraction repair may be necessary.

18.10.4 Unsatisfactory Eyelid Contour or Eyelid Crease Asymmetry

Unsatisfactory eyelid contour or eyelid crease asymmetry may require revision surgery or modification with hyaluronic acid fillers such as Restylane (off-label use).

18.10.5 Wound Infection

Wound infection is rare due to eyelid vascularity and generally can be managed by oral antibiotics. If an abscess forms, it must be drained.

18.10.6 Retrobulbar Hemorrhage

Retrobulbar hemorrhage is a rare but serious complication with risk of permanent vision loss.

- If there is tense hematoma, urgently reopen the incisions as a primary intervention to allow decompression.

- If intraocular and orbital pressures are still elevated, emergent canthotomy and cantholysis need to be performed. The release is sufficient once the lower lid can be easily pulled away from the globe, and the pressure on the globe is decreased.
- The patient should continue to be monitored by checking visual acuity and intraocular pressure. In rare circumstances, additional medical and surgical intervention may be required.

18.11 Conclusion

ELA is an excellent and efficient way to address aponeurotic ptosis in a reliable and reproducible way to improve eyelid opening and enhance facial appearance.

References

[1] Part II Periocular Soft Tissues. 11 Periocular malpositions and involutional changes. In: Foster JA, eds. Basic and Clinical Science Course (BCSC), Section 07: Orbit, Eyelids, and Lacrimal System. American Academy of Ophthalmology; 2016–2017:209–221

[2] Dortzbach RK, Sutula FC. Involutional blepharoptosis. A histopathological study. Arch Ophthalmol. 1980; 98(11):2045–2049

[3] Frueh BR. The mechanistic classification of ptosis. Ophthalmology. 1980; 87 (10):1019–1021

[4] McCulley TJ, Kersten RC, Kulwin DR, Feuer WJ. Outcome and influencing factors of external levator palpebrae superioris aponeurosis advancement for blepharoptosis. Ophthal Plast Reconstr Surg. 2003; 19(5):388–393

[5] Older JJ. Levator aponeurosis surgery for the correction of acquired ptosis. Analysis of 113 procedures. Ophthalmology. 1983; 90(9):1056–1059

[6] Bassin RE, Putterman AM. Full-thickness eyelid resection in the treatment of secondary ptosis. Ophthal Plast Reconstr Surg. 2009; 25(2):85–89

[7] Wang Y, McCulley TJ, Doyle JJ, Chang J, Lee MS, McClelland CM. Brown syndrome following upper eyelid ptosis repair. Neuroophthalmology. 2017; 42 (1):49–51

19 Small Incision Anterior Levator Advancement

Mark J. Lucarelli

Abstract

Aponeurotic blepharoptosis is a commonly encountered problem in patients with functional and/or cosmetic concerns. Both external levator repair and conjunctival mullerectomy are time-honored surgical approaches. A subset of patients with upper eyelid ptosis are good candidates for external levator repair through a modified incision. Initially, small incision external levator repair was described through an 8-mm incision. This chapter describes a useful modification of small incision external levator repair through a slightly larger incision.

Keywords: blepharoptosis, external levator repair, small incision external levator repair, minimally invasive ptosis repair

19.1 Introduction

A frequent argument at oculofacial surgical conferences debates whether conjunctival mullerectomy (CML) or external levator repair is superior. In fact, both are excellent surgical options and should be part of the surgical armamentarium of any experienced oculofacial surgeon. Each of these operations has its advantages and disadvantages.

This chapter will focus on external levator repair through a limited eyelid crease incision.[1-7] When upper blepharoplasty is not desired, a small incision may be advantageous in terms of time, efficiency, reduced postoperative edema and ecchymosis, and possibly increased accuracy. The main disadvantage to this small incision variation is the reduced exposure. The modified external levator repair described in this chapter strikes a balance between full-incision ptosis repair (i.e., in the setting of upper eyelid blepharoplasty) and the previously described small incision external levator advancement performed through an 8-mm eyelid crease incision. For surgeons experienced in full-incision external levator repair, this modified approach is easily learned.

19.2 Goals/Indications

- Elevation of the upper eyelid (i.e., increase the margin reflex distance 1).
- Improved visual function and visual field for patients with visually significant blepharoptosis.
- Improved cosmesis.
- Avoidance of complications such as overcorrection or undercorrection.

19.3 Risks of the Procedure

- Hemorrhage.
- Infection.
- Upper eyelid asymmetry.
- Eyelid crease abnormalities.
- Overcorrection/undercorrection.
- Exposure keratopathy/worsening of dry eye symptoms.
- Lagophthalmos.

19.4 Benefits of the Procedure

- Improvement of visual field and visual function.
- Improvement of periocular aesthetics.

19.5 Contraindications

19.5.1 Absolute Contraindications

- Poor levator excursion:
  - For levator excursion 5 mm or less, frontalis suspension is usually recommended.
  - For levator excursion between 5 and 10 mm, a full-incision open approach is often preferable.
- The eyelid that has had many surgeries.

19.5.2 Relative Contraindications

- Patients at risk for ocular surface decompensation (i.e., corneal anesthesia, poor blink, poor Bell's phenomenon, or very severe dry eyes).

19.6 Informed Consent

- Careful discussion of the risks and benefits as described above.
- It is important that the patient understands that he or she will need to awaken, sit up, and look up and down during the surgery to allow eyelid height adjustment. This intraoperative assessment helps improve the accuracy of the procedure.

19.7 The Procedure

19.7.1 Instruments Needed

- Marking pen.
- Ruler.
- Corneal protective shield.
- Incisional devices such as scalpel, Westcott scissors, and monopolar unit with microdissection needle.
- Tissue forceps (0.5-mm forceps).
- Sutures:
  - The 6–0 Prolene, blue, for advancement of the levator aponeurosis onto the anterior tarsus.
  - The 7–0 Vicryl for orbicularis closure.
  - A 6–0 fast-absorbing or 6–0 Prolene suture for skin closure.

19.7.2 Preoperative Checklist

- Informed consent.
- Instrumentation available.

19.7.3 Operative Technique

- With the patient supine and looking straight up at the ceiling, mark the position of the pupil on the skin near the upper eyelid margin.
- With the patient in primary gaze, mark the lid crease from the position of the medial limbus to the lateral limbus. A 12-mm incision allows a reasonably comfortable working space and preserves the small incision nature of the technique (▶ Fig. 19.1).
- Local anesthetic (2% lidocaine with 1:100,000 epinephrine mixed in equal parts with 0.5% Marcaine with 1:100,000 epinephrine) is injected superficially into the eyelid in the area of the lid crease marking. Typically, 0.5 mL of the local anesthetic mixture is injected.
- Incision of the skin along the marked area of eyelid crease is performed (▶ Fig. 19.2).
- With gentle retraction directed inferiorly by an assistant, dissection is carried out through the orbicularis muscle and through the orbital septum to reach the levator complex. The preaponeurotic fat should be identified. Blunt dissection can be helpful during this step. In patients with a deep superior sulcus (for whom this technique is especially useful), the preaponeurotic fat may be quite scant and somewhat difficult to identify. The musculoaponeurotic junction should also be identified (▶ Fig. 19.3). No specific release of the levator aponeurosis or dissection between levator and Müller's muscle is necessary.
- The superior third of the anterior tarsus in the area of the incision is identified (▶ Fig. 19.4). Westcott scissors are often useful for clearing the fine attachments of connective tissue off the tarsus.
- A single-armed 6–0 Prolene suture is then directed inferiorly through the musculoaponeurotic junction. It is then passed in a partial-thickness fashion horizontally through the anterior

superior tarsus at the position where the pupil was previously marked on the eyelid skin. Next, the suture is returned superiorly and passed from underneath the levator aponeurosis through the musculoaponeurotic junction. This suture is then tied in a temporary fashion. A second similarly passed suture of 6–0 Prolene is placed lateral to the first suture to help establish proper lateral contour of the eyelid.

- With the patient in the seated position and no significant sedation on board, eyelid height and contour are inspected in primary gaze, upgaze, and downgaze. Attempted closure is

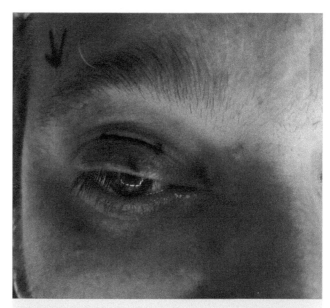

Fig. 19.2 A lid crease incision extending 12 mm provides adequate working space and preserves the small incision nature of the technique.

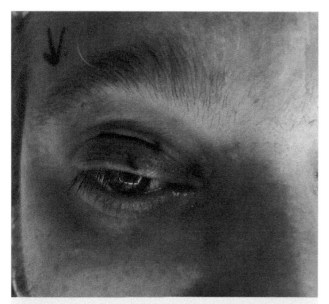

Fig. 19.1 The position of the incision is centered over the pupil with the patient in primary gaze.

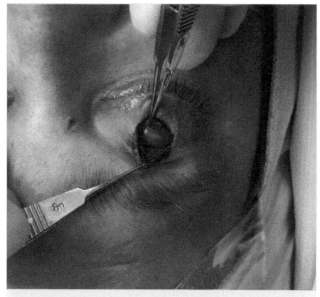

Fig. 19.3 With careful dissection, the levator complex and the musculoaponeurotic junction are clearly identified.

also assessed. The Prolene sutures are then adjusted as needed using smooth tying forceps. If needed, a medial suture can be placed, but this is rarely needed.

- The Prolene sutures are tied in a permanent fashion over a curved needle holder.
- The orbicularis is reapproximated with one buried interrupted suture of 7–0 Vicryl.
- The skin is closed in a running fashion using 6–0 fast-absorbing plain gut suture.
- The patient is seen 1 to 2 weeks postoperatively. In the event of significant overcorrection or undercorrection, the operated eyelid(s) can be adjusted in the office in the 2-week period, following the first postoperative week.

19.8 Expert Tips/Pearls/Suggestions

- Patient selection is best reserved for patients with none or mild dermatochalasis or those patients for whom avoiding

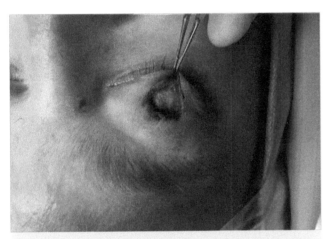

Fig. 19.4 The superior third of the tarsus is exposed with standard dissection techniques, and the external levator repair is then completed in typical fashion.

any upper eyelid skin excision is preferable (▶ Fig. 19.5, ▶ Fig. 19.6).

- If the procedure is performed under monitored sedation, the anesthesia team needs to understand the timeline for when patient will need to be wide awake and sitting up. Propofol is an excellent drug for this purpose.
- Surgeons should be familiar and experienced with external levator repair through a standard upper eyelid blepharoplasty incision prior to performing this small incision technique.
- In cases where significant scarring is anticipated (such as multiply operated upper eyelid or status post significant lacerating trauma), a standard external levator repair is probably more appropriate.

19.9 Postoperative Care Checklist

- Ice-cold gauze is applied to the operative site for the first 48 hours while the patient is awake.
- Head of bed elevation is recommended.
- Steroid antibiotic ointment is applied to the incision wounds three times a day for 1 week. In patients with multiple allergies, Vaseline or white petroleum jelly is used on the incision line.

19.10 Complications and Their Management

- Overcorrection or undercorrection is best prevented by assessing the eyelid height carefully in the operating room with the patient awake and minimal to no sedation on board.
- In the event of undercorrection or overcorrection, revision is performed in the office in the second or third postoperative week. After 3 weeks, revision is difficult and is better deferred until complete healing has occurred.

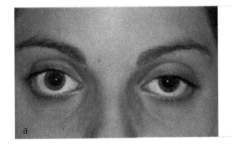
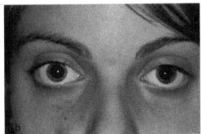

Fig. 19.5 (a, b) Pre- and postoperative results in a patient with unilateral blepharoptosis and minimal dermatochalasis.

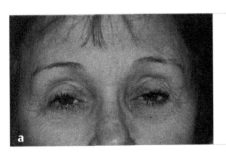
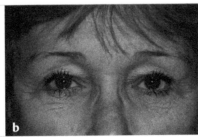

Fig. 19.6 (a, b) Pre- and postoperative results in a patient with bilateral blepharoptosis and prominent superior sulcus. Note the improvement of both the superior sulcus contour and the blepharoptosis.

References

[1] Lucarelli MJ, Lemke BN. Small incision external levator repair: technique and early results. Am J Ophthalmol. 1999; 127(6):637–644

[2] Lucarelli MJ, Cook BE Jr, Lemke BN. Small-incision external levator repair. In: Brazzo BG, ed. Complications in Ophthalmic Plastic Surgery. New York, NY: Springer; 2003:103–112

[3] Baroody M, Holds JB, Sakamoto DK, Vick VL, Hartstein ME. Small incision transcutaneous levator aponeurotic repair for blepharoptosis. Ann Plast Surg. 2004; 52(6):558–561

[4] Frueh BR, Musch DC, McDonald HM. Efficacy and efficiency of a small-incision, minimal dissection procedure versus a traditional approach for correcting aponeurotic ptosis. Ophthalmology. 2004; 111(12):2158–2163

[5] Bernardini FP, de Conciliis C, Devoto MH. Mini-invasive ptosis surgery. Orbit. 2006; 25(2):111–115

[6] McDonald H. Minimally invasive levator advancement: a practical approach to eyelid ptosis repair. Semin Plast Surg. 2007; 21(1):41–46

[7] Lucarelli MJ. Small incision external levator repair. In: Harstein M, Holds J, Massry G, eds. Pearls and Pitfalls in Cosmetic Oculoplastic Surgery. New York, NY: Springer; 2008:494–496

20 Müller's Muscle–Conjunctival Resection

Allen M. Putterman

Abstract

The Müller's muscle–conjunctival resection (MMCR) ptosis procedure is recommended for patients with blepharoptosis whose upper eyelids elevate to a normal level when 10% phenylephrine drops are applied to the upper ocular fornix. Candidates usually have minimal congenital ptosis and varying degrees of aponeurotic ptosis. The advantage over the Fasanella–Servat and external levator advancement procedures is that MMCR preserves the tarsus and produces predictable results with excellent upper eyelid contour.

Keywords: Müller's muscle–conjunctival resection, ptosis, ptosis surgery

20.1 Introduction

Early in my career, Dr. Martin Urist and I developed a procedure to treat thyroid upper eyelid retraction. It consisted of dissecting conjunctiva from the Müller's muscle and then doing a graded severing of Müller's muscle from superior tarsal border with dissection of Müller's muscle from its loose attachments to the levator aponeurosis.

Shortly after this procedure was developed, I decided to prove that the Fasanella procedure corrected blepharoptosis by its resection of Müller's muscle rather than resection of levator as Fasanella thought. I approached this with the same technique I used for thyroid lid retraction and found that the Müller's muscle resection corrected upper eyelid ptosis. As the dissection of conjunctiva from Müller's muscle was difficult for many residents and some ophthalmologists to do, Urist and I simplified the procedure to the Müller's muscle–conjunctival resection (MMCR).[1,2] It is an ideal procedure for patients that have aponeurotic ptosis, defined by decreased palpebral fissure, decreased palpebral fissure on downgaze, decreased margin reflex distance 1 (MRD1), increased margin crease and fold distances, and levator excursion > 10 mm with a positive phenylephrine test.

20.2 Special Preoperative Considerations

Eyelid measurements guide surgical management. The two key indicators in deciding on whether to perform MMCR are the MRD1 and response to phenylephrine testing.

20.2.1 Margin Reflex Distance 1

Before performing the phenylephrine test, it is important to assess the upper eyelid levels with the MRD1 measurement (▸ Fig. 20.1).[3] The surgeon holds a muscle light at eye level and shines it onto the patient's eyes. The distance from the corneal light reflex to the central upper lid margin is the MRD1, measured in positive millimeters. If the eyelid is below the middle of the pupil, the surgeon elevates the lid until the light reflex is first seen; the estimated number of millimeters the lid is lifted is the MRD1, in negative millimeters. The difference in the MRD1, on the normal side compared with the ptotic side, indicates the degree of ptosis. The normal MRD1 is approximately 4.5 mm; this number is used as a reference in bilateral cases. The MRD1 measurement has the advantage of measuring the ptosis and not the palpebral fissure width. This is preferred because there is a Müller's muscle in the lower lid that can also respond to the phenylephrine. Measuring the palpebral fissure width would lead to erroneous interpretation of the upper lid level after phenylephrine instillation.

20.2.2 Phenylephrine Test[4]

To avoid precipitating any side effects, such as myocardial infarction, hypertension, and acute glaucoma, it is important to make sure that the patient does not have a cardiac problem or shallow anterior chamber before instilling phenylephrine drops. The patient's head is tilted backward, the upper eyelid is lifted, and the patient is instructed to gaze downward. Several drops of 10% phenylephrine are dropped between the upper eyelid and the globe. During drop installation, the canaliculi are compressed with the examiner's finger for 10 seconds to minimize the excretion of phenylephrine into the nasal cavity and the potential side effect of systemic absorption. This is repeated immediately two more times. One minute later, two additional drops are applied. Two to four minutes after instillation of the phenylephrine, the MRD1 is measured (▸ Fig. 20.2).

20.2.3 Determining the Amount of Müller's Muscle–Conjunctival Resection

The amount of the MMCR is guided by the response to the phenylephrine test. If the upper eyelid elevates to a normal level or to the level of the opposite side, and if only a unilateral procedure is to be performed, I will do an 8.5-mm resection. If the phenylephrine test leads to the lid being above or below the desired level, then I will vary the resection from 6 mm to 10 mm or even to 10 mm with 1- to 2-mm resection of superior tarsus.[5] In general, experience with the MMCR procedure will lead to the surgeon getting a feel for the amount of resection.

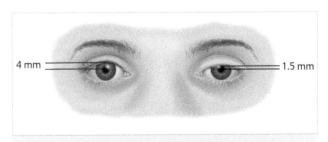

Fig. 20.1 Measurement of the margin reflex distance 1 (MRD1) is performed with a light shining straight ahead and the contralateral eyelid lifted. It is the distance between the light reflex and eyelid margin.

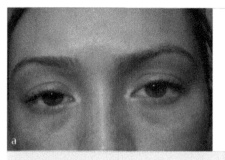 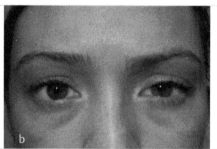 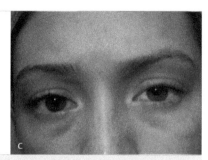

Fig. 20.2 **(a)** A patient with right upper eyelid ptosis. **(b)** After phenylephrine on the right side, the right upper eyelid lifts and the contralateral eyelid falls. **(c)** Eyelid height after installation of phenylephrine in the left eye is equal.

20.3 Risks

- Overcorrection.
- Undercorrection.
- Corneal abrasion.
- Bleeding.
- Conjunctival scarring and eye discomfort.

20.4 Benefits

- Predictable and reproducible eyelid lift.
- Easily done in an outpatient or office-based surgery setting.

20.5 Informed Consent

- Include risks and benefits.

20.6 Contraindications

- Cicatrizing conjunctival disease, i.e., mucous membrane pemphigoid.
- Severe dry eye with exposure keratopathy.
- Myopathic or neurogenic ptosis with poor response to phenylephrine.
- Prior glaucoma surgery in patients with large avascular superior conjunctival blebs.

20.7 Instrumentation

- Castroviejo needle driver.
- Forceps.
- Desmarres retractor.
- #15 blade.
- Caliper.
- Putterman ptosis clamp.
- Hemostat.
- Sutures:
  - 4–0 silk G-3, double-armed.
  - 5–0 plain catgut, S-14 needle, double-armed.
  - 6–0 silk suture, S-14 needle, double-armed.

20.8 Preoperative Checklist

- Informed consent.

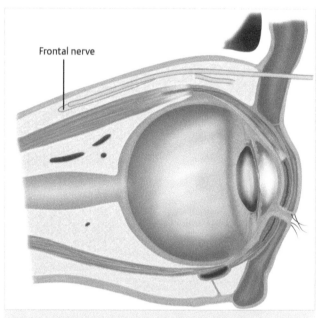

Frontal nerve

Fig. 20.3 Frontal nerve block injection given for patient comfort during local or monitored anesthesia.

- Instrumentation on hand.
- Preoperative clinical photographs to verify the site of surgery.
- Preoperative and postphenylephrine measurements and photographs.

20.9 Operative Technique

The procedure can be performed under local, monitored, or general anesthesia in an office-based procedure room, ambulatory operating room, or hospital-based setting.

- Local anesthesia injection:
  - A frontal nerve block is used with local anesthesia to avoid swelling of the upper eyelid by local infiltration, which would make the operation more difficult and inexact. A 23-gauge retrobulbar-type needle is inserted into the superior orbit, entering just under the middle of the superior orbital rim (▶ Fig. 20.3).
    - The needle should hug the roof of the orbit during insertion and is advanced until a depth of 4 cm is reached.
    - Approximately 1.5 mL of 2% lidocaine with epinephrine is injected.

○ Another 0.25 mL is injected subcutaneously over the center upper eyelid, just above the eyelid margin (▶ Fig. 20.4).
- A 4–0 black silk traction suture is inserted through skin, orbicularis muscle, and superficial tarsus 2 mm above the eyelashes at the center of the upper eyelid (▶ Fig. 20.5).
- A large- to medium-sized Desmarres retractor everts the upper eyelid and exposes the palpebral conjunctiva from the superior tarsal border to the superior fornix. In an awake patient, topical tetracaine drops are applied over the upper palpebral conjunctiva.
- A caliper set at the desired amount of MMCR, with one arm at the superior tarsal border, facilitates insertion of a 6–0 black silk suture through the conjunctiva above the superior tarsal border (▶ Fig. 20.6). One passage centrally and two others, approximately 7 mm nasal and temporal to the center, mark the site.

○ I usually place the suture 8.25 mm above the superior tarsal border, but it may be placed 6 to 10 mm above it if the response of the upper eyelid level to the phenylephrine test is slightly more or less than desired, respectively.
- A toothed forceps grasps conjunctiva and Müller's muscle between the superior tarsal border and marking suture and separates Müller's muscle from its loose attachment to the levator aponeurosis (▶ Fig. 20.7).

○ This maneuver is possible because Müller's muscle is firmly attached to conjunctiva but only loosely attached to the levator aponeurosis.
- One blade of a specially designed clamp (Putterman MMCR clamp, Storz Company, Manchester, MO) is placed at the level of the marking suture. Each tooth of this blade engages each

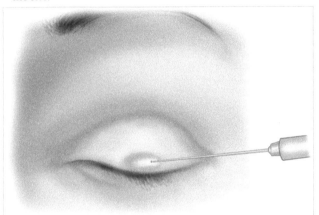
Fig. 20.4 Local anesthesia into the central upper eyelid.

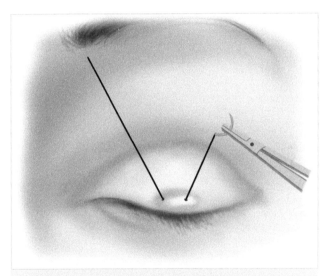
Fig. 20.5 Placement of a 4–0 silk traction suture through skin, orbicularis, and partial-thickness tarsus, 2 mm above the eyelid margin.

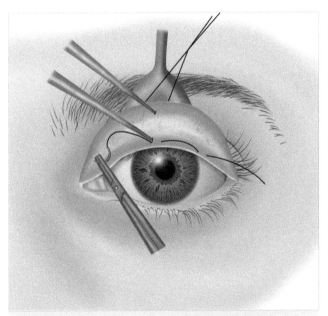
Fig. 20.6 Placement of a 6–0 silk marking suture at the location of the resection, measured in millimeters with a Castroviejo caliper. The amount of the resection is planned in preoperative patient evaluation.

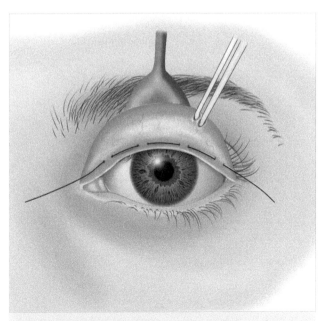
Fig. 20.7 Conjunctiva and Müller's muscle are pulled away from the underlying levator aponeurosis with a toothed forceps.

suture bite that passes through the palpebral conjunctiva (► Fig. 20.8a, b). The Desmarres retractor is then slowly released as the outer blade of the clamp engages conjunctiva and Müller's muscle adjacent to the superior tarsal border (► Fig. 20.8a, b). Any entrapped tarsus is pulled out of the clamp with the surgeon's finger (► Fig. 20.9). The clamp is compressed, and the handle is locked, incorporating conjunctiva and Müller's muscle between the superior tarsal border and the marking suture.

- The upper eyelid skin is then pulled in one direction while the clamp is pulled simultaneously in the opposite direction (► Fig. 20.10).
  - If the surgeon feels a sense of attachment between the skin and clamp during this maneuver, the levator aponeurosis has been inadvertently trapped in the clamp. If this occurs, the clamp should be released and reapplied in its proper position.

  - This maneuver is possible because the levator aponeurosis sends extensions to orbicularis muscle and skin to form the lid crease.
- With the clamp held straight up, a 5–0 double-armed plain catgut mattress suture is run 1.5 mm below the clamp along its entire width in a temporal to nasal direction in a horizontal mattress fashion, through the upper margin of the tarsus, and through Müller's muscle and conjunctiva on the other side and vice versa (► Fig. 20.11a, b).
  - The sutures are placed approximately 2 to 3 mm apart.
- A #15 surgical blade is used to excise the tissues held in the clamp by cutting between the sutures and the clamp (► Fig. 20.12).
  - The knife blade is rotated slightly, with its sharp edge hugging the clamp. As the tissues are excised from the clamp, the surgeon and assistant watch to ensure that the suture on each side is not cut.

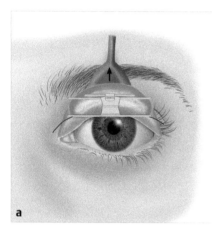
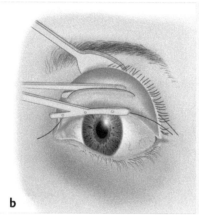

a   **b**

Fig. 20.8 The Desmarres retractor is removed as the clamp is applied to the tissue **(a)** by everting the retractor **(b)**. The superior conjunctiva is engaged prior to Desmarres retractor eversion.

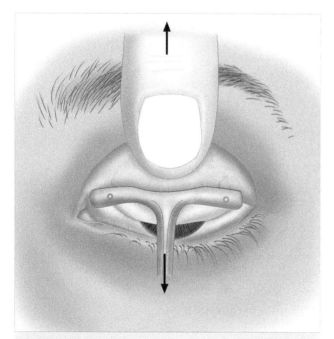

Fig. 20.9 If tarsus is entrapped in the clamped material, the clamp is gently released and a finger is used to remove the clamped tarsus before reapplying the clamp.

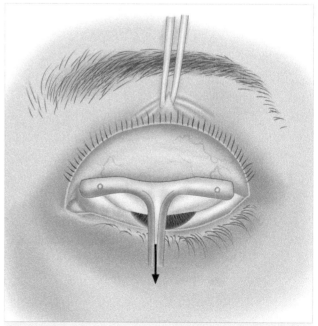

Fig. 20.10 The upper eyelid skin and orbicularis are pulled away from the underlying clamped material to ensure the levator aponeurosis is not inadvertently ensnared in the clamped material.

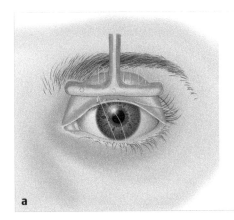
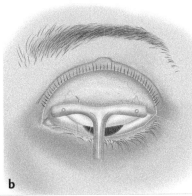

Fig. 20.11 A 5–0 double-armed plain catgut suture is run from the temporal aspect of the wound to the nasal aspect in a horizontal mattress fashion as seen on the conjunctival side (a) and tarsal conjunctival side (b).

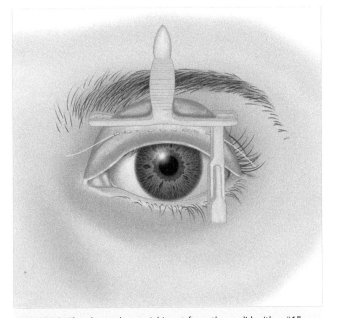

Fig. 20.12 The clamped material is cut from the eyelid with a #15 blade after suture placement.

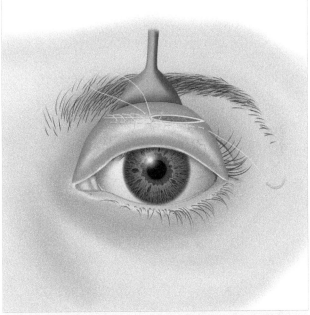

Fig. 20.13 The Desmarres is reapplied and the 5–0 plain suture is run from the nasal aspect temporally, reattaching conjunctiva–Müller's muscle to the superior tarsal border. This internally advances the levator aponeurosis.

- The Desmarres retractor again everts the eyelid while gentle traction is applied to the 4–0 black silk centering suture. The nasal end of the suture is then run continuously in a temporal direction; the stitches should be approximately 2 mm apart as they pass through the edges of superior tarsal border, Müller's muscle, and conjunctiva (▶ Fig. 20.13).
  - The surgeon must be careful to avoid cutting the original mattress suture during this continuous closure. Towards this end, the surgeon uses a small suture needle (S-14 spatula), observing the mattress suture position during each bite, and the assistant applies continuous suction along the incision edges.
- Once each arm of the suture reaches the temporal end of the eyelid, it is passed through each side of the conjunctiva and Müller's muscle before it exits through the temporal end of the incision (▶ Fig. 20.14). The suture arms are then tied with approximately four to five knots, and the ends are cut close to

the knot, thus burying the knot subconjunctivally upon eyelid re-eversion to lessen the risk of postoperative keratopathy from suture/cornea rub.

20.10 Expert Tips/Pearls/Suggestions[6]

- Most of my cases involve patients with bilateral upper eyelid ptosis. Many of these patients think they only have unilateral ptosis but when their most ptotic lid is elevated with my finger or with the phenylephrine test, the contralateral lid drops, according to Hering's law of equal innervation (▶ Fig. 20.2). Therefore, in these cases, I recommend bilateral MMCR.
- To determine how much Müller's muscle/conjunctiva to resect in bilateral cases, the MRD1 and phenylephrine test

measurements are important. It is critical to measure the MRD1 on each side while elevating the contralateral lid with the examiner's finger to eliminate the effect of Hering's law of equal innervation.

- In general, I will do a 2-mm difference of resection for each 1-mm difference in MRD1. For example, if there is a 0.5-mm difference in the MRD1 between the two eyelids, I will do a 1-mm difference in resection. A 1-mm difference leads to a 2-mm difference in resection; a 1.5-mm difference, a 3-mm difference in resection; and a 2-mm difference, a 4-mm difference in resection.

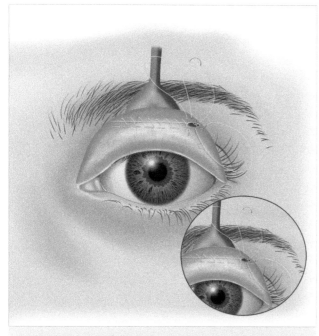

Fig. 20.14 Each arm of the 5–0 gut suture is passed through conjunctiva and into the wound. Once tied and the eyelid re-everted, the knot is buried on the inside of the upper eyelid.

- With small amounts of resection, 6.25 to 7.25 mm, it is sometimes challenging to apply the clamp without incorporating superior tarsus. In these cases, after placement of the marking suture, two 6–0 double-armed sutures are placed through conjunctiva and the Müller's muscle between the superior tarsal border and the marking suture nasal centrally and temporal centrally (▶ Fig. 20.15**a**). These sutures are left long, and each arm of the double-armed suture is tied to the other arm. After engaging the three teeth of the blade of the clamp into the marking suture bites on the conjunctiva, the two double-armed sutures are pulled together by the assistant, as the surgeon releases the Desmarres retractor (▶ Fig. 20.15**b**), and the clamp blades are closed and secured (▶ Fig. 20.15**c**). The two double-armed sutures are removed or are cut short, and the suturing and resection are performed as usual.
- Elevating the ptotic eyelid with the MMCR procedure commonly leads to an increase in the upper eyelid skin and a decrease in the distance from the eyelid margin to the upper lid fold in primary position of gaze (▶ Fig. 20.16). This upper eyelid skin crowding develops because the patient ceases to raise the brow up to see, the upper eyelid is in an elevated position, and the eyelid crease is lowered due to the internal advancement of the levator aponeurosis. This makes one aspect of the patient look better (the elevated lid) and another aspect look worse (the increase in the upper eyelid excess skin). In these cases, excision of upper eyelid skin, with or without orbicularis and fat, and reconstruction of the upper lid crease are commonly done in addition to the MMCR ptosis procedure (▶ Fig. 20.17, ▶ Fig. 20.18).[7]

20.11 Postoperative Management

- A topical antibiotic such as erythromycin is placed on the eye.
- Cold compresses are applied to the eyelid for 24 hours.
- Topical antibiotic ointment is applied to the eyes twice a day for 1 week and once a day for a second week.

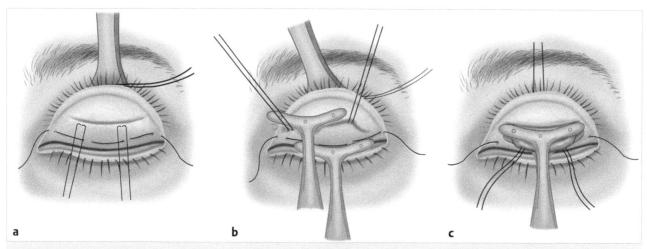

Fig. 20.15 With small eyelid resections, which are technically more challenging, an alternative way to apply the clamp can be performed. Two sutures are placed midway between the marking suture and superior tarsal border (**a**). The clamp is applied while the assistant pulls on the midway sutures (**b**). The clamp blades are closed (**c**). This technique is discussed in further detail in Chapter 21.

20.12 Complications and Their Management[8]

- Postoperative corneal abrasion caused by the catgut mattress suture: Placing the suture bites closer together on the tarsal surface and further apart on the conjunctival surface decreases the incidence of this complication. Should it occur, a soft contact lens can be worn for 2 to 7 days postoperatively until the suture dissolves.
- Eyelid malposition: There is an approximately 3 to 5% chance of an over- or undercorrection with this procedure.
  - If an overcorrection occurs, downward massage of the eyelid can be used during the immediate postoperative period. The eyebrow is held upward while the upper lid is pushed in and downward several times each day. The eyelid usually attains its final level 3 to 6 weeks postoperatively. Should the overcorrection persist, it can be treated with a levator recession procedure.[9]
  - If an undercorrection occurs, the next line of treatment would be a levator aponeurosis advancement, tuck, and resection ptosis procedure. However, I have performed a secondary MMCR in many patients who respond to the phenylephrine test.
- Exposure keratopathy: This can be treated with artificial tears and/or topical ointments.

20.13 Acknowledgment

▶ Fig. 20.1, ▶ Fig. 20.3, ▶ Fig. 20.4, ▶ Fig. 20.5, ▶ Fig. 20.6, ▶ Fig. 20.7, ▶ Fig. 20.13, ▶ Fig. 20.8, ▶ Fig. 20.9, ▶ Fig. 20.10, ▶ Fig. 20.11, ▶ Fig. 20.12, ▶ Fig. 20.14, ▶ Fig. 20.14, ▶ Fig. 20.15 are being published with permission from my chapter in Levine's fourth edition of Manual of Oculoplastic Surgery that was published by Slack Incorporated.

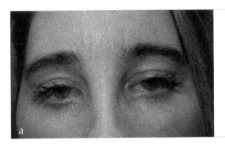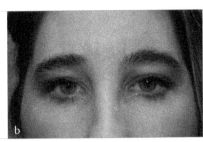

Fig. 20.16 A typical patient before (a) and after (b) MMCR. Note the improved MRD1 and increased bilateral upper eyelid excess skin, correlating with a decrease in the margin fold distance.

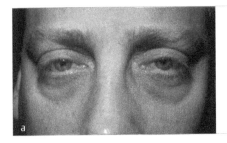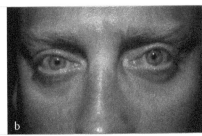

Fig. 20.17 A typical male patient pre- (a) and post- (b) MMCR with four eyelid blepharoplasty performed for aesthetic enhancement.

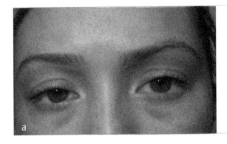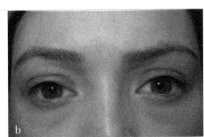

Fig. 20.18 The patient in ▶ Fig. 20.2 before (a) and after (b) right > left MMCR and bilateral upper eyelid blepharoplasty.

References

[1] Putterman AM. How the Müller's muscle-conjunctival resection ptosis procedure was developed. Ophthal Plast Reconstr Surg. 2016; 32(2):156–157

[2] Putterman AM, Urist MJ. Müller muscle-conjunctiva resection. Technique for treatment of blepharoptosis. Arch Ophthalmol. 1975; 93(8):619–623

[3] Putterman AM. Margin reflex distance (MRD) 1, 2, and 3. Ophthal Plast Reconstr Surg. 2012; 28(4):308–311

[4] Glatt HJ, Fett DR, Putterman AM. Comparison of 2.5% and 10% phenylephrine in the elevation of upper eyelids with ptosis. Ophthalmic Surg. 1990; 21(3):173–176

[5] Patel RM, Aakalu VK, Setabutr P, Putterman AM. Efficacy of Müller's muscle and conjunctiva resection with or without tarsectomy for the treatment of severe involutional blepharoptosis. Ophthal Plast Reconstr Surg. 2017; 33(4):273–278

[6] Putterman AM. Pearls for Müller's muscle-conjunctival resection ptosis procedure combined with upper blepharoplasty. In: Hartstein ME, Massry GG, Holds JB, eds. Pearls and Pitfalls in Cosmetic Oculoplastic Surgery, 2nd ed. New York: Springer; 2015:655–657

[7] Putterman AM. Müller's muscle-conjunctival resection-ptosis procedure combined with upper blepharoplasty. In: Putterman AM, ed. Chapter in Cosmetic Oculoplastic Surgery, 2nd ed. Philadelphia, PA: W.B. Saunders; 1993:168–186

[8] Putterman AM, Fett DR. Müller's muscle in the treatment of upper eyelid ptosis: a ten-year study. Ophthalmic Surg. 1986; 17(6):354–360

[9] Putterman AM. Eyelid finger manipulation in the treatment of overcorrected blepharoptosis and postblepharoplasty ectropion-retraction. Plast Reconstr Surg. 2015; 135(6):1073e–1074e

21 Dresner's Modification of Müller's Muscle–Conjunctival Resection

Steven C. Dresner, Margaret L. Pfeiffer

Abstract

Müller's muscle–conjunctival resection is a surgical procedure to correct 1 to 3 mm of ptosis from a posterior approach. This procedure was originally described by Putterman and Urist to correct minimal to moderate ptosis in patients with good levator excursion. Since then, there have been several nomograms developed by other surgeons. Here, we discuss Dresner's modifications to the procedure and nomogram.

Keywords: Müller's muscle–conjunctival resection, ptosis, ptosis surgery

21.1 Introduction

Müller's muscle–conjunctival resection (MMCR) is a surgical procedure for correction of 1 to 3 mm of ptosis from a posterior approach. This procedure was originally described by Putterman and Urist to correct minimal to moderate ptosis in patients with good levator excursion.[1,2] Modified techniques have been described by Weinstein and Buerger, Guyuron and Davies, and Dresner.[3-5]

21.2 Indications

Candidates for this procedure have minimal to moderate ptosis, ranging from 1 to 3 mm of ptosis, good levator excursion (> 10 mm), normal contour, and a positive phenylephrine test (▶ Fig. 21.1). Preoperatively, the margin reflex distance 1 (MRD1) is measured in both upper eyelids. Phenylephrine (2.5%) is applied to the ptotic eye or eyes. The MRD1 is then rechecked in both eyes in 3 to 5 minutes. A response of 2 mm or more upper eyelid elevation is a positive result, and one can proceed with surgical planning.

A nomogram has been developed that gives accurate guidelines for how much Müller's muscle and conjunctiva to resect for the measured amount of ptosis (▶ Fig. 21.2). For 1 mm of ptosis, a 4-mm resection of Müller's muscle is planned. For 1.5 mm of ptosis, a 6-mm resection is planned. For 2 mm of ptosis, an 8-mm resection is planned. If 3 mm of ptosis is present, a 10-mm resection can be performed; however, the nomogram is less predictable in larger amounts of ptosis.

21.3 Risks

- Overcorrection.
- Undercorrection.
- Corneal abrasion.
- Bleeding.

21.4 Benefits

- Predictable amount of eyelid lift.
- Easily performed in office setting with minimal patient discomfort.

21.5 Informed Consent

- Include risks and benefits.

21.6 Contraindications

- Cicatrizing conjunctival disease like mucous membrane pemphigoid.
- Severe dry eye and exposure keratopathy may lead the surgeon to do a smaller eyelid elevation.
- Prior glaucoma surgery in the superior conjunctiva and, in particular, large trabeculectomy blebs are a relative contraindication.

21.7 Instrumentation

- Castroviejo needle driver.
- Forceps.
- Desmarres retractor.
- A #15 blade.
- Caliper.
- Sterile marking pen.
- Ptosis clamp (Putterman clamp or a modified MMCR clamp).
- Hemostat.
- Sutures:
  - Two 4–0 silk G-3 double-armed per side.
  - 6–0 Prolene P-3.

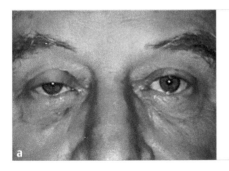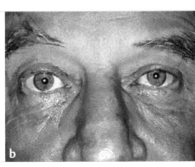

Fig. 21.1 Photographs of a patient upon presentation (a) and 5 minutes after phenylephrine instilled into the right eye (b).

21.8 Preoperative Checklist

- Informed consent.
- Instrumentation on hand.
- Preoperative clinical photographs to verify the site of surgery and measurements pre- and postphenylephrine.

21.9 Operative Technique

The procedure can be performed under local, monitored, or general anesthesia in an office-based procedure room, ambulatory operating room, or hospital-based setting.

- The pupillary axis is marked with the patient in the upright position.

- With the patient in the supine position, the upper lid is infiltrated subcutaneously with 1% lidocaine with epinephrine with hyaluronidase in the preseptal area.
- Topical tetracaine is applied to the conjunctival surface.
- After prepping and draping, a 4–0 silk suture is placed through the lid margin in the previously marked pupillary axis.
- The eyelid is everted over a Desmarres retractor. Marks are made medially, centrally, and laterally on the palpebral conjunctiva at the halfway point of the total resection amount.
- Another mark is made at the location for the total resection amount centrally (▶ Fig. 21.3).
- Three 4–0 silk sutures are placed through the conjunctiva and Müller's muscle at the marked halfway points (▶ Fig. 21.4).

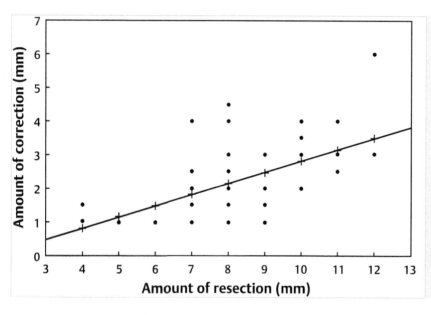

Fig. 21.2 Nomogram developed by Dresner that gives accurate guidelines for how much Müller's muscle–conjunctiva to resect for the measured amount of ptosis.

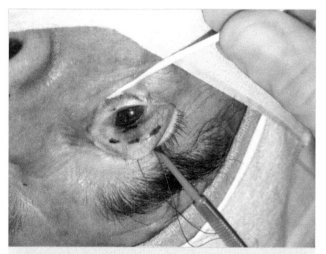

Fig. 21.3 With the eyelid everted over a Desmarres retractor, marks are made medially, centrally, and laterally on the palpebral conjunctiva at the halfway point of the total resection amount. Another mark is made at the location for the total resection amount centrally.

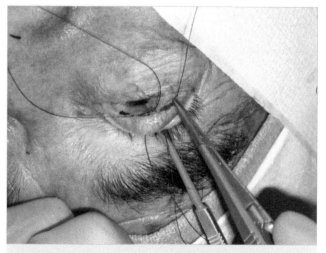

Fig. 21.4 Three 4–0 silk sutures are placed through the conjunctiva and Müller's muscle at the marked halfway points. The sutures are tied into two bundles.

- The Desmarres retractor is removed and the lid margin suture is clamped superiorly on the drape with a hemostat.
- The sutures are gathered in two bundles and elevated by the surgeon and assistant (▶ Fig. 21.5).
- The clamp is placed over the tissues (▶ Fig. 21.6).
- A 6–0 Prolene suture is placed under the clamp, beginning exteriorly through the pretarsal eyelid.
- The suture is passed multiple times approximately 1 mm below the clamp, ending exteriorly through the pretarsal eyelid (▶ Fig. 21.7).
- A #15 blade is used to cut between the clamp and the sutures (▶ Fig. 21.8). No cautery is necessary.
- The Prolene suture is tied on itself in the pretarsal area (▶ Fig. 21.9).
- The traction suture in the lid margin is removed. No patch is required.

21.10 Expert Tips/Pearls/Suggestions

- Always check in the wound for remnant silk suture, which can be inadvertently cut with the #15 blade.
- The suture does not need to be tightly tied in the pretarsal area. We prefer to tie the suture so that the knot is resting on the pretarsal skin without too much tension. This allows for eyelid swelling.
- Counsel patients that bloody tears are common after this procedure and will improve with pressure on the closed eyelid and ice.

21.11 Results

Accurate results can be achieved for 1, 1.5, and 2 mm of ptosis (▶ Fig. 21.10). MMCR can be combined with upper lid blepharoplasty.[6]

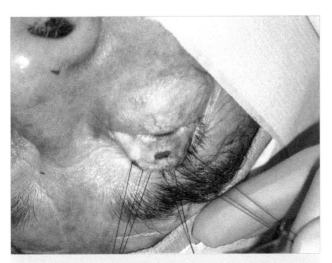

Fig. 21.5 After removing the Desmarres retractor and clamping the lid margin suture on the drape, the sutures are gathered in two bundles and elevated by the surgeon and assistant.

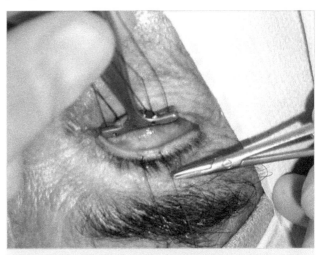

Fig. 21.6 The ptosis clamp is placed over the tissues in line with the central marking.

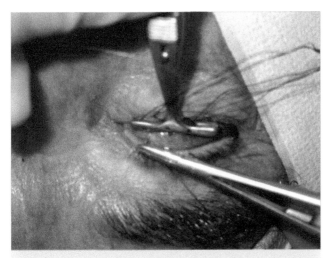

Fig. 21.7 A 6–0 Prolene suture is passed multiple times approximately 1 mm below the clamp beginning and ending exteriorly through the pretarsal eyelid.

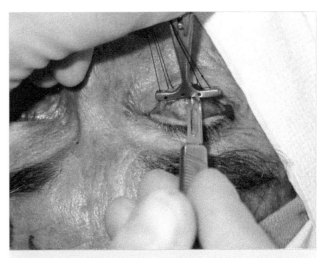

Fig. 21.8 A #15 blade is used to cut between the clamp and the sutures.

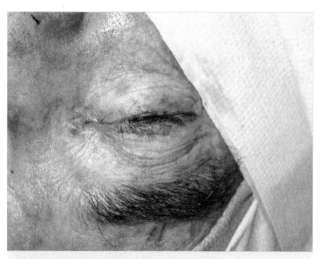

Fig. 21.9 The Prolene suture is tied on itself in the pretarsal area.

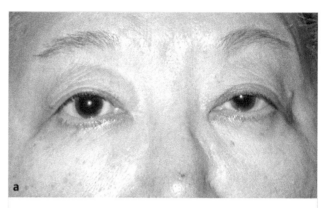

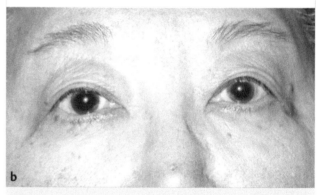

Fig. 21.10 Typical preoperative (a) and postoperative (b) results after left upper eyelid Müller's muscle–conjunctival resection (MMCR).

21.12 Complications and Their Management

Complications include undercorrection, overcorrection, and rarely a corneal abrasion. Overcorrection can be managed by removing the suture, followed by digital massage. Rarely, Müller's muscle can be recessed with a cotton swab if necessary. Undercorrections should be observed until all edema has resolved. Reoperation usually will require a Fasanella–Servat procedure or levator repair. Corneal abrasions can be managed with a bandage contact lens.

21.13 Conclusion

The MMCR is an excellent procedure with predictable results and minimal recovery in patients with ptosis and a positive phenylephrine test. It can be easily combined with upper blepharoplasty and performed in an office setting.

References

[1] Putterman AM, Urist MJ. Müller's muscle-conjunctival resection ptosis procedure. Ophthalmic Surg. 1978; 9(3):27–32

[2] Putterman AM, Urist MJ. Müller muscle-conjunctiva resection. Technique for treatment of blepharoptosis. Arch Ophthalmol. 1975; 93(8):619–623

[3] Weinstein GS, Buerger GF, Jr. Modification of the Müller's muscle-conjunctival resection operation for blepharoptosis. Am J Ophthalmol. 1982; 93(5):647–651

[4] Guyuron B, Davies B. Experience with the modified Putterman procedure. Plast Reconstr Surg. 1988; 82(5):775–780

[5] Dresner SC. Further modifications of the Müller's muscle-conjunctival resection procedure for blepharoptosis. Ophthal Plast Reconstr Surg. 1991; 7(2):114–122

[6] Brown MS, Putterman AM. The effect of upper blepharoplasty on eyelid position when performed concomitantly with Müller muscle-conjunctival resection. Ophthal Plast Reconstr Surg. 2000; 16(2):94–100

22 Posterior White Line Advancement

Katja Ullrich, Raman Malhotra

Abstract

The posterior white line advancement technique and the levator-pexy for congenital ptosis derived from it are two approaches of posterior ptosis repair. They are useful for mild to severe involutional ptosis and for congenital ptosis, respectively. The white line advancement can be performed on thinned tarsus and has consistently predictable results when modifying the technique according to preoperative measurements.

Keywords: ptosis, surgical technique, posterior approach ptosis correction, levatorpexy, white line advancement

22.1 Introduction

The Müller's muscle–conjunctival resection (MMCR) procedure is considered an evolution to the Fasanella–Servat procedure and has traditionally been used for patients with a positive phenylephrine test and mild to moderate ptosis as well as good levator function (LF). It does not involve a tarsectomy. It was described by Putterman and Urist in 1975.[1]

The mechanism of posterior Müller's muscle resection appears to work by the aponeurosis being splinted forward. This observation helps explain the concept of isolated posterior approach levator advancement developed by Collin,[2] and later modified as the white line advancement by Malhotra.[3] The difference between Collin's levator advancement and Malhotra's white line advancement is that the white line advancement technique advances the exposed posterior surface of the aponeurosis and does not breach the orbital septum or include a tarsectomy.

We prefer the posterior approach for severe involutional ptosis because the attenuated and retracted levator aponeurosis in the deeper orbit can be more difficult to find when approached anteriorly, and it requires more dissection, which can result in more trauma compared to the posterior approach. The thinned tarsus in severe involutional ptosis may be difficult to suture and the risk of full-thickness needle pass exists. In avoiding full-thickness needle passes, partial-thickness bites in thinned tarsus may be more vulnerable to early dehiscence.

The white line advancement technique for aponeurotic ptosis was subsequently modified into the *levatorpexy* procedure for congenital ptosis. The levatorpexy procedure plicates levator palpebrae superioris (LPS) to mimic levator resection, contributing to improved margin reflex distance 1 and decreased margin fold distance. This fold creates volume and contributes to improved cosmesis by adding fullness to the preseptal eyelid. Depending upon the LF, the position of suture placement varies, allowing the surgeon to make precise modifications in the surgical approach based on the individual patient needs.[4]

22.2 Relevant Anatomy

Müller's muscle is a smooth muscle that together with the LPS forms the upper lid retractors. Müller's origin is situated on the underside of the levator aponeurosis and is sympathetically innervated.

Anatomically, Müller's muscle inserts into the superior border of the tarsal plate.[5] It extends medially and laterally, as far as the medial rectus and lateral rectus pulleys, respectively. Along its lateral course, the extension of Müller's muscle passes through the lacrimal gland fascia and can appear more attenuated. Müller's muscle has, therefore, been described as a component of the peribulbar smooth muscle network rather than an isolated anatomical structure.[6]

The LPS originates from the lesser wing of the sphenoid and transitions into its aponeurosis after approximately 36 mm.[7] At the musculotendinous transition, Whitnall's ligament suspends the LPS and acts as its pulley.[8] Whitnall's ligament extends from the lateral aspect of the trochlea and Whitnall's tubercle (on the lateral orbital wall), passing between the orbital and the palpebral part of the lacrimal gland laterally.

The levator aponeurosis originates from the LPS and anatomically consists of two layers. Both of those layers—anterior and posterior—contain smooth muscle.[9] The anterior layer contains thick fibrous tissue, whereas the posterior layer consists of thin fibrous tissue and a much larger proportion of smooth muscle.[9]

The postlevator aponeurosis fat pad has been known about for some time, initially reported in the late 1980s.[10] However, only a recent study confirmed these findings and conducted a detailed macroscopic and microscopic histological assessment.[11] This fat pad is a distinct entity in the postaponeurotic space, located between Müller's muscle and the posterior layer of the levator aponeurosis with its associated smooth muscle. Macroscopically, the fat is located between the two layers of smooth muscle situated posterior to the aponeurosis, which has previously been described by Kakizaki and colleagues.[9] The postlevator aponeurosis fat tends to be central and medially located, where it overlies Müller's muscle and commonly continues posterior to the aponeurosis up to the levator muscle. The fat pad tends to be diffuse with some more discreet, multi-lobulated areas[11] and it has been described in both adults and children.[4,11]

The postaponeurotic fat pad is a significant landmark for ptosis surgery and will inform the oculoplastic surgeon to guide dissection of Müller's muscle and the LPS aponeurosis. One has to avoid mistaking it for the preaponeurotic fat pad anterior to it.

22.3 Indications

- All types of involutional ptosis, mild to severe.
- Congenital ptosis, especially when a posterior approach with absence of a skin incision and creation of a skin crease is desired.

22.4 Risks

- Corneal abrasion.
- Undercorrection.
- Overcorrection.
- Eyelid contour abnormalities.

22.5 Benefits

- Absence of skin incision, no external scar.
- Predictable results and eyelid contour outcomes.[3,12-15]
- Suture placement is independent of pupil position in primary gaze and is guided by the superior tarsal contour.
- Avoids violation of the septum, particularly medially, avoiding disruption of the medial fibers of the medial horn of the LPS that continue anteriorly as the septum.[16,17]
- May be combined with skin-only or skin–muscle flap blepharoplasty.
- May be performed under local, monitored, or general anesthesia in adults and children.[14,15,18]

22.6 Informed Consent

- Discussion of the aim of the procedure.
- Benefits of the procedure, as above.
- Risks of the procedure, as above.
- Alternatives to white line advancement like MMCR or external levator advancement in aponeurotic ptosis.
- Alternatives to levatorpexy like levator resection in congenital ptosis with diminished levator excursion (< 4–10 mm).

22.7 Contraindications

There are a few relative contraindications for the white line advancement technique. These include:

- Individuals with conjunctival scarring disease (pemphigoid, Stevens–Johnson syndrome, and fornix contraction).
- Glaucoma patients either with blebs or those in whom conjunctival scarring is to be avoided (i.e., those being considered for filtration surgery).

22.8 Instrumentation

- Surgical skin marker.
- Local anesthesia:
  ○ Approximately 0.5% bupivacaine with 1:200,000 adrenaline.
  ○ Syringe and needle, prefer 25 to 27 gauge.
- Surgical skin preparation, for example, povidone-iodine.
- Surgical drapes.
- Routine suture tray with curved and straight needle holder, toothed forceps, and scissors.
- Diathermy/cautery.
- A #15 Bard-Parker blade.
- Sutures:
  ○ The 4–0 silk traction sutures.
  ○ Double-armed x 5–0 Vicryl suture (the authors prefer an S-24, 8.0-mm, ¼ circle, spatulated needle).
- Antibiotic ointment.

22.9 Preoperative Checklist

A routine preoperative checklist should be performed including:

- Patient name.
- Patient hospital record number/identifier.
- Patient date of birth.
- Procedure to be performed.
- Left or right eye or bilateral procedure.
- Any patient allergies.
- Any surgical/anesthetic/nursing concerns.
- Patient's signature on the consent form for surgical and anesthetic consents.

22.10 Operative Technique

The authors have developed a transconjunctival levator advancement procedure for involutional ptosis ("white line advancement"), which then developed into a levator tuck procedure or levatorpexy for congenital ptosis, to advance and plicate the levator to the tarsal plate posteriorly.[4] This technique has all the advantages of posterior approach ptosis surgery, including the absence of skin incision and predictable and excellent lid contour, while avoiding tissue resection.

22.10.1 The White Line Advancement for Aponeurotic Ptosis

The white line advancement technique has been described in detail and is summarized below.[3,18,19] The white line advancement technique advances the exposed posterior surface of the aponeurosis to correct ptosis and also helps restore a more defined skin crease in the process.

- Using 0.5% bupivacaine with 1:200,000 adrenaline, infiltrate 1 ml subcutaneously to eyelid skin crease and in the midpupil pretarsal region and 0.5 ml subconjunctivally (▶ Fig. 22.1**a, b**).
- Place a 4–0 silk traction suture in the grey line and evert the eyelid over a Desmarres retractor (▶ Fig. 22.1**c**).
- Apply gentle diathermy over the proposed conjunctival incision site (▶ Fig. 22.1**d**).
- Incise the conjunctiva using a #15 Bard-Parker blade along but above the superior border of tarsus (▶ Fig. 22.1**e**).
- Dissect Müller's muscle and conjunctiva as composite flap to expose the white line, which represents the posterior border of the levator aponeurosis (▶ Fig. 22.1**f**).
- Dissect further between the posterior surface of the levator aponeurosis and the conjunctiva to expose the postaponeurotic fat pad and the posterior surface of the LPS muscle (▶ Fig. 22.1**g**).
- Pass a double-armed 5–0 Vicryl suture (5–0 Ethicon coated Vicryl), polyglactin 910, undyed, S-24, 8.0-mm, ¼ circle, spatulated needle at a point in a vertical line with the central peak of the tarsal plate through the most proximal white line at its junction with the LPS (▶ Fig. 22.1**h**).
- Then pass the suture through the conjunctival surface of the tarsal plate, 1 mm below its superior border, and then through the skin (▶ Fig. 22.1**i, j**).
- Ensure the suture is passed through the skin at the level of the lid crease (▶ Fig. 22.1**k**).
- Take care to pass both double-armed needles through the same exit skin site to facilitate burying of the eventually tied suture knot.
- Assess the lid height and eyelid contour and tie the suture in a bow (▶ Fig. 22.1**l**).

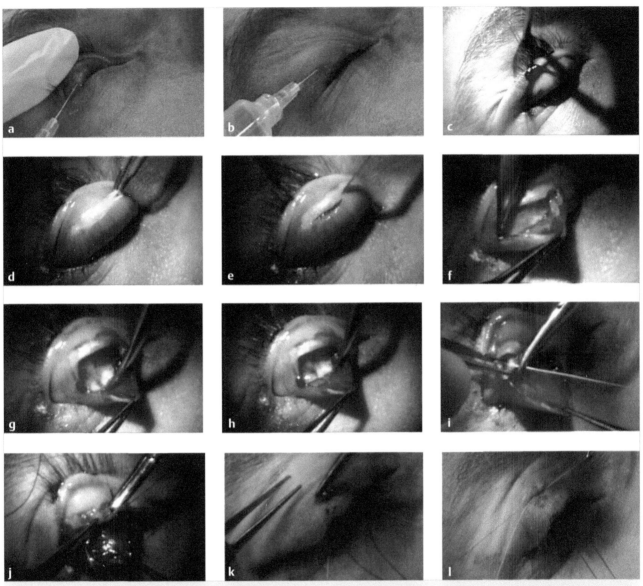

Fig. 22.1 White line advancement technique. **(a, b)** Approximately 1 ml of subcutaneous infiltration in the midpupil pretarsal region upon eversion and skin crease using 0.5% bupivacaine with 1:200,000 adrenaline. **(c)** A 4–0 silk traction suture placed in the grey line of the upper eyelid, everted over a Desmarres retractor. **(d)** Gentle diathermy applied to the conjunctiva immediately above and at the superior tarsal border. **(e)** Conjunctival incision made with a #15 Bard-Parker blade along but above the superior border of the tarsus. **(f, g)** Müller's muscle and conjunctiva dissected off as a composite flap until the white line, representing the posterior border of the levator aponeurosis. **(h–j)** A double-armed 5–0 Vicryl suture was placed centrally through the posterior surface of the white line **(h)**, in a forehand manner and was then passed through the conjunctival surface of the tarsal plate, 1 mm below its superior border **(i)**, and then through to the skin **(j)**. **(k)** The suture was captured through the skin in the region of the skin crease. **(l)** The final lid height and contour at the end of the procedure.

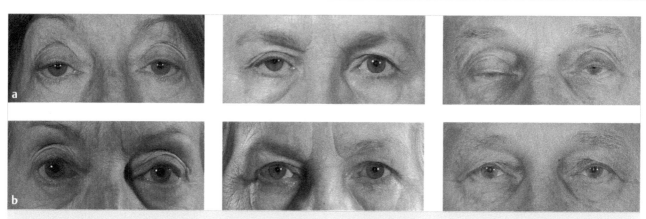

Fig. 22.2 (a) Preoperative and (b) postoperative photographs at 3-month follow-up of three patients who underwent bilateral posterior approach white line advancement for aponeurotic ptosis.

- If the lid height is too low after the first suture, relax it and pass a second suture higher through the white line and again the tarsal plate and the skin.
- If the upper eyelid contour appears peaked after the first suture, then relax it (i.e., tie it loosely only) and place a second suture more centrally to the position of the peak. This way, the position of the second suture can alter and adjust the lid position without having to remove the initial suture.
- In the majority of cases, the use of the second suture avoids the need to remove the initial suture. This can be tied gently as "support" rather than "cardinal suture."
- The sutures can be left to dissolve and the composite flap of Müller's muscle and conjunctiva can be left to heal.
- The above method can be combined with a skin-only or skin–muscle blepharoplasty, avoiding breach of the septum.
- Apply antibiotic ointment and a pressure dressing as needed.
- Excellent symmetric results may be achieved with this surgical technique (▶ Fig. 22.2).

22.10.2 Levatorpexy for Congenital Ptosis

Levatorpexy is a useful option in congenital ptosis with poor to good levator excursion (< 4–10 mm).[4,20,21] The procedure can obtain similar results to those procedures done by an anterior approach.[22-24] The levatorpexy procedure can be performed under general or local anesthesia, depending on surgeon preference.

22.11 Expert Tips/Pearls/ Suggestions

- During white line advancement surgery and levatorpexy, it is essential to distinguish between white line and "pseudo white line." The levator aponeurosis has two layers, and the anterior layer is thick with less muscle fibers and reflects superiorly to the tarsus to become continuous with the orbital septum. The posterior layer has more smooth muscle

fibers and inserts into the lower one-third of tarsus and subcutaneous tissue. It is possible to mistakenly place the suture in the "pseudo white line," that is, that anterior section of levator that becomes the orbital septum. Here, the postaponeurotic fat pad is a helpful landmark: when dissecting the composite conjunctiva and Müller's muscle flap using the described technique, one encounters the postaponeurotic fat pad, which lies on anterior Müller's muscle. The postaponeurotic fat pad is a distinct thin diffuse sheet fat in the postaponeurotic space, located between Müller's muscle and the posterior smooth muscle layer of the aponeurosis. Dissection then should continue to identify the healthy white sheet of the posterior surface of posterior surface of aponeurosis. The sutures are placed into this healthy white sheet rather than the orbital septum. If placed into the pseudo white line, undercorrection will likely occur.
- The suture placement is essential for determining the outcome and is based on preoperative evaluation (▶ Table 22.1). Once dissection between the posterior surface of the levator aponeurosis and the conjunctiva has been performed and the posterior surface of the levator muscle is reached, the initial suture can be placed.
  ○ For involutional ptosis with LF better than 10 mm, the initial suture is placed into the healthy aponeurosis if phenylephrine test is positive. If phenylephrine testing is negative, the initial suture needs to be located at the junction of the white line aponeurosis and LPS.
  ○ For congenital ptosis, the placement is somewhat more variable.
- Remove the Desmarres retractor on commencing the Müller's muscle–conjunctiva flap to improve exposure. Ask your assistant to maintain traction of the flap in a caudal direction.
- The surgeon must ensure to pass the needle carefully making two small bites, each taking a partial bite of the aponeurosis to avoid incarcerating orbital septum. For congenital ptosis, where a levatorpexy is required, the needle is passed higher through the LPS muscle, again taking care not to incarcerate the orbital septum.

1 Local anesthetic injection (bupivacaine 0.25% with 1:200,000 adrenaline) into the subcutaneous tissue along the upper lid crease and pretarsal area. Further subconjunctival injection to the region superior to the tarsal plate is performed after everting the upper lid (see the image in the next column).

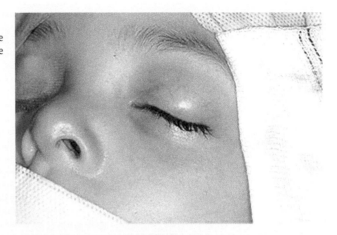

2 A 4–0 silk traction suture is placed into the grey line of the upper lid, and the lid is then everted over a Desmarres retractor (see the image in the next column).

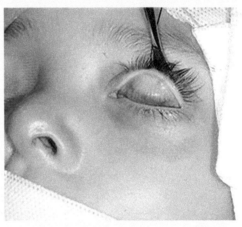

3 Application of gentle diathermy to the conjunctiva at and above the superior tarsal border to minimize bleeding when sutures are placed (see the image in the next column).

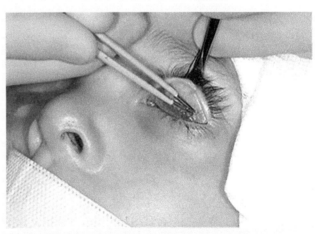

4 A conjunctival incision is made using a #15 blade scalpel, taking care to incise the conjunctiva just superior to the border of the tarsus (see the image in the next column).

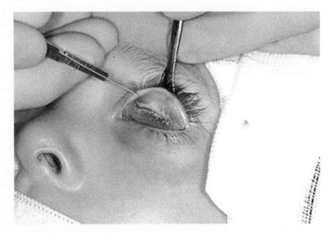

5   Following the incision, a composite flap containing the Müller's muscle and conjunctiva is dissected off until the white line is identified, which represents the posterior border of the levator aponeurosis. It is here, where the surgeon will often encounter the postaponeurotic fat pad, guiding the dissection. Further dissection to identify the undersurface of the levator muscle is (see the image in the next column).

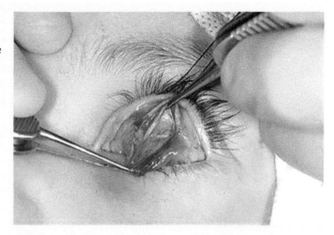

6   A double-armed 5–0 Vicryl suture, undyed, with a ¼ circle spatulated needle. This suture is placed (forehand) through the posterior surface of the levator muscle about 1 mm from the superior edge of the levator aponeurosis, in line with the central peak of the tarsal plate (see the image in the next column).

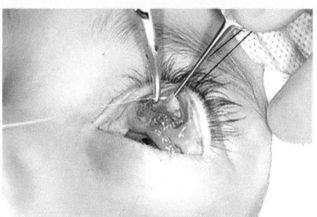

7   Placement of the suture is critical and the needle should be passed twice, each taking a partial bite of the levator muscle. The suture is then placed through the conjunctival surface of the tarsal plate, at less than 1 mm below its superior border, followed by passing through the skin and exiting at the area of the usual lid crease. Both needles of the double-armed suture are placed in the same fashion and should exit in close proximity to allow burying of the suture once tied (▶ Fig. 22.3, also see the image in the next column).

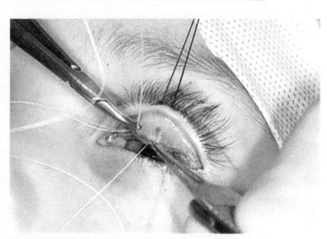

8   Placement of the suture is critical and the needle should be passed twice, each taking a partial bite of the levator muscle. The suture is then placed through the conjunctival surface of the tarsal plate, at less than 1 mm below its superior border, followed by passing through the skin and exiting at the area of the usual lid crease. Both needles of the double-armed suture are placed in the same fashion and should exit in close proximity to allow burying of the suture once tied (▶ Fig. 22.3, also see the image in the next column).

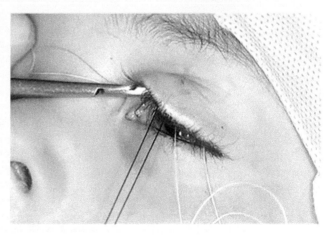

9   A second suture is placed through levator in the same manner as described above. This suture should be located at the same vertical height as the first suture but within 2 mm and medial to the first suture. Again, it is passed through the tarsal plate within 2 mm and medial to the first suture and then through the skin, where it should exit immediately medial to the first suture (see the image in the next column).

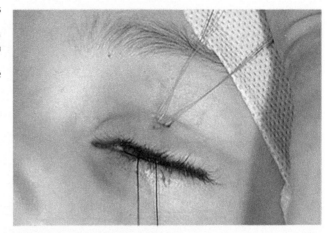

10   The sutures can be tied in a bow and then tied off on the skin once the placement is satisfactory. The sutures are not removed and the Müller's muscle–conjunctiva flap is left to heal spontaneously. An antibiotic ointment is applied at the end of the procedure (Please see image in the next column).
     a. Typical pre- and postoperative photographs of congenital ptosis (mean LF 11 mm, range 5–15 mm) corrected with levatorpexy may be seen in ▶ Fig. 22.4.

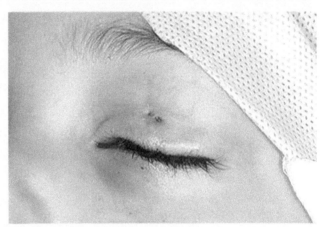

Table 22.1 Placement of the initial suture

Levator excursion	Congenital ptosis		Involutional ptosis	
	Phenyl positive	Phenyl negative	Phenyl positive	Phenyl negative
LF > 10 mm	Suture at the junction of white aponeurosis and LPS	Just above the junction, that is, < 1 mm above	Suture into healthy aponeurosis	Suture at the junction of the LPS and aponeurosis and be prepared to adjust based upon response
LF > 8 mm	Pass suture through the junction of the superior edge of the white aponeurosis and LPS	Pass suture 2 mm superior to the junction of the aponeurosis and LPS	–	–
LF < 4 mm	–	Place suture 4 + mm above the junction of aponeurosis and LPS into the levator muscle. If under general anesthesia, aim for desired palpebral aperture	–	–

Abbreviations: LF, levator function; LPS, levator palpebrae superioris.

- The suture is then passed through the conjunctival surface of the tarsal plate, less than 1 mm below its superior border, and then through the skin emerging at or slightly below the skin crease (▶ Fig. 22.3).
  - Avoid capturing orbital septum while the eyelid is everted.
  - The needle should emerge through to the skin in the region of the eyelid skin crease and less than 10 mm from the lid margin. If it emerges higher, in the preseptal region, assume that septum has been incarcerated and redo this suture pass.
  - Any breach of the medial septum and hence the medial horn may contribute to the occasional medial droop seen following involutional ptosis correction. Small incision anterior approach surgery also claims to have good contour results, again likely due to its septal-sparing nature.[16,17]
- After the initial suture placement, the suture is tied in a bow to assess lid height and contour.
  - If the lid height is too low after the first suture, relax it and pass a second suture higher through the white line and again the tarsal plate and the skin.
  - If the upper eyelid contour appears peaked after the first suture, then relax it and place a second suture more centrally to the position of the peak. This way, the position of the second suture can alter and adjust the lid position without having to remove the initial suture.

22.12 Complications and Their Management

The white line advancement and levatorpexy have minimal complications. A peaked lid contour can be avoided with careful intraoperative assessment. The final lid position may not be certain until 6 to 8 weeks postprocedure, especially if significant edema or hematoma is present.

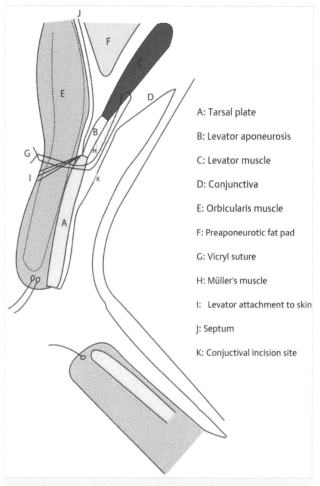

A: Tarsal plate

B: Levator aponeurosis

C: Levator muscle

D: Conjunctiva

E: Orbicularis muscle

F: Preaponeurotic fat pad

G: Vicryl suture

H: Müller's muscle

I: Levator attachment to skin

J: Septum

K: Conjuctival incision site

Fig. 22.3 Pathway of correct suture placement in anatomical cross section.

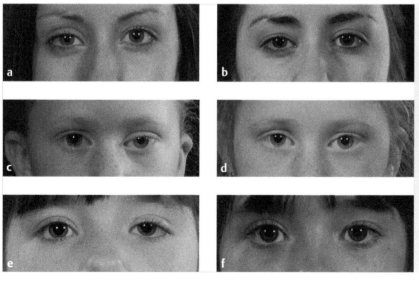

Fig. 22.4 Levatorpexy for congenital ptosis. Preoperative (**a, c, e**) and postoperative (**b, d, f**) photographs at 6-month follow-up.

- Corneal abrasion: The correct suture placement has been discussed above and care should be taken to avoid placing any suture full thickness through the tarsus to avoid corneal abrasions. If a corneal abrasion does occur, it should be treated symptomatically with antibiotic ointment until it heals, as long as there is no full-thickness tarsal suture bite. A bandage contact lens may be placed, and the removal of suture should rarely be required.
- Wound infection: Wound infection should be treated in the standard way, and the patient (especially younger children) must be monitored for the development of secondary orbital cellulitis.
- Undercorrection: Undercorrection may settle as perioperative edema resolves; however, ongoing undercorrection may necessitate further surgery after approximately 3 months.
- Overcorrection: Overcorrection should be rare with proper preoperative measurements. Mild overcorrection may settle with gentle massage. In the setting of severe overcorrection, the release of the sutures may be required.
- Eyelid contour abnormalities: Contour abnormalities are uncommon with this type of procedure. Any peaking of the eyelid can be identified intraoperatively. If the upper eyelid contour appears peaked after the first suture, then relax it and place a second suture more centrally to the position of the peak. This way, the position of the second suture can alter and adjust the lid position without having to remove the initial suture.
- Worsening dry eye: Worsening dry eye is a risk after any type of ptosis surgery. Encourage frequent and deliberate blink closure throughout the day. Frequent lubricating drops can be prescribed. Symptoms usually improve within a few weeks.

22.13 Conclusions

The white line advancement technique can be used for all types of involutional ptosis, ranging from severe to mild. It is possible to modify the technique depending on the results of phenylephrine testing. The levatorpexy is useful for congenital ptosis, especially when a posterior approach with the absence of a skin incision, but the creation of a skin crease is desired. Both procedures lead to consistent results, with excellent cosmesis of the lid contour and upper lid tarsal show.

References

[1] Putterman AM, Urist MJ. Müller muscle-conjunctiva resection. Technique for treatment of blepharoptosis. Arch Ophthalmol. 1975; 93(8):619–623

[2] Collin JR. A ptosis repair of aponeurotic defects by the posterior approach. Br J Ophthalmol. 1979; 63(8):586–590

[3] Patel V, Salam A, Malhotra R. Posterior approach white line advancement ptosis repair: the evolving posterior approach to ptosis surgery. Br J Ophthalmol. 2010; 94(11):1513–1518

[4] Al-Abbadi Z, Sagili S, Malhotra R. Outcomes of posterior-approach 'levatorpexy' in congenital ptosis repair. Br J Ophthalmol. 2014; 98(12):1686–1690

[5] Kakizaki H, Malhotra R, Selva D. Upper eyelid anatomy: an update. Ann Plast Surg. 2009; 63(3):336–343

[6] Kakizaki H, Takahashi Y, Nakano T, et al. Müller's muscle: a component of the peribulbar smooth muscle network. Ophthalmology. 2010; 117(11):2229–2232

[7] Ng SK, Chan W, Marcet MM, Kakizaki H, Selva D. Levator palpebrae superioris: an anatomical update. Orbit. 2013; 32(1):76–84

[8] Kakizaki H, Lay-Leng S, Asamoto K, Nakano T, Selva D, Leibovitch I. Dissection of the eyelid and orbit with modernised anatomical findings. Open Anat J 2010;2:5–24

[9] Kakizaki H, Zako M, Nakano T, Asamoto K, Miyaishi O, Iwaki M. The levator aponeurosis consists of two layers that include smooth muscle. Ophthal Plast Reconstr Surg. 2005; 21(5):379–382

[10] Bartley GB, Waller RR. Retroaponeurotic fat. Am J Ophthalmol. 1989; 107(3):301

[11] Malhotra R, Mahadevan V, Leatherbarrow B, Barrett AW. The post-levator aponeurosis fat pad. Ophthal Plast Reconstr Surg. 2015; 31(4):313–317

[12] Choudhary MM, Chundury R, McNutt SA, Perry JD. Eyelid contour following conjunctival müllerectomy with or without tarsectomy blepharoptosis repair. Ophthal Plast Reconstr Surg. 2016; 32(5):361–365

[13] Peter NM, Khooshabeh R. Open-sky isolated subtotal Muller's muscle resection for ptosis surgery: a review of over 300 cases and assessment of long-term outcome. Eye (Lond). 2013; 27(4):519–524

[14] Malhotra R, Salam A, Then SY, Grieve AP. Visible iris sign as a predictor of problems during and following anterior approach ptosis surgery. Eye (Lond). 2011; 25(2):185–191

[15] Antus Z, Salam A, Horvath E, Malhotra R. Outcomes for severe aponeurotic ptosis using posterior approach white-line advancement ptosis surgery. Eye (Lond). 2018; 32(1):81–86

[16] Frueh BR, Musch DC, McDonald HM. Efficacy and efficiency of a small-incision, minimal dissection procedure versus a traditional approach for correcting aponeurotic ptosis. Ophthalmology. 2004; 111(12):2158–2163

[17] Gire J, Robert PY, Denis D, Adenis JP. [Small-incision, minimal dissection procedure (Frueh's procedure) in correction of involutional and congenital ptosis: A retrospective study of 119 cases]. J Fr Ophtalmol. 2011; 34(7):439–447

[18] Malhotra R, Salam A. Outcomes of adult aponeurotic ptosis repair under general anaesthesia by a posterior approach white-line levator advancement. Orbit. 2012; 31(1):7–12

[19] Patel V, Malhotra R. Transconjunctival blepharoptosis surgery: a review of posterior approach ptosis surgery and posterior approach white-line advancement. Open Ophthalmol J. 2010; 4:81–84

[20] Feldman I, Brusasco L, Malhotra R. Improving Outcomes of Posterior Approach Levatorpexy for Congenital Ptosis With Reduced Levator Function. Ophthal Plast Reconstr Surg. 2018; 34(5):460–462

[21] Lee JH, Aryasit O, Kim YD, Woo KI, Lee E, Johnson ON, III. Maximal levator resection in unilateral congenital ptosis with poor levator function. Br J Ophthalmol. 2017; 101(6):740–746

[22] Krohn-Hansen D, Haaskjold E. A modified technique for levator resection in congenital ptosis. J Plast Surg Hand Surg. 2013; 47(4):243–247

[23] Skaat A, Fabian D, Spierer A, Rosen N, Rosner M, Ben Simon GJ. Congenital ptosis repair-surgical, cosmetic, and functional outcome: a report of 162 cases. Can J Ophthalmol. 2013; 48(2):93–98

[24] Jordan DR, Anderson RL. The aponeurotic approach to congenital ptosis. Ophthalmic Surg. 1990; 21(4):237–244

23 The Fasanella–Servat Procedure

Steven C. Dresner, Margaret L. Pfeiffer

Abstract

The Fasanella–Servat procedure was originally described by Fasanella and Servat to correct small to medium amounts of ptosis in patients with normal levator excursion. This procedure has fallen out of favor in recent years because of complications that include contour abnormalities, corneal abrasions, and the inability to grade the resections with an accurate nomogram. A modified Fasanella–Servat procedure has been described by Samimi et al, with the goal of minimizing contour abnormalities and corneal abrasions.

Keywords: ptosis, ptosis surgery, Fasanella–Servat

23.1 Introduction

A modified Fasanella–Servat procedure has been described by Samimi, Erb, Lane, and Dresner to correct small to medium amounts of ptosis in patients with normal levator excursion (> 10 mm).[1] This procedure has fallen out of favor in recent years because of complications that include contour abnormalities, corneal abrasions, and the inability to grade the resections with an accurate nomogram. A modified Fasanella–Servat procedure has been described by Samimi et al.[2] The modified Fasanella–Servat eliminates the use of two hemostats as originally described and utilizes a Putterman clamp or a modified Putterman clamp, such as the Dresner/Uzcategui clamp (▶ Fig. 23.1). The use of these clamps minimizes the chance of contour abnormalities. A 6-0 Prolene pullout suture is also utilized instead of a plain gut suture to minimize the possibility of corneal abrasions. A nomogram has been described that accurately guides the surgeon on the amount of resection necessary for the amount of ptosis present: for every 1 mm of ptosis, 2 mm of tarsus is resected along with the accompanying Müller's muscle and conjunctiva.[2]

23.2 Indications

The Fasanella–Servat procedure is an excellent procedure for between 1 and 2.5 mm of ptosis in patients with normal levator excursion, normal eyelid contour, and a negative phenylephrine test. The Müller's muscle–conjunctival resection procedure is preferable in patients with minimal to moderate ptosis with a positive phenylephrine test. In patients with a negative phenylephrine test, this procedure is ideal. It is also useful in patients undercorrected after Müller's muscle–conjunctival resection or external levator repair. It can be combined with upper blepharoplasty.

23.3 Risks

- Overcorrection.
- Undercorrection.
- Corneal abrasion.
- Bleeding.

23.4 Benefits

- Predictable amount of eyelid lift.
- Easily performed in office setting with minimal patient discomfort.
- Excellent option as a second procedure to correct residual ptosis after external levator advancement or Müller's muscle–conjunctival resection.

23.5 Informed Consent

- Include risks and benefits.

23.6 Contraindications

- Severe dry eye and exposure keratopathy may lead the surgeon to do a smaller eyelid elevation.

23.7 Instruments Needed

- Castroviejo needle driver.
- Forceps.

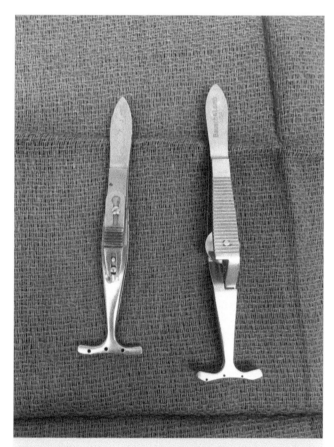

Fig. 23.1 The Putterman ptosis clamp (*left*) and the Dresner/Uzcategui clamp (*right*).

- Desmarres retractor.
- A #15 blade.
- Caliper.
- Sterile marking pen.
- Ptosis clamp (Putterman clamp or a modified Müller's muscle–conjunctival resection clamp).
- Sutures:
  ○ One 4–0 silk G-3 double-armed, cut in half, per side.
  ○ 6–0 Prolene P-3.

23.8 Preoperative Checklist

- Informed consent.
- Instrumentation on hand.

23.9 Operative Technique

This procedure can be done under local, monitored, or general anesthesia in an office-based procedure room, ambulatory operating room, or hospital-based setting.

- The pupillary axis is marked on the pretarsal skin with the patient in the upright position.
- Local anesthesia consisting of 1% lidocaine with epinephrine and hyaluronidase is injected into the upper fornix. Topical tetracaine is applied to the ocular surface.
- The upper lid is reflected over a Desmarres retractor, and a mark is made with a sterile marking pen on the tarsus, designating the amount of total resection. The total amount of resection is measured from the superior tarsal margin, and the mark is made in line with the pupillary axis (► Fig. 23.2).
- A double-armed 4–0 silk suture is cut in half, and each end is placed medially and laterally on the superior tarsal margin to act as a traction suture (► Fig. 23.3).
- Each suture is tied to itself to form a loop.
- The Desmarres retractor is removed and the traction sutures are elevated by the surgeon and assistant (► Fig. 23.4).
- The ptosis clamp is placed over the tissues to be excised in line with the marking on the tarsus (► Fig. 23.5).

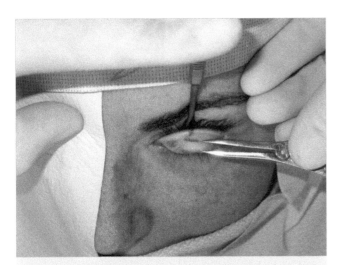

Fig. 23.2 With the upper eyelid reflected over a Desmarres retractor, the total amount of resection is marked from the superior tarsus in line with the pupillary axis.

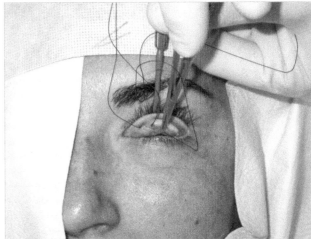

Fig. 23.3 A double-armed 4–0 silk suture is cut in half, and one end is placed medially and laterally on the superior tarsal border. Each suture is tied to itself to form a loop. These act as traction sutures.

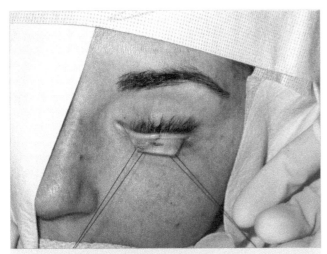

Fig. 23.4 The Desmarres retractor is removed and the traction sutures are elevated by the surgeon and assistant.

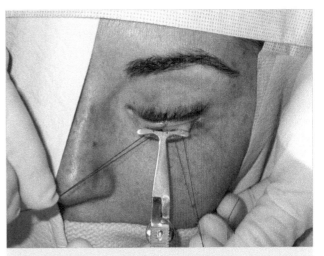

Fig. 23.5 The ptosis clamp is placed over the tissues to be excised in line with the marking on the tarsus.

- A 6–0 Prolene suture is passed multiple times approximately 1 mm below the clamp beginning and ending exteriorly through the pretarsal eyelid (▶ Fig. 23.6).
- A #15 blade is used to excise the tissues between the clamp and the suture (▶ Fig. 23.7). No cautery is necessary.
- The eyelid is reflected back in the anatomic position and the suture is tied in the pretarsal area (▶ Fig. 23.8). No patch is required.

23.10 Expert Tips/Pearls/Suggestions

- If there is difficulty maintaining eversion of the eyelid over the Desmarres retractor, one can pass the silk sutures prior to marking the total amount of resection. Once passed, the assistant can elevate the traction sutures, which allows the surgeon to mark.
- The larger P-3 needle on the Prolene suture is easier to pass than a smaller needle, particularly on the initial pass from the pretarsal skin to the clamped tissue and on the final pass from the clamped tissue to the pretarsal skin.
- The suture does not need to be tightly tied in the pretarsal area. We prefer to tie the suture so that the knot is resting on the pretarsal skin without too much tension. This allows for eyelid swelling.

23.11 Results

Excellent results can be obtained for 1, 1.5, and 2 mm of ptosis (▶ Fig. 23.9).[2] Because of limitations of tarsal resection, 2.5 mm

of ptosis is the greatest amount of ptosis that can be corrected with this technique.

23.12 Complications and Their Management

Contour abnormalities are rare with this modified technique. Although overcorrection is unlikely, it can be addressed by

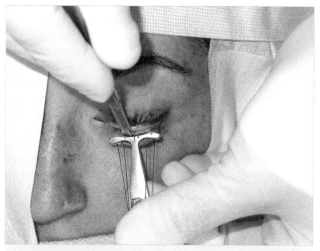

Fig. 23.7 A #15 blade is used to excise the tissues between the clamp and the suture.

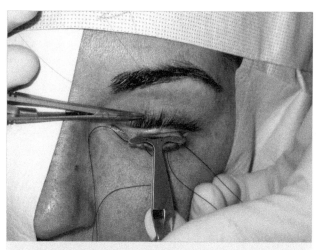

Fig. 23.6 A 6–0 Prolene suture is passed multiple times approximately 1 mm below the clamp beginning and ending exteriorly through the pretarsal eyelid.

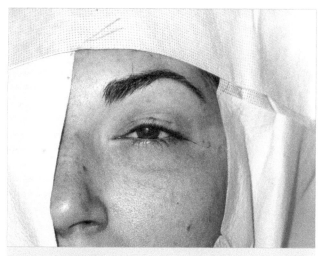

Fig. 23.8 The eyelid is reflected back in the anatomic position and the suture is loosely tied on itself in the pretarsal area.

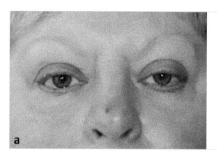
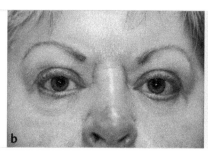

Fig. 23.9 Preoperative (a) and postoperative (b) photographs after bilateral Fasanella–Servat procedure in a phenylephrine negative patient.

removing the suture and applying digital massage. Undercorrection needs levator repair and can be easily accomplished in spite of the previous tarsal resection. The Prolene suture is well tolerated by the cornea, and keratopathy is rarely seen.

23.13 Conclusion

The modified Fasanella–Servat procedure is a useful procedure to add to the surgical armamentarium. It is an excellent procedure for ptosis that does not respond to phenylephrine or undercorrected ptosis after levator repair or Müller's muscle–

conjunctival resection. It can be easily combined with upper blepharoplasty and performed in an office setting. Using our nomogram, we are able to obtain predictable results.

References

[1] Fasanella RM, Servat J. Levator resection for minimal ptosis: another simplified operation. Arch Ophthalmol. 1961; 65:493–496

[2] Samimi DB, Erb MH, Lane CJ, Dresner SC. The modified Fasanella-Servat procedure: description and quantified analysis. Ophthal Plast Reconstr Surg. 2013; 29(1):30–34

24 Combined Upper Blepharoplasty and Ptosis Repair

Steven C. Dresner, Eric B. Hamill, Margaret L. Pfeiffer

Abstract

Many patients who present for upper blepharoplasty have concurrent myogenic ptosis; similarly, many who present for ptosis repair have excess skin. Recognition and evaluation of ptosis preoperatively is important to postoperative success and patient happiness. The surgeon may easily combine upper blepharoplasty with Müller's muscle–conjunctival resection, Fasanella–Servat, and/or levator aponeurotic repair.

Keywords: ptosis, ptosis surgery, blepharoplasty, Fasanella–Servat, Müller's muscle–conjunctival resection

24.1 Introduction

Many patients who present for upper blepharoplasty have ptosis that may or may not be evident to the patient. Usually, the ptosis is minimal (2 mm or less) and the levator excursion is within normal limits (> 10 mm). When performing blepharoplasty, there are various methods for simultaneous ptosis repair, including Müller's muscle–conjunctival resection (MMCR), Fasanella–Servat, or levator aponeurotic repair.

24.2 Clinical Evaluation and Indications for Surgery

The initial exam should evaluate visual acuity, ocular surface health, presence or absence of dry eye, extraocular motility, and the anterior segment. Brow position, amount of dermatochalasis, and distribution of herniated orbital fat should be noted. The margin reflex distance 1 (MRD1) should be assessed. Levator excursion, Bell's phenomenon, amount of lagophthalmos, and degree of lower lid laxity are also documented. Though not uniformly performed during the upper eyelid ptosis consultation, the margin reflex distance 2 often provides helpful information to the oculoplastic surgeon.

After the initial assessment outlined above, a phenylephrine test is performed on patients undergoing evaluation for ptosis correction. A drop of phenylephrine is placed on the ocular surface of the ptotic eye or eyes. It is important to document an MRD1 prior to drop installation. The patient is reexamined 5 minutes after installation of phenylephrine, and the MRD1 is documented in both eyes. An elevation of 2 mm or more in the medicated eye is considered a positive response and indicates that an MMCR is a good option for ptosis repair. A negative phenylephrine test indicates that an MMCR is not viable, and the patient would be better served with either a Fasanella–Servat procedure or levator repair. In the case of a negative phenylephrine test, the Fasanella–Servat procedure is a good option if the amount of ptosis is 2.5 mm or less on each side. If the ptosis is greater than 2.5 mm or the ptosis is exceedingly asymmetric, levator repair is preferable.

Though ptosis is often bilateral, there are cases in which the ptosis initially appears unilaterally. In these patients, a positive phenylephrine test in the ptotic eye may induce a contralateral ptosis in the fellow eye due to Hering's law of equal innervation. The development of contralateral ptosis should be assessed and documented. Consideration should be given to bilateral repair in these instances, and the type of surgical procedure and amount of correction should be determined according to previously discussed algorithms.

It is important to consider patient age and ability to cooperate intraoperatively. A poorly cooperative patient would not be an ideal candidate for levator repair, as this is best done with the patient's cooperation under local or monitored anesthesia care. Patients who desire general anesthesia are better served with an MMCR or Fasanella–Servat combined with upper blepharoplasty as these procedures require no intraoperative patient cooperation.

24.3 Combined Müller's Muscle–Conjunctival Resection and Blepharoplasty

This procedure can be performed under local, monitored, or general anesthesia. No patient cooperation is required. The amount of Müller's muscle and conjunctiva to resect is determined according to standard nomograms (see Chapter 21), and no adjustment is made when performed in conjunction with blepharoplasty. Prior to administering anesthesia, the pupillary axis is marked on the upper eyelid with the patient in a seated position. The amount of skin to be resected is marked. Local anesthesia is injected. The order of repair is arbitrary; we prefer performing the MMCR first. The procedure is performed in a standard fashion (see Chapter 21). The blepharoplasty is best performed as a skin-only excision, preserving the underlying orbicularis muscle. The medial and central fat pads can be accessed through a medial buttonhole. Care must be taken not to cut the MMCR suture when performing the upper blepharoplasty. No patch is necessary postoperatively.

24.4 Combined Fasanella–Servat and Blepharoplasty

This procedure can also be performed under local, monitored, or general anesthesia. No patient cooperation is required. The amount of tarsus to resect is determined according to standard nomograms (see Chapter 23), and no adjustment is made when performed in conjunction with blepharoplasty. The eyelids are marked as previously described. The Fasanella is performed in a standard fashion and can be performed prior to or after the blepharoplasty (see Chapter 23). We prefer performing the Fasanella first. During blepharoplasty, again, the orbicularis muscle is preserved to avoid dry eye and allow for adequate eyelid closure. Care must be taken not to cut the Fasanella suture. No patch is necessary postoperatively.

24.5 Combined Levator Aponeurotic Advancement and Blepharoplasty

This procedure is usually performed under local or monitored anesthesia. General anesthesia precludes patient cooperation and is therefore undesirable for optimal results. Unlike the MMCR and Fasanella, in which ptosis repair is performed prior to blepharoplasty, blepharoplasty is performed first when combined with levator repair. This sequence allows for better ease of dissection both down to the tarsal plate and through the orbital septum.

24.5.1 Indications

- Aponeurotic ptosis with normal levator function.

24.5.2 Contraindications

- Severe dry eye.

24.5.3 Instrumentation

- Castroviejo needle driver.
- Forceps.
- A #15 blade scalpel.
- Westcott scissors.
- Monopolar and high-temperature cautery.
- Two rakes.
- Corneal protector.
- Sterile tetracaine on field.
- Sutures:
  - One 5–0 polyglactin S-14 double-armed per side.
  - 6–0 Prolene P-1 for skin closure.

24.5.4 Preoperative Checklist

- Informed consent.
- Instrumentation on hand.
- Preoperative clinical photographs to verify the site of surgery and measurements.

24.5.5 Operative Technique

Combined levator repair and upper blepharoplasty is best performed under local or local-monitored anesthesia care to allow patient cooperation at setting the upper eyelid heights.

- The pupillary axis is marked on the pretarsal skin with the patient in the seated position.
- The patient is placed in the supine position and the lower part of the incision is marked. Usually, this is in the patient's normal eyelid crease but can be moved lower, especially in men. A modified "pinch" technique is performed to assess the upper border of the blepharoplasty incision.
- Local anesthesia consisting of lidocaine with epinephrine is injected subcutaneously. Hyaluronidase is usually avoided to prevent inadvertent paralysis of the levator muscle. A corneal protector is placed over the ocular surface.
- The incision is begun with a #15 blade or diamond blade. A pure skin flap is developed, preserving the orbicularis oculi muscle (▶ Fig. 24.1).
- With the assistant providing inferior traction, dissection is carried out through the orbicularis down to the tarsal plate with Westcott scissors (▶ Fig. 24.2).
- Dissection proceeds suborbicularis to the orbital septum. With the assistant providing inferior and superior traction, the orbital septum is incised with Westcott scissors, revealing the underlying preaponeurotic fat and levator aponeurosis (▶ Fig. 24.3).
- A high-temperature cautery is used to create a free edge of the levator and dissect between the levator and Müller's

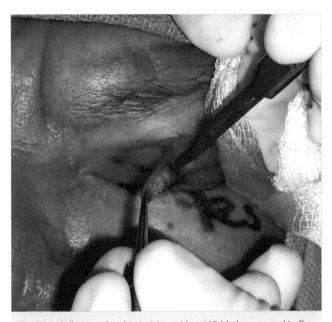

Fig. 24.1 Following the skin incision with a #15 blade, a pure skin flap is developed, preserving the orbicularis oculi muscle.

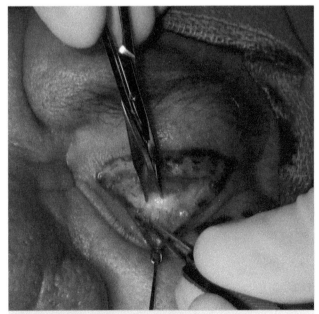

Fig. 24.2 Dissection is carried out through the orbicularis down to the tarsal plate with Westcott scissors.

muscle towards Whitnall's ligament. Topical tetracaine can be applied to the surgical field to aid in anesthesia (▸ Fig. 24.4).

- A double-armed 5–0 polyglactin suture on an S-14 needle is placed partial thickness in two broad bites through the superior third of the tarsus at the previously marked pupillary line (▸ Fig. 24.5). Each end is then passed superiorly through the levator aponeurosis (▸ Fig. 24.6).

- With the assistant providing inferior traction on the levator aponeurosis, the suture is tied temporarily and the patient is examined for height and contour (▸ Fig. 24.7). The patient can be raised to the sitting position if desired. A slight overcorrection is necessary to obtain the desired final result.

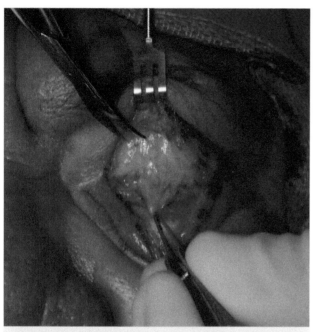

Fig. 24.3 The orbital septum is incised with Westcott scissors, revealing the underlying preaponeurotic fat and levator aponeurosis.

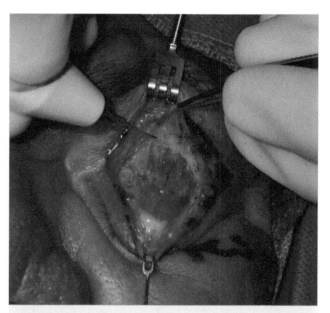

Fig. 24.4 A high-temperature cautery is used dissect between the levator and Müller's muscle towards Whitnall's ligament.

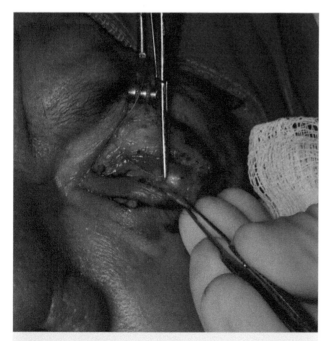

Fig. 24.5 A double-armed 5–0 polyglactin suture on an S-14 needle is placed through the superior third of the central tarsus in two broad bites.

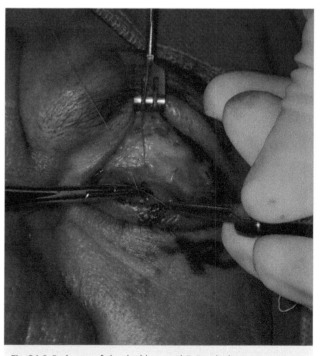

Fig. 24.6 Each arm of the double-armed 5–0 polyglactin suture is passed superiorly through the levator aponeurosis.

- If an adjustment to eyelid height or contour is necessary, the suture can be pulled out of the aponeurosis and repassed. No additional sutures are required.
- The suture is tied permanently and the excess aponeurosis is trimmed with Westcott scissors or a high-temperature cautery (▶ Fig. 24.8).
- The orbital fat can be addressed and debulked as desired, and the skin is closed using a 6–0 Prolene suture on a P-1 needle with supratarsal fixation of every other bite.

- Typical pre- and postoperative results of combined levator advancement and blepharoplasty are presented in ▶ Fig. 24.9, ▶ Fig. 24.10, and ▶ Fig. 24.11.

24.6 Expert Tips/Pearls/Suggestions

- Often, the polyglactin suture will need to be adjusted several times before the appropriate height and contour are obtained. We often check eye's eyelid position in the supine and seated position.

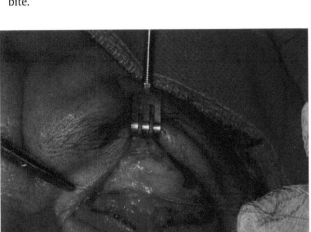

Fig. 24.7 The suture is tied temporarily and the patient is examined for height and contour.

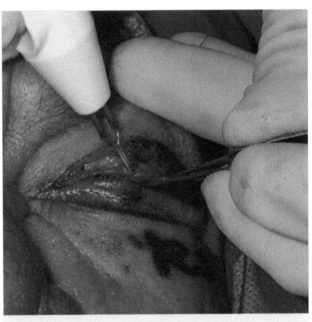

Fig. 24.8 After the suture is tied permanently, the excess aponeurosis is trimmed with a high-temperature cautery or Westcott scissors.

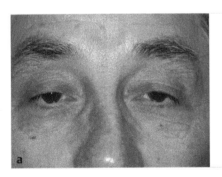
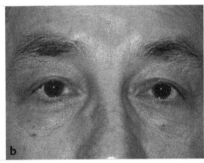

a

b

Fig. 24.9 **(a)** Preoperative external photograph of the patient undergoing combined blepharoplasty and levator aponeurotic repair. **(b)** Postoperative external photograph of the patient undergoing combined blepharoplasty and levator aponeurotic repair.

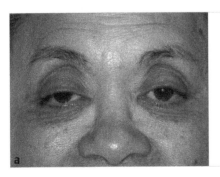
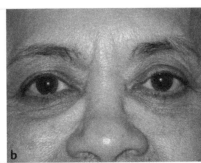

a

b

Fig. 24.10 **(a)** Preoperative external photograph of the patient undergoing combined blepharoplasty and levator aponeurotic repair. **(b)** Postoperative external photograph of the patient undergoing combined blepharoplasty and levator aponeurotic repair.

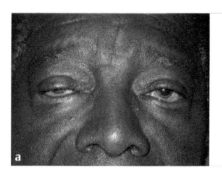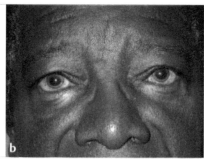

Fig. 24.11 (a) Preoperative external photograph of the patient undergoing combined blepharoplasty and levator aponeurotic repair. (b) Postoperative external photograph of the patient undergoing combined blepharoplasty and levator aponeurotic repair.

- Avoid injecting too much local anesthetic and try to inject a symmetric amount on each eyelid. Topical tetracaine provides good supplemental anesthesia when desired, particularly during dissection of the levator aponeurosis.

24.7 Postoperative Management

The patient uses a combination antibiotic–steroid ointment on the wound three times per day. Sutures are removed at postoperative week 1.

24.8 Complications and Their Management

Complications include undercorrection, overcorrection, contour abnormalities, and tarsal kink. Undercorrection can be managed with a Fasanella–Servat or repeat levator advancement, but we prefer the former. Contour abnormalities typically require repeat levator repair but can be managed as well with full-thickness eyelid resection. Overcorrection can be initially managed by downward massage but may require levator recession.

25 Floppy Eyelid Syndrome Repair with Concomitant Ptosis Repair

Krishnapriya Kalyam, John B. Holds

Abstract

The lax eyelids in patients with floppy eyelid syndrome demonstrate a number of anatomic defects, including horizontal lid laxity, eyelash ptosis, and blepharoptosis. Successful correction of eyelid ptosis and ocular irritation in these patients often requires horizontal tightening of the eyelids in addition to aponeurotic advancement.

Keywords: floppy eyelid syndrome, ptosis repair

25.1 Introduction

Floppy eyelid syndrome (FES), initially described in 1981,[1] is characterized by chronic eye irritation due to increased laxity of the eyelids that can be easily everted by applying minimal traction (▶ Fig. 25.1). The etiology of FES is multifactorial with depletion of elastin fibers and upregulation of matrix metalloproteinases.[2] The superior tarsus is flaccid, malleable, rubbery, and easily everted, especially in the temporal area. Aponeurotic blepharoptosis, eyelash ptosis, and entropion or ectropion are commonly found causing visual obstruction and ocular irritation (itching, redness, mucous discharge, foreign body sensation, and photosensitivity). FES is associated with obstructive sleep apnea (OSA), obesity, papillary conjunctivitis, and keratoconus.[3] Sleep apnea evaluation is warranted in patients with FES due to the morbidity and mortality associated with OSA.

In mild cases, FES is most often treated with topical agents such as artificial tears and lubricating ointment at bedtime combined with eyelid shielding or taping.[4] In moderate cases, conservative treatment can be combined with an eyelid tightening procedure with a full-thickness wedge resection. Severe cases of FES often require multiple procedures, including full-thickness wedge resection, aponeurotic advancement, and eyelash ptosis repair. Full-thickness wedge resection alone may correct horizontal eyelid laxity, eyelid ptosis, and eyelash ptosis.

With progressive symptoms, multiple surgical strategies are used to address eyelid laxity and blepharoptosis with good short-term success rates but some tendency to relapse over months to years. Surgical correction of blepharoptosis or horizontal lid tightening alone may be not successful if not combined. For 24 years, the senior author has treated this condition by combining upper lid tightening at the canthal angle with upper eyelid ptosis repair. Horizontal laxity is addressed by lateral shortening and reinserting the lateral canthal tendon to the orbital rim. Aponeurotic ptosis is corrected with anterior levator advancement/reinsertion. Eyelash ptosis is corrected by rotational crease fixation sutures.

25.2 Goals of Intervention/ Indications

- Elevate eyelid to improve visual obstruction due to ptosis.
- Decrease ocular irritation and discomfort due to FES.
- Relief from eyelid taping and patching at bedtime.

25.2.1 Risks of the Procedure

- Bleeding.
- Infection.
- Scarring, especially at the lateral canthus.
- Recurrence due to underlying pathology, patient sleeping on the surgical side, and patient eyelid rubbing.

25.2.2 Benefits of the Procedure

- Stopping nocturnal eyelid eversion.
- Improvement in ocular comfort.
- Relief from nighttime patching and ocular lubrication.
- Address blepharoptosis and eyelash ptosis at the same time, improving visual obstruction and eyelash ptosis, respectively.

25.3 Informed Consent

- Include risks and benefits (as above).
- Discussion of need for revision surgery due to recurrence, undercorrection, or overcorrection. Overcorrection is extremely rare.

25.4 Contraindications

- Medical status precluding surgery.

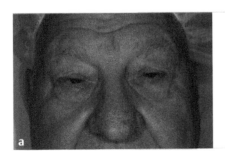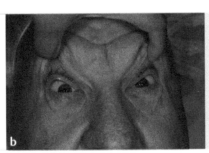

Fig. 25.1 (a, b) External photographs of the patient showing ptosis and eyelid laxity.

25.5 Preoperative Assessment

- Preoperative assessment should be performed in an upright position with facial muscles in relaxed state.
- Marginal reflex distance 1 should be assessed for degree of blepharoptosis.
- Redundant eyelid tissue should be assessed by lateral traction to see how easily the eyelid everts (▶ Fig. 25.1).
- Excess skin should be measured.
- A slit lamp examination should be performed to evaluate for papillary conjunctivitis, conjunctival irritation, and corneal exposure keratopathy.

25.6 Operative Technique

This procedure can be done under local or monitored anesthesia in an office-based procedure room, ambulatory operating room, or hospital-based setting. Often, corrective surgery is performed bilaterally.

25.6.1 Instruments Needed

- Westcott scissors.
- Castroviejo needle drivers.
- A # 15 Bard-Parker blade and handle.
- Paufique forceps.
- Desmarres eyelid retractor.
- Knapp four-prong retractor.
- Sutures:
  - A 6–0 silk G-1 needle (Ethicon).
  - A 5–0 Polysorb P-21 needle (Covidien) or 5–0 Vicryl P-2 needle (Ethicon).
  - A 6–0 polypropylene P-3 needle (Ethicon).
- Local anesthetic:
  - Bupivacaine 0.5% with 1:100,000 units of epinephrine.
  - Lidocaine 2% with 1:100,000 units of epinephrine.

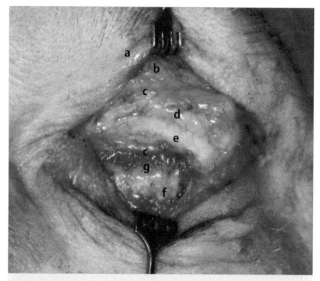

Fig. 25.2 Photograph demonstrates upper eyelid anatomy. a, skin; b, orbicularis oculi muscle; c, cut edges of orbital septum; d, preaponeurotic fat pad; e, levator aponeurosis; f, tarsus; g, Müller's muscle.

25.6.2 Surgical Technique

- Upper eyelids are marked to create the eyelid crease and denote the excess skin to be removed. This amount is generally significantly less than one would excise in an otherwise uncomplicated ptosis repair with blepharoplasty. A diagonal line extending from lateral canthus to the upper eyelid crease incision is also marked.
- Dilute anesthetic (0.03% lidocaine w/epinephrine) is injected into the marked areas under sedation followed by 2% lidocaine with 1:100,000 w/epinephrine after the prepping and draping the patient.
- A #15 blade is used to make a skin incision. Westcott scissors are used to remove skin and a central strip of orbicularis muscle.
- Scissor dissection opens the orbital septum, exposing the levator aponeurosis (▶ Fig. 25.2).
- Thinned and redundant levator aponeurosis is excised near the upper tarsus.
- Bipolar cautery is applied for hemostasis.
- A #15 blade is used to make a transverse groove in the tarsus 2 mm below its upper edge to 30 to 50% tarsal depth.
- The distinct levator aponeurosis is advanced to the upper tarsus and sutured with interrupted 6–0 silk sutures. The identical procedure is performed on the opposite side. Height and contour are checked in the supine and sitting position. Additional 6–0 silk sutures are placed. After final adjustments of the silk sutures, these are tied down (▶ Fig. 25.3).
- A #15 blade is then used to make an incision through skin and orbicularis muscle along the line angling superiorly from the lateral canthus to the eyelid crease incision (▶ Fig. 25.4).
- The upper lid lateral canthal tendon is released (▶ Fig. 25.5). A tarsal strip is fashioned, horizontally incising the tarsus approximately 4 mm above the eyelid margin. This strip is then sharply released from the anterior lamella (▶ Fig. 25.6). Unlike the normal lower eyelid where only 1 to 4 mm of lateral tarsus is excised, the tarsus is shortened 4 to 12 mm. Care is taken to avoid damage to lacrimal ductules.
- The lateral canthal tendon is reattached to inner orbital rim using 5–0 Polysorb P-21 needle (Covidien) or 5–0 Vicryl P-2 needle (Ethicon) sutures (▶ Fig. 25.7).
- Deep crease fixation sutures are placed by attaching skin and orbicularis muscle to the levator aponeurosis in interrupted fashion using 6–0 polypropylene (P-13 needle, Surgipro, Covidien or P-3 needle, Prolene, and Ethicon) sutures, lifting

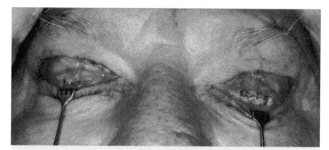

Fig. 25.3 Photograph demonstrating bilateral ptosis repair. After resecting the appropriate amount of aponeurosis, 6–0 silk sutures are used to attach aponeurosis to tarsus in an interrupted fashion. Lid height is checked before tying sutures down.

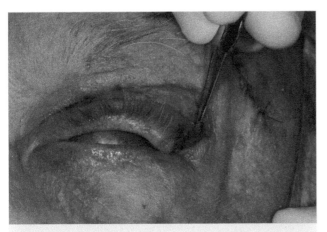

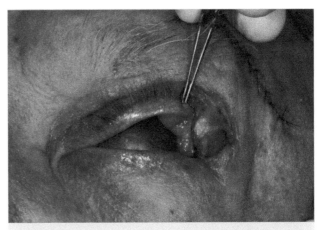

Fig. 25.4 A #15 blade is used to create a skin incision from lateral canthus to the blepharoplasty wound. Westcott scissors are used to cut through orbicularis muscle.

Fig. 25.5 A lateral upper lid cantholysis is performed using Westcott scissors. Care is taken to avoid damage to the lacrimal gland.

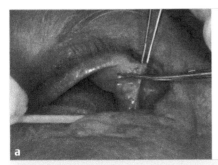
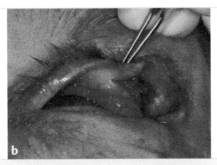
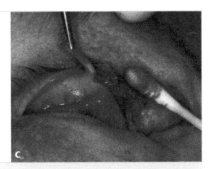

Fig. 25.6 A lateral tarsal strip is fashioned. Care is taken to avoid damage to lacrimal ductules.

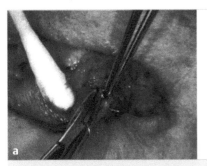
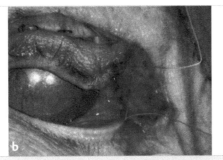
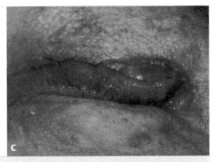

Fig. 25.7 Lateral tarsal strip is reattached to the orbital rim using 5–0 Polysorb sutures. The lateral canthal angle is reformed with 5–0 Polysorb sutures.

the anterior lamella to allow eyelash margin rotation (▶ Fig. 25.8).

- The skin is closed with running 6–0 polypropylene sutures. The redundant skin is temporally excised, rearranged, and closed with same suture (▶ Fig. 25.9, ▶ Fig. 25.10).

25.7 Expert Tips/Pearls/Suggestions

- Care is taken to avoid damage to lacrimal ductules by releasing the tarsus 4 mm above the lid margin.

- The mechanism that induces these changes may recur, requiring three to four very solid sutures between tarsus and aponeurosis in the ptosis repair.
- Avoid excess local anesthetic until after the blepharoptosis ptosis repair.

25.8 Postoperative Care Checklist

- Ice is applied to the operative sites as tolerated for 48 hours.
- The patient is advised to sleep with the head of the bed elevated.

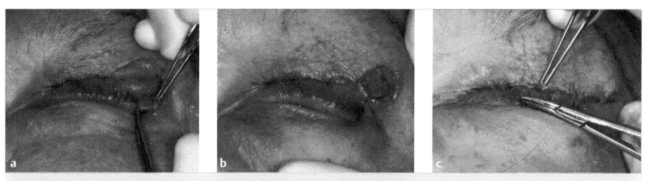

Fig. 25.8 Excess skin and orbicularis are excised. The skin is rearranged and closed with 7–0 polypropylene sutures in interrupted and running fashion.

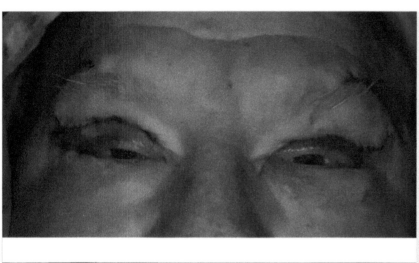

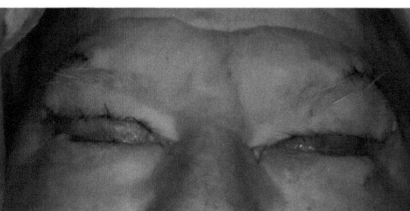

Fig. 25.9 Immediate postoperative result.

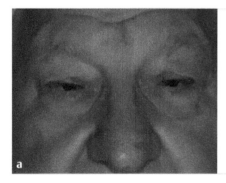

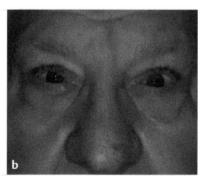

Fig. 25.10 (a, b) Typical preoperation and 3-month postoperation result.

- Postoperative medications are given:
  - Antibiotic ointment (Neosporin or erythromycin) three times a day.
  - Oral pain medication, typically acetaminophen/hydrocodone, 5 mg/325 mg.
- Postoperative wound check at 8 to 13 days for suture removal.

25.9 Complications

- Eyelid hematoma may be treated by blood evacuation.
- Wound infection may be treated as needed.

- Undercorrection or overcorrection, generally in ptosis repair element, may be treated in the same fashion as other aponeurotic ptosis adjustments.

References

[1] Culbertson WW, Ostler HB. The floppy eyelid syndrome. Am J Ophthalmol. 1981; 92(4):568–575

[2] Schlötzer-Schrehardt U, Stojkovic M, Hofmann-Rummelt C, Cursiefen C, Kruse FE, Holbach LM. The Pathogenesis of floppy eyelid syndrome: involvement of matrix metalloproteinases in elastic fiber degradation. Ophthalmology. 2005; 112(4):694–704

[3] Young T, Peppard PE, Gottlieb DJ. Epidemiology of obstructive sleep apnea: a population health perspective. Am J Respir Crit Care Med. 2002; 165(9):1217–1239

26 Management of Lacrimal Gland Prolapse

John D. Ng, Jennifer Murdock

Abstract

Prolapse of the lacrimal gland is an involutional change where the lacrimal gland descends into the anterior orbit. It can cause a mechanical ptosis of the eyelid along with an unattractive cosmetic appearance. This can be managed with suture repositioning in an outpatient surgical setting. Other disorders of the eyelid can mask lacrimal gland prolapse, and it is important to identify this problem as a possible incidental finding during other surgical procedures.

Keywords: lacrimal gland prolapse, dacryoadenopexy, blepharoplasty

26.1 Introduction and Anatomy

The lacrimal gland is positioned within the lacrimal fossa of the frontal bone and secured in place with suspensory ligaments in addition to lateral extensions of Whitnall's ligament. These suspensory ligaments also anatomically separate the lacrimal gland into orbital and palpebral lobes. The orbital lobe has excretory ducts that pass through and join with the ducts of the palpebral lobe, which lies more proximal to the eye. In a normal position, the palpebral lobe can often be seen through the conjunctiva of the superotemporal fornix when the eyelid is everted. Similar to other structures in the body that fall victim to gravity during the aging process, the suspensory ligaments of the lacrimal gland can become lax, resulting in lacrimal gland prolapse (LGP).

Disorders that affect eyelid and periorbital laxity such as sleep apnea and floppy eyelid syndrome, mechanical manipulation, and recurrent periocular edema often due to allergies can predispose patients to LGP. LGP can also be seen in congenital disorders with weak periorbital tissues as seen in congenital ptosis and craniosynostosis.[1]

Often, LGP is found with other involutional changes of the eyelid, such as blepharoptosis in older patients or blepharochalasis in younger patients. Management of the LGP can be combined with a blepharoplasty or ptosis repair. Clinically identifiable LGP was initially reported in about 15% of patients who presented for blepharoplasty evaluation. However, studies of older patient populations, with a mean age of 78, have shown LGP in 60% of cases when examined surgically.[2]

LGP often presents as a periocular mass or bulging of the soft tissue (► Fig. 26.1, ► Fig. 26.2). The palpebral lobe can be seen through the conjunctiva with eyelid eversion, while the orbital lobe presents as soft tissue fullness in the superotemporal eyelid. The prolapsed lacrimal gland can be differentiated from herniated fat by the former being firmer in texture with palpation.

26.2 Goals of Intervention

- Repositioning of the lacrimal gland into proper position in the lacrimal gland fossa.
- Improving cosmesis by correcting LGP and minimizing scarring with a superior eyelid crease incision.
- Recovering superior visual field by reversing mechanical ptosis from LGP.

26.3 Risks

- Bleeding/hematoma.
- Injury to lacrimal gland resulting in decreased tear production and dry eyes.
- Recurrence of LGP and need for additional surgery.

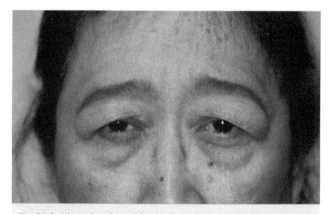

Fig. 26.2 Bilateral prolapsed lacrimal gland noted in conjunction with other involutional changes, including temporal eyebrow ptosis, aponeurotic ptosis, and upper dermatochalasis. (This image is provided courtesy of Michael A. Burnstine, MD.)

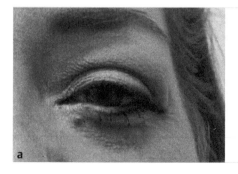 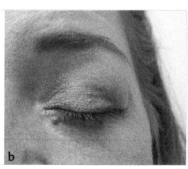

Fig. 26.1 Lacrimal gland prolapse (LGP) seen in anterior superotemporal orbit is exhibited by enlargement of the lateral upper eyelid. Temporal orbital fullness is noted in primary gaze **(a)** and downgaze **(b)**.

26.4 Benefits

- Improved superior visual field if affected at preoperative evaluation.
- Improved cosmesis of the upper eyelids.

26.5 Contraindications

- Lacrimal gland malignancy.
- Caution is recommended to avoid injury of the lacrimal gland if the patient has a history of severe dry eyes.

26.5.1 Surgical Procedure

The surgical procedure can be performed in an office-based procedure room or ambulatory surgery center.

26.5.2 Instruments Needed

- Incision: #15 Bard-Park blade or incisional laser.
- Retraction: Two-prong skin hook, four-prong rake, and Demarres retractor.
- Dissection: Cautery or sharp tenotomy scissors.
- Bishop or Manhattan toothed forceps.
- Castroviejo needle driver.
- Sutures:
  - Repositioning: A 5–0 or 6–0 nonabsorbable monofilament or absorbable braided suture.
  - Orbicularis closure: A 6–0 absorbable braided suture.
  - Skin closure: A 6–0 or 7–0 nonabsorbable monofilament or absorbable gut suture.

26.5.3 Operative Technique: Step by Step

- A lid crease incision is marked, and the upper eyelids are infiltrated with local anesthetic. A combination of lidocaine with epinephrine and bupivacaine works well to anesthetize the area and provide local vasoconstriction.
- A lid crease incision is made with either a #15 Bard-Parker blade or incisional laser. When the laser is used, eye protection should be ensured with laser-safe corneal shields.

- Retraction can be achieved with a two-pronged skin hook, four-pronged rake, and Desmarres retractor to optimize visualization. Dissection with cautery or scissors is carried through the orbicularis oculi muscle and the orbital septum until the prolapsed gland is visualized in the superotemporal anterior orbit (▶ Fig. 26.3). Palpation of the globe can help to prolapse the gland anteriorly for better visualization (▶ Fig. 26.4).
  - Often, there can be expansion of fat from the central fat pad overlying the gland, and most surgeons recommend resection of this fat with cautery or excision with scissors before manipulation of the lacrimal gland.[3]
- Treatment is based on the degree of LGP:
  - If mild prolapse, 2 mm or less, is seen when the lacrimal gland is identified, cautery of the surrounding capsule and soft tissues allow a small amount of retraction of the lacrimal gland.[2]
  - If moderate (3–5 mm) to severe (6 mm or more) LGP is found, suture repositioning is recommended.
    - Either a 5–0 or 6–0 nonabsorbable monofilament (Ethilon nylon) or absorbable braided suture (Polysorb or Vicryl) is used to make two passes through the orbital lobe of the lacrimal gland (▶ Fig. 26.5).
    - The suture is passed through the periosteum of the lacrimal fossa, posterior to orbital rim (▶ Fig. 26.6).
    - The suture is tied off to secure and to reposition the lacrimal gland (▶ Fig. 26.7).
    - Retropulsion of the globe with demonstrated reduced gland prolapse can be used to confirm proper suture suspension and gland repositioning.
- Once the suture repositioning is achieved, the upper eyelid skin is redraped in the proper position. The orbicularis oculi muscle can be closed with a 6–0 absorbable suture. The eyelid skin incision is closed with a running or interrupted absorbable gut or nonabsorbable suture (▶ Fig. 26.8).

26.6 Expert Tips/Pearls/ Suggestions

- Basal tear secretion test is recommended at preoperative evaluation to document baseline tear production.

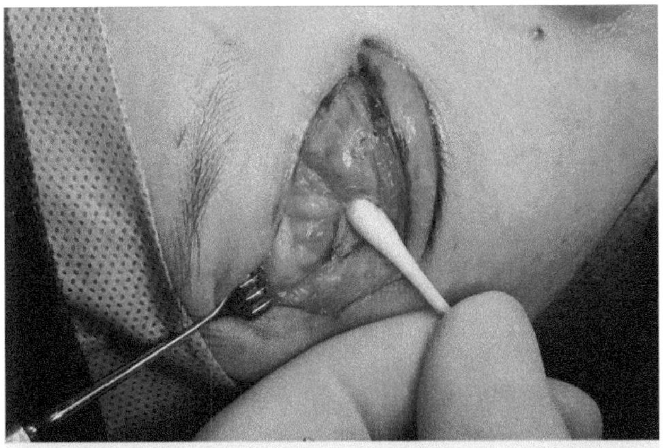

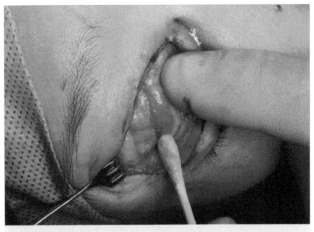

Fig. 26.3 Careful dissection through a superior eyelid crease incision and posterior to the orbital septum with adequate retraction reveals a prolapsed lacrimal gland.

Fig. 26.4 Palpation of the globe results in further anterior prolapse of the lacrimal gland and aids with visualization.

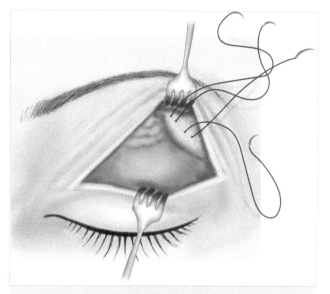

Fig. 26.5 One or two sutures (nylon or polypropylene) are placed through the tip of the orbital portion of the lacrimal gland.

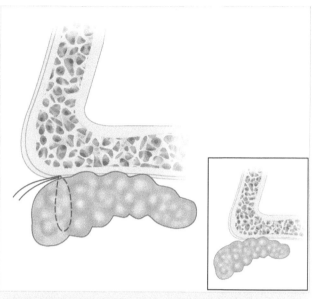

Fig. 26.7 When the suture is tied, the lacrimal gland is reposited back into the orbit.

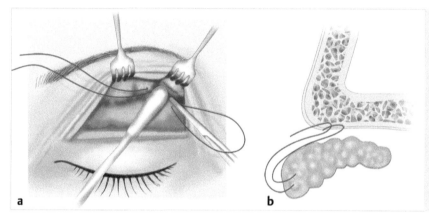

Fig. 26.6 The suture is passed through the periosteum of the lacrimal gland fossa behind the orbital rim. Retraction of the gland to reposit it (a) and plicate it within the orbital rim (b).

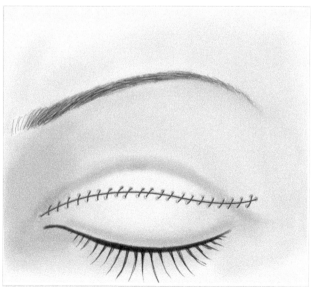

Fig. 26.8 The upper eyelid wound is closed in the standard fashion.

- Similar to other surgeries where an opening in the orbital septum is created, care must be taken to achieve judicious hemostasis to prevent postoperative orbital hemorrhage.
- Because of its anatomic proximity to the globe, the globe can be gently palpated intraoperatively to prolapse the lacrimal gland anteriorly for easier identification (▸ Fig. 26.4).
- Once the fixation suture has been passed through to secure the anterior tip of the lacrimal gland, the gland can be retracted into the orbit with a small ribbon retractor or the handle of a forceps to make passage of the suture needle through the interior edge of the superotemporal orbital rim periosteum easier (▸ Fig. 26.6).

26.7 Postoperative Management and Complications (▸ Fig. 26.9)

- Ice is applied to the operative site for 48 hours, and ophthalmic ointment is applied to the incision.
- Care must be taken to observe for postoperative hemorrhage, which could potentially form in the retrobulbar space and

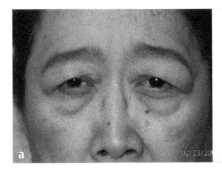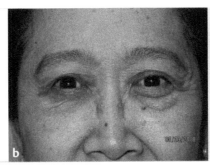

Fig. 26.9 A 78-year-old woman before (a) and after (b) lacrimal gland repositioning and bilateral upper eyelid ptosis repair, blepharoplasty, and AIRO eyebrow elevation. (These images are provided courtesy of Michael A. Burnstine, MD.)

cause permanent vision loss. It is imperative to review postoperative precautions of worsening pain or vision loss with the patient so that any emergencies can be identified and treated as soon as possible.

- Eye rubbing should be avoided in the postoperative period, and often protective eye shields at night are recommended to avoid dehiscence of the sutures in the patients' sleep. This is especially important in patients with sleep apnea who have increased periorbital laxity of the soft tissues.

References

[1] Jordan DR, Germer BA, Anderson RL, Morales L. Lacrimal gland prolapse in craniosynostosis syndromes and poor function congenital ptosis. Ophthalmic Surg. 1990; 21(2):97–101

[2] Massry GG. Prevalence of lacrimal gland prolapse in the functional blepharoplasty population. Ophthal Plast Reconstr Surg. 2011; 27(6):410–413

[3] Beer GM, Kompatscher P. A new technique for the treatment of lacrimal gland prolapse in blepharoplasty. Aesthetic Plast Surg. 1994; 18(1):65–69

Section IV Myogenic Ptosis

4

27 Myogenic Ptosis: Etiology and Management

Jessica R. Chang

Abstract

Myogenic ptosis refers to a process intrinsic to the levator palpebrae superioris muscle, as opposed to its innervation or connective tissue (aponeurosis). This chapter introduces static and progressive forms of myogenic ptosis and an overview of their evaluation and management, with more detailed exploration in the following chapters.

Keywords: myogenic (myopathic) ptosis, congenital ptosis

27.1 Introduction

Myogenic ptosis, also known as myopathic ptosis, refers to a process intrinsic to the retractor muscle of the upper eyelid, the levator palpebrae superioris (LPS), as opposed to its innervation or connective tissue (aponeurosis). There are both static and progressive forms of myogenic ptosis, which generally correlate with congenital and acquired, respectively (▶ Table 27.1). In each form, the palpebral fissure and margin reflex distance 1 (MRD1) are diminished. The upper eyelid crease may be absent, but when present, the margin crease distance (from upper eyelid margin to crease in downgaze) is generally normal and the margin fold distance (from eyelid margin to fold in primary gaze [MFD]) is increased. The palpebral fissure on downgaze is increased in congenital ptosis, and the Bell phenomenon (upward movement of the eye with eyelid closure) is affected in progressive myopathic ptosis. This chapter highlights the

more common specific etiologies of myogenic ptosis in each of these two groups and briefly reviews their presentation and management.

27.2 Static Myogenic Ptosis

Simple congenital ptosis, an isolated developmental abnormality in the levator muscle, is by far the most common presentation of static myogenic ptosis, affecting up to 0.18% of the population.[1] It may be bilateral, but most cases are unilateral, with a slight left-sided predominance (55%).[2] Most often congenital ptosis is sporadic, but it may also be familial.[1,2] Histopathology shows fibrosis of the LPS with decreased muscle fibers, although the exact pathogenesis remains unclear. Theories include disordered muscle development and/or innervation or even birth trauma–induced levator dehiscence.[1,3]

Congenital ptosis may also be associated with congenital abnormalities in other extraocular muscles, for example, in monocular elevation deficiency (previously known as double elevator palsy), and congenital fibrosis of the extraocular muscles (CFEOM).

Congenital ptosis also forms one component of blepharophimosis ptosis epicanthus inversus syndrome and may be present in several other developmental craniofacial syndromes such as Noonan syndrome, Saethre–Chotzen syndrome, and lymphedema–distichiasis syndrome (see Chapter 32).[4]

The management of congenital ptosis depends on many factors, including the severity and laterality of the ptosis, the function of the levator muscle (levator excursion), and the presence or risk of amblyopia. Unilateral ptosis poses a great risk for deprivational or anisometropic amblyopia, but bilateral ptosis may still cause significant astigmatism and amblyopia. Surgical repair is guided primarily by levator excursion and includes conjunctivomullerectomy for levator excursion greater than 10 mm, external levator advancement/resection for levator excursion greater than 4 mm, and frontalis suspension procedures for levator excursion less than 4 mm (▶ Table 27.1). If the Bell phenomenon is compromised, such as in CFEOM, more conservative surgery is indicated.

27.3 Progressive Myogenic Ptosis

Acquired forms of myogenic ptosis that progress over time consist mostly of genetic diseases. The levator, orbicularis, and extraocular muscles have slightly different physiology than other striated skeletal muscles; therefore, only certain myopathies cause ptosis, and many common muscular dystrophies do not affect eyelid or eye movements.[5] When suspecting a progressive myogenic ptosis, it is important to obtain a family

Table 27.1 Summary of myogenic ptosis

Myogenic ptosis	Static (congenital)	Progressive
Palpebral fissure (primary gaze)	Decreased	Decreased
Palpebral fissure (downgaze)	Increased	Variable
MRD1	Decreased	Decreased
MCD	Normal or absent crease	Normal
MFD	Increased	Increased
Bell's phenomenon	Usually normal[a]	Decreased
Surgical options LE < 4 mm	FS	FS or SB
LE 4–10 mm	LR or LA	LA, LR, or SB
LE > 10 mm	LA or MMCR	LA, MMCR, or SB

Abbreviations: FS, frontalis suspension; LA, levator advancement; LE, levator excursion; LR, levator resection; MCD, margin crease distance, in downgaze; MFD, margin fold distance, in primary gaze; MMCR, Müller's muscle–conjunctival resection; MRD1, margin reflex distance 1; SB, supramaximal blepharoplasty.

[a]Some congenital cases have associated ophthalmoplegia as well and also have reduced Bell's phenomenon.

history, although variable penetrance may obscure a hereditary pattern or mutations may be sporadic. Rarely, toxic processes affecting muscles have also been noted to cause a progressive myogenic ptosis, such as HIV medication–induced myopathy.[6,7] Myositis is similarly rare as a cause of acquired myogenic ptosis and can be distinguished by associated pain, timing of onset, and imaging findings.[8] Most commonly, progressive myogenic ptosis results from chronic progressive external ophthalmoplegia (CPEO), oculopharyngeal muscular dystrophy (OPMD), and myotonic dystrophy type 1 (MD1).

CPEO results from a variety of genetic defects that affect mitochondrial function. Patients typically present in young adulthood (age 18–40 years) with progressive weakening of the extraocular muscles, levator, and orbicularis oculi. Pupil reactivity is preserved. CPEO most often results from a sporadic mutation in genes affecting mitochondrial function. The condition may also be hereditary, showing a maternal inheritance pattern when the mitochondrial DNA is affected or autosomal inheritance (recessive or dominant) when the nuclear DNA is affected. Diagnosis is confirmed by muscle biopsy, classically showing ragged red fibers and cytochrome c oxidase deficiency.[9]

CPEO may occur in isolation or as part of a mitochondrial syndrome (sometimes called "PEO plus"). Kearns–Sayre syndrome, for example, features a pigmentary retinopathy, cardiac conduction defects, elevated cerebrospinal fluid protein, and cerebellar ataxia.[9] Other forms of CPEO feature pigmentary retinopathy as well, and some may also have optic neuropathy. Peripheral neuropathy is a feature of certain named syndromes, including sensory ataxic neuropathy, dysarthria, and ophthalmoplegia,[10,11] and mitochondrial neurogastrointestinal encephalomyopathy (MNGIE). In addition to ptosis and ophthalmoplegia, MNGIE presents with gastrointestinal dysmotility, peripheral demyelinating neuropathy, and leukoencephalopathy.[12] There has also been report of CPEO symptoms associated with certain mutations in OPA1, the gene involved in dominant optic atrophy, another mitochondrial disease.[9]

OPMD is an autosomal dominant or recessive condition associated with trinucleotide expansion in the PABPN1 gene.[13] Patients present in middle age with progressive ptosis, dysphagia, and characteristic dysphonia. Onset prior to age 45 may indicate a more severe course, and some patients also have proximal limb weakness. Diagnosis is confirmed with genetic testing. Although approximately 60% have reduced supraduction and 40% have facial weakness, most have an adequate Bell's phenomenon.[13]

MD1, also known as Steinert disease, is also associated with a trinucleotide expansion mutation, but, unlike OPMD, it is always autosomal dominant. Genetic testing of the DMPK gene confirms the diagnosis. The number of trinucleotide repeats ranges from 50 to > 1,000 and roughly correlates with severity and age of onset.[14] There are many systemic features, including myotonia, cardiac conduction defects, and balding. The most severe cases present at birth, and these patients may additionally have intellectual disability, respiratory compromise, and marked facial weakness.[14] The classic ophthalmic finding is the "Christmas tree" cataract, affecting nearly all patients with MD1, but approximately half may also have ophthalmoplegia and ptosis.[5,15]

When a patient presents with progressive myogenic ptosis, appropriate work-up may include referral to other specialists and systemic testing, for example, to evaluate for potentially life-threatening cardiac arrhythmias in patients with Kearns–Sayre syndrome, or a swallow evaluation in OPMD patients.

Surgical repair of progressive myogenic ptosis is guided by the degree of ptosis, ability to protect the cornea, and levator excursion (▶ Table 27.1). For severe progressive myopathic ptosis with levator excursion less than 4 mm, management generally consists of frontalis sling procedures or upper eyelid skin-only blepharoplasty, or nonsurgical correction with ptosis crutches on spectacles.[16–18] Surgical treatment of progressive myopathic ptosis is limited by the weakened orbicularis oculi and a poor Bell's phenomenon that puts these patients at risk of lagophthalmos and exposure keratopathy, particularly in CPEO and also in MD1. Adjunctive techniques such as raising the lower eyelids to reduce lagophthalmos have also been proposed.[17,19] The following chapters explore the evaluation and management of both static and progressive myogenic ptoses in more detail.

References

[1] SooHoo JR. Davies BW, Allard FD, Durairaj VD. Congenital ptosis. Surv Ophthalmol. 2014; 59:483–492

[2] Griepentrog GJ, Diehl NN, Mohney BG. Incidence and demographics of childhood ptosis. Ophthalmology. 2011; 118(6):1180–1183

[3] Bosley TM, Abu-Amero KK, Oystreck DT. Congenital cranial dysinnervation disorders: a concept in evolution. Curr Opin Ophthalmol. 2013; 24(5):398–406

[4] Dollfus H, Verloes A. Dysmorphology and the orbital region: a practical clinical approach. Surv Ophthalmol. 2004; 49(6):547–561

[5] Aring E, Ekström AB, Tulinius M, Sjöström A. Ocular motor function in relation to gross motor function in congenital and childhood myotonic dystrophy type 1. Acta Ophthalmol. 2012; 90(4):369–374

[6] Chapman KO, Lelli G. Blepharoptosis and HAART related mitochondrial myopathy. Orbit. 2014; 33(6):459–461

[7] Pfeffer G, Côté HCF, Montaner JS, Li CC, Jitratkosol M, Mezei MM. Ophthalmoplegia and ptosis: mitochondrial toxicity in patients receiving HIV therapy. Neurology. 2009; 73(1):71–72

[8] Court JH, Janicek D. Acute unilateral isolated ptosis. BMJ Case Rep. 2015; 2015:2015

[9] Fraser JA, Biousse V, Newman NJ. The neuro-ophthalmology of mitochondrial disease. Surv Ophthalmol. 2010; 55(4):299–334

[10] Van Goethem G, Martin JJ, Dermaut B, et al. Recessive POLG mutations presenting with sensory and ataxic neuropathy in compound heterozygote patients with progressive external ophthalmoplegia. Neuromuscul Disord. 2003; 13(2):133–142

[11] Weiss MD, Saneto RP. Sensory ataxic neuropathy with dysarthria and ophthalmoparesis (SANDO) in late life due to compound heterozygous POLG mutations. Muscle Nerve. 2010; 41(6):882–885

[12] Hirano M. Mitochondrial neurogastrointestinal encephalopathy disease. In: Adam MP, Ardinger HH, Pagon RA, et al, eds. GeneReviews® [Internet]. Seattle, WA: University of Washington, Seattle; 2005 [Updated January 14, 2016]. Available at: https://www.ncbi.nlm.nih.gov/books/NBK1179/

[13] Trollet C, Gidaro T, Klein P, et al. Oculopharyngeal Muscular Dystrophy. In: Adam MP, Ardinger HH, Pagon RA, et al, eds. GeneReviews® [Internet]. Seattle (WA): University of Washington, Seattle; 2001 [Updated February 20, 2014]. Available at: https://www.ncbi.nlm.nih.gov/books/NBK1126/

[14] Bird TD. Myotonic dystrophy type 1. In: Adam MP, Ardinger HH, Pagon RA, et al, eds. GeneReviews® [Internet]. Seattle (WA): University of Washington, Seattle; 1999 [Updated October 22, 2015]. Available at: https://www.ncbi.nlm.nih.gov/books/NBK1165/

[15] Ikeda KS, Iwabe-Marchese C, França MC, Jr, Nucci A, Carvalho KM. Myotonic dystrophy type 1: frequency of ophthalmologic findings. Arq Neuropsiquiatr. 2016; 74(3):183–188

[16] Burnstine MA, Putterman AM. Upper blepharoplasty: a novel approach to improving progressive myopathic blepharoptosis. Ophthalmology. 1999; 106 (11):2098–2100

[17] Doherty M, Winterton R, Griffiths PG. Eyelid surgery in ocular myopathies. Orbit. 2013; 32(1):12–15

[18] Vemuri S, Christianson MD, Demirci H. Correcting myogenic ptosis accompanying extraocular muscle weakness: The "Bobby Pin" procedure. Orbit. 2016; 35(5):267–270

[19] Holck DE, Dutton JJ, DeBacker C. Lower eyelid recession combined with ptosis surgery in patients with poor ocular motility. Ophthalmology. 1997; 104(1): 92–95

28 Static Myogenic Ptosis: Evaluation and Management

Jeremy Tan, Jill A. Foster

Abstract

Static myogenic ptosis can be caused by a variety of congenital or syndromic conditions that have levator muscle maldevelopment. The most common type of static myogenic ptosis is congenital ptosis, which is present at birth. Other causes include blepharophimosis ptosis epicanthus inversus syndrome, congenital fibrosis of the extraocular muscles, monocular elevation deficiency syndrome (formerly known as double elevator palsy), Marcus Gunn jaw-winking ptosis, Duane retraction syndrome, and traumatic ptosis. Here, we discuss evaluation and surgical management.

Keywords: congenital ptosis, amblyopia, frontalis suspension, levator resection, blepharophimosis

28.1 Introduction

Static myogenic ptosis is a unilateral or bilateral condition characterized by a stable decreased vertical palpebral fissure (PF) and margin reflex distance 1 (MRD1) present at birth. The margin crease distance (MCD) and margin fold distance (MFD) may be less distinct, absent, or elevated (▶ Fig. 28.1) compared to normal eyelid findings. A characteristic of the congenitally ptotic eyelid is that the eyelid is typically elevated in downgaze compared to the less affected or normal eyelid (▶ Fig. 28.2). There is a significant decrease in levator excursion (LE) leading to a lowered position of the upper eyelid in upgaze and diminished inferior corneal limbus to margin (margin limbal distance: MLD) (▶ Fig. 28.3). Histopathologic investigation demonstrates displacement of normal striated muscle fibers by fibrous and fatty tissue, leading to poor contraction and reduced elasticity of the levator palpebrae superioris (LPS) muscle complex.[1] Ultimately, the position of the eyelid in primary gaze, the integrity of the ocular movements, and the severity of the levator complex dysgenesis and resultant diminished levator muscle excursion dictate management.

Management of static myogenic ptosis deserves special consideration due to the young age of the affected patients. The congenitally ptotic eyelid puts the affected eye at risk of amblyopia. Congenital ptosis may induce astigmatism leading to refractive amblyopia or may occlude the visual axis causing deprivational amblyopia. Additionally, as congenital ptosis may lead to a compensatory chin-up position, these patients are at risk for ocular torticollis and postural problems. Correction of ptosis protects visual development, enlarges the visual field, and improves cosmesis.

28.2 Causes and Syndromic Associations of Static Myopathic Ptosis

Static myopathic ptosis may be separated into isolated congenital ptosis, static myopathic ptoses with associated periocular abnormalities, and aberrant innervation syndromes. Clinicians should be aware of these associated syndromes as they may require adjustment of treatment plans, offering genetic counseling, and management of systemic complications. This section discusses each of these static myopathic ptoses. Progressive myopathic syndromes are discussed in Chapter 32.

28.2.1 Isolated Congenital Ptosis

The most common cause of a static congenital ptosis is idiopathic maldevelopment of the LPS muscle, as in simple congenital ptosis. Congenital ptosis occurs in as many as 1 out of 842 births with the left side more commonly affected at 55%.[2] The

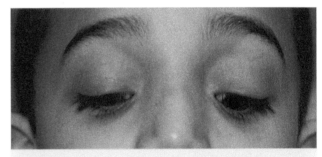

Fig. 28.2 Congenital left upper blepharoptosis in downgaze. Note the increased palpebral fissure (PF) in downgaze on the left.

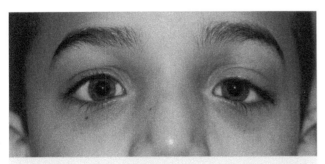

Fig. 28.1 Left upper eyelid congenital ptosis in primary gaze. Note the decreased left palpebral fissure (PF), decreased left margin reflex distance 1 (MRD1), increased left margin fold distance (MFD), and frontalis activation left greater than right.

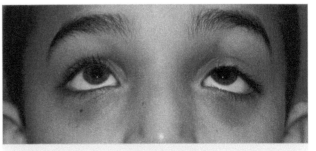

Fig. 28.3 Congenital ptosis in upgaze. The levator excursion (LE) was 16 mm on the right side and 6 to 7 mm on the involved left side. The left margin limbal distance (MLD) is diminished.

degree of upper eyelid ptosis and LE varies. While most cases of isolated congenital ptosis are sporadic, both autosomal dominant and X-linked inheritance patterns have been described for isolated congenital ptosis.[3,4] Management depends on the degree of ptosis, LE, and corneal protective mechanisms.

28.2.2 Static Myopathic Ptosis with Associated Periocular Anomalies

These disorders include blepharophimosis ptosis epicanthus inversus syndrome (BPES), congenital fibrosis of the extraocular muscles (CFEOM), and monocular elevation deficiency. The periocular anomalies can be further titrated as BPES is associated with other eyelid and midface anomalies, whereas CFEOM and monocular elevation deficiency are associated with disorders of the extraocular muscles.

Blepharophimosis Ptosis Epicanthus Inversus Syndrome

BPES is an inherited constellation of midface abnormalities accompanying ptosis. The prevalence is unknown. People with this condition have a narrowed horizontal eyelid opening (horizontal phimosis), ptosis, vertical shortening of the lower eyelid, and an upward fold of the skin of the lower eyelid near the inner corner of their eye (epicanthus inversus). In addition, there is telecanthus, an increased distance between the medial canthi (▶ Fig. 28.4). People with BPES may also have a broad nasal bridge, low set ears, or shortened distance between the nose and lip (short philtrum).

A mutation in the *FOXL2* gene causes BPES types I and II.[5] The *FOXL2* gene creates a protein that is active in the eyelids and ovaries, and it is likely involved in the normal development of the eyelid muscles. Mutations that lead to the complete loss of FOXL2 protein function often cause BPES I. These more severe mutations impair the regulation of eyelid development and various activities in the ovaries, which result in the above eyelid abnormalities and accelerated ovarian cell maturation and premature death of the egg cells. Type II mutations, which result in partial loss of the FOXL2 protein function, present with the eyelid abnormalities with no premature ovarian failure.[5] Genetic counseling should be considered for affected individuals of childbearing age, and reproductive fertility counseling may be an additional consideration depending on subtypes identified.

Because the ptosis is typically severe, surgical intervention for amblyopia-inducing ptosis is encouraged as an early intervention to improve visual development. In rare cases, the medial canthal position may also limit horizontal visual fields. Medial canthoplasties may be considered in a simultaneous or a staged fashion with ptosis correction. When ptosis repair and medial canthal repositioning are performed simultaneously, the traction on the medial canthal area may compete with the vertical vector to lift the eyelids.

While some aspects of surgical reconstruction are best accomplished at younger ages, there are also times when it is prudent to allow tissues to grow and develop prior to cosmetic alteration while operating to optimize visual function in the more immediate setting. The surgeon makes an individual judgment for each patient on whether to perform the surgeries simultaneously or sequentially.

Congenital Fibrosis of the Extraocular Muscles

CFEOM is a condition that presents with congenital ptosis and decreased ocular motility. There are five presentations: CFEOM types 1, 2, 3, Tukel syndrome, and CFEOM3 with polymicrogyria. Furthermore, there are at least eight genetically identified strabismus syndromes (CFEOM1A, CFEOM1B, CFEOM2, CFEOM3A, CFEOM3B, CFEOM3C, Tukel syndrome, and CFEOM3 with polymicrogyria). CFEOM1 is the most common and affects 1 in 230,000 people. CFEOM types 1 and 3 are autosomal dominant. In CFEOM1A and CFEOM3B, the problem is a pathogenic variant in the gene *KIF21A*. *KIF21A* is responsible for kinesin, which is an essential cellular transport protein with a pivotal role in the development of the nerves in the face and head.[6] In CFEOM1B and the other CFEOM3 variants (A, C, and type 3 with polymicrogyria), problems with the *TUBB3* and *TUBB2B* genes have been identified.[6–8] CFEOM type 2 is inherited in an autosomal recessive pattern and associated with mutations in the *PHOX2A* gene, which is involved in the development of cranial nerves III and IV.[9] Tukel syndrome's inheritance is consistent with an autosomal recessive pattern; however, no definitive pathogenic genetic loci have been elucidated. Current research suggests the problem lies in chromosome 21.[10]

Clinically, the syndromes affect both eyes to varying degrees, are congenital and nonprogressive, most often involve the superior rectus, and demonstrate variable limitation of horizontal

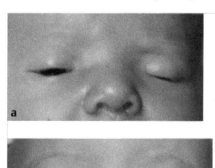
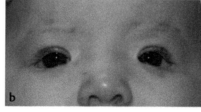
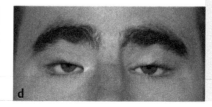

Fig. 28.4 (a–c) Initial presentation of BPES in female infant, 1-week postoperative appearance after bilateral frontalis sling, 8 weeks postoperative appearance. **(d)** The same patient's father who had previous surgeries.

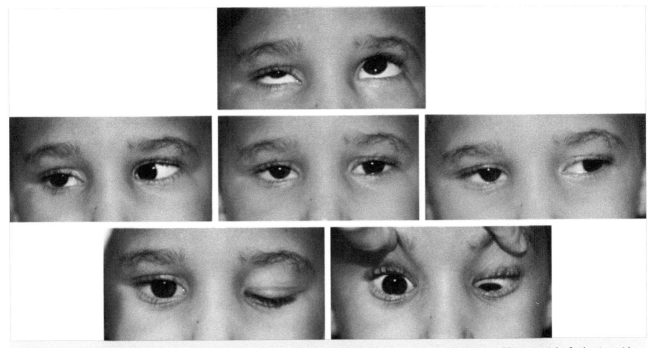

Fig. 28.5 Congenital fibrosis of the extraocular muscles. Note the motility deficits of the right eye in abduction, adduction, and infraduction with relatively full supraduction. In primary gaze, there is relatively symmetric PF, MRD1, and MRD2. The asymmetry in appearance lies in increased inferior scleral show and more obstructed right cornea due to a right hypertropia in primary gaze. LE is minimal on the right.

gaze (▶ Fig. 28.5). Ocular alignment and head posture are variable, but often the affected eye(s) are held in a more downward gaze in primary position causing a chin-up posture due to the relatively unopposed inferior rectus. Type 1 has no other associated findings, while type 2 may also have retinal dysfunction. Type 3 CFEOM may present with more asymmetry between the two eyes as well as variable intellectual and social disability, facial weakness, vocal cord paralysis, Kallmann syndrome, cyclic vomiting, spasticity, and progressive sensorimotor axonal polyneuropathy. Tukel syndrome presents like type 3 CFEOM along with postaxial (towards the ulnar fifth digit) oligodactyly or oligosyndactyly. Finally, CFEOM type 3 with polymicrogyria will also present with intellectual disability, polymicrogyria, and microcephaly.[10]

As eyelid position may change with the alteration of extraocular muscles, strabismus surgery should precede eyelid surgery in patients with CFEOM. Ptosis repair is conservative because poor LE, limited extraocular motility, and poor Bell's phenomenon increase the risk for postoperative corneal exposure.

Monocular Elevation Deficiency

Monocular elevation deficiency, previously known as double elevator palsy, is another form of strabismus that can affect eyelid position. First described by White and coined as double elevator palsy by Dunlap, this disorder of ocular motility is characterized by the inability of the affected eye to elevate in any field of gaze.[11,12] The initial etiology was thought to be from paresis of the superior rectus and the inferior oblique (the eyelid elevators), leading to the disorder's moniker. Further studies have demonstrated a component of fibrosis of the ipsilateral inferior rectus muscle, and thus, the name monocular elevation deficiency is more descriptive.[13] There may also be a supranu-

clear basis of the motility dysfunction.[13] The condition is not known to be hereditary. The ptosis present in this syndrome is often a combination of pseudoptosis and true ptosis, as the eyelid position often follows the hypotropic eye.[14] Surgical treatment of the underlying strabismus should, therefore, be addressed prior to elevating the eyelid.[15] When the abnormal lid position is purely pseudoptosis from the relative hypotropia of the involved eye, strabismus correction may obviate the need for eyelid repositioning.

28.2.3 Congenital Ptosis with Aberrant Innervation

Found in association with congenital ptosis, there are two syndromes that involve aberrant innervation (miswiring of cranial nerve function). These include Marcus Gunn jaw-winking (MGJW) and Duane retraction syndrome (DRS). Both are discussed below.

Marcus Gunn Jaw-Winking Syndrome

This phenomenon was first described by Robert Marcus Gunn in 1883 as unilateral ptosis associated with synkinetic eyelid movement with either the internal or, more commonly, the external pterygoid muscle.[16] This clinical finding is most likely due to a cross-wiring of cranial nerve III with the motor branches of the mandibular division of cranial nerve 5 (V3) (▶ Fig. 28.6).[17] Most histopathologic studies of the LPS support the aberrant innervation hypothesis as the cause of ptosis, as most studies show normal striated muscle rather than fatty infiltration as in the other forms of static ptosis.[1]

Management of MGJW ptosis is nuanced. Reducing visual axis occlusion and resulting amblyopia is paramount. However, addressing the jaw-wink phenomenon takes further discussion

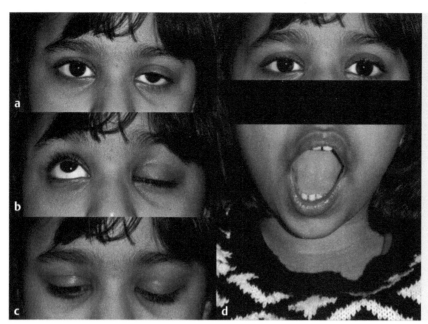

Fig. 28.6 Marcus Gunn jaw-wink. **(a)** Primary gaze, **(b)** upgaze, and **(c)** downgaze displaying the affected side lid position without activation of the jaw muscles. **(d)** Position of the involved lid elevates with jaw opening and deviation to the contralateral side, revealing the synkinesis with the ipsilateral left external pterygoid muscle.

because eliminating or decreasing the "wink" can only be accomplished by weakening the contraction of the levator complex, a seeming contradiction in an eyelid that is already ptotic.

Some surgeons favor leaving the jaw-wink mechanism intact as some patients adapt subtle jaw movements to mitigate the eyelid movement. Here, the goal would be better symmetry of eyelid height in primary gaze when the pterygoid is at rest. However, as the new position of the eyelid is "set higher," when pterygoid is activated, overelevation of the eyelid occurs with a fluttering of increased superior scleral show. If this is the treatment chosen, good preoperative counseling must be given to set appropriate expectations. In the child whose eyelid is in an amblyogenic position, and when the family is reluctant to take on the risks of more anatomically disturbing (but potentially more cosmetically appealing) surgeries, this choice is an appropriate compromise.

On the other hand, if decreasing synkinetic movement is a definite goal of the patient and family, disabling of the levator muscle must be incorporated into the surgery. There are surgical options to disable the levator, including release and recession of the levator aponeurosis from the tarsal plate, myectomy above Whitnall's ligament, or full extirpation of the levator aponeurosis complex.[18] These choices are influenced by the magnitude of the wink and surgeon preference.

Some authors favor operating solely on the aberrant side by disabling the affected levator muscle and inserting a frontalis sling. This limits surgery to the affected eyelid. This would lessen the synkinetic movement in the affected eye by creating unilateral ptosis with poor LE, and then treating the ptosis with a frontalis suspension. However, symmetry in movement and possibly contour may be less than desired when one lid is controlled by the levator complex and the other by the frontalis muscle. The shortcomings of unilateral frontalis sling surgery will be discussed in Chapter 30.

There are also surgeons who prefer bilateral levator disabling with frontalis sling surgery with the goal of complete patient control and symmetry.[17] However, the surgeon and family must accept sacrificing the normal levator muscle on the unaffected side and causing an iatrogenic ptosis in order to achieve this endpoint. The final outcome, though maximally symmetric in facial movement, is still bilaterally abnormal in eyelid function.

The decision-making in surgical management is based on the degree of ptosis and potential amblyopia, magnitude of jaw-winking, and thorough discussion with the patient and family to assess their goals.

Duane Retraction Syndrome

This synkinetic strabismus phenomenon has been described as early as the 19th century, but it was in 1905 that Alexander Duane reported a case series of 54 patients with possible etiologies and management strategies.[19] It is a congenital anomaly of eye movements with variable horizontal deficits, narrowing of the PF due to globe retraction on attempted adduction, with variable upshoots or downshoots. It has most recently been categorized as a congenital cranial dysinnervation disorder (CCDD) with a problem in the abducens nerve communication with the lateral rectus muscle.[20] This may be the primary absence of innervation leading to fibrosis of the receiving muscle or a secondary problem due to aberrant innervation from other cranial nerves. CCDDs are nonprogressive and often have abnormal bony associations.[21]

There are several classifications of DRS based on abnormal cocontractions, electromyogram analysis, or overall clinical presentation.[20] There are three types of clinical presentations:
- Type 1 absent to markedly limited abduction with relatively normal adduction.
- Type 2 absent to markedly limited adduction with relatively normal abduction.
- Type 3 absent to markedly limited abduction and adduction.

Variably present is a primary esotropia or exotropia with compensatory head turn. Moreover, variably present is the globe retraction with upshoots and downshoots, though always in attempted adduction. From the ptosis perspective, it is the globe retraction that induces narrowing of the PF. Isenberg and

Urist found that about 52% of all DRS had lowering of the upper lid along with the elevation of the lower lid.[22] Kekunnaya et al describe a grading system for the retraction from 0 (no narrowing) to 4 (≥ 75% narrowing).[23]

Surgical goals in the treatment of DRS are improvement of ocular alignment in primary gaze, correction of head posture, improvement of duction limitations, decrease in globe retraction along with upshoots or downshoots, and expansion of the field of binocularity.[20] Focusing on the lid malpositions, direct surgery on the levator (or lower lid retractors) is generally not indicated as it is the cocontraction of the medial and lateral rectus muscles that pulls the globe inward and draws the lids together. Therefore, recession of these muscles helps relieve the retraction leading to less draw on the lids. The amount of recession needed may be large and possibly require fixation to the surrounding periosteum.[24] Correction of primary position imbalance must also be considered while performing these recessions. Adults may need larger recessions due to fibrosis of the muscles due to the longer presence of synkinetic cocontraction.[25]

28.2.4 Trauma

Traumatic injuries to the levator muscle may also cause static myogenic ptosis. In these cases, accompanying tissue injuries should be evaluated in the context of a full ophthalmic examination. Poor visual acuity, pupillary abnormalities, or increased intraocular pressures may suggest intracranial, orbital, optic nerve, or globe compromise. Extraocular motility evaluation may elicit potential cranial neuropathies or orbital fractures with entrapment. Careful inspection of the globe for lacerations or other associated injuries must be performed.

The severity of the damage to the levator muscle may have a wide range of effect on eyelid position, from minor cosmetic asymmetry to complete ptosis. The underlying pathophysiology of traumatic ptosis is variable and may result from direct avulsion of the levator muscle or aponeurosis, alterations in the action of the muscle from anatomic disruption due to fractures of the orbital roof or orbital foreign bodies, postcontusional ptosis, cicatricial changes, neurogenic injury, or postsurgical ptosis.[26] In the adult patient with traumatic ptosis, surgery should be delayed until the eyelid position and LE have stabilized, which may take 6 to 12 months. In the pediatric patient, traumatic ptosis may put the patient at risk for amblyopia, which necessitates careful monitoring of vision. Part-time occlusive therapy may help to prevent amblyopia while waiting for surgical correction decisions (▶ Fig. 28.7, ▶ Fig. 28.8).

28.3 History

Obtaining a thorough history of present illness, including birth history, and family history of ptosis is critical to the comprehensive management of congenital ptosis to help make the correct diagnosis.

28.3.1 Personal History of Ptosis

Evaluation of pediatric ptosis begins with collecting information about the onset, degree, duration, and stability of the eyelid changes. A systemic history, particularly of other congenital anomalies in the child, or family history of congenital anomalies is useful. Although static congenital ptosis is present at birth, it may not become obvious until the child grows and becomes more interactive. Review of historical photographs may display subtle changes that can be helpful to point out to parents. Progression or extreme variability in eyelid position points away from static congenital ptosis, and the surgeon should investigate for other etiologies of ptosis.

28.3.2 Family History of Ptosis

A family history of ptosis may be present or may be directly observed in a parent, as in BPES. Birth and medical history should also be reviewed, as these may suggest a traumatic etiology or alert the clinician to other systemic issues that would complicate surgery or anesthesia such as congenital heart anomalies.[27]

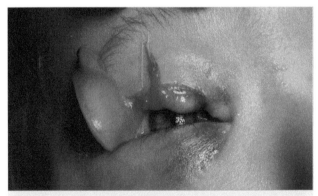

Fig. 28.7 Traumatic avulsion of the right upper eyelid. Note prolapse of orbital fat and free edge of tarsus for nearly 75% of the upper eyelid. Urgent repair was performed with reattachment of the levator edge to the superior tarsus, reanastomosis of the anterior medial canthal tendon with medial canthopexy to reapproximate the posterior limb of the avulsed tendon to the periosteum.

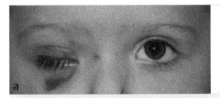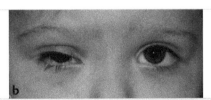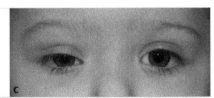

Fig. 28.8 (a) One-week postoperative result after repair of complex lid avulsion in ▶ Fig. 28.7. Right MRD1 of – 3 mm with flick of LE noted. (b) Six weeks postrepair with returning LE (3–4 mm) and improved MRD1 of 0 mm. (c) The 4 months postinitial repair with improved MRD1 of 1 mm and LE of 6 to 8 mm. Further observation is planned.

28.4 The Physical Examination

In addition to a thorough history, a complete eyelid and eye examination is performed.

28.4.1 The Eyelid and Adnexal Examination

Evaluation of a pediatric patient can be challenging for those clinicians who do not evaluate children often. With the help of a toy, with or without gentle stabilization of the head, encourage the patient to visually engage with an object. This is often facilitated by lights, color, and sound. When the patient is given an interesting visual task, the clinician will be better able to judge the adaptive mechanisms of the child.

Head Positioning

An adaptive head positioning will likely be present and further drawn out by the visual target. This posture and head positioning should not be discouraged prior to surgical correction as it may be facilitating binocular development and stereoscopic vision. Alternatively, if there is no adaptive positioning and an eyelid is in an occlusive position, the impetus to proceed with surgery is hastened and likely occlusive patching of the contralateral eye will be necessary. The examiner will look for synkinetic movements, namely, a Marcus Gunn jaw-wink by having the patient wiggle the mandible from side to side, chew, or suck. Finally, observe the motility of the frontalis muscle. If there is any underlying weakness or preference noted, the surgical plan for a frontalis sling may need adjustment.

Eyelid Measurements

Standard periocular measurements for ptosis are important for evaluation, including PF, palpebral fissure in downgaze, LE measured in isolation of the frontalis muscle, MRD1 (when appropriate, before and after the instillation of phenylephrine), MCD, and MFD. As noted at the beginning of the chapter, the position of the eyelid in downgaze in the patient with static congenital ptosis may be higher due to the fibrotic changes in the levator muscle complex, limiting the elasticity of the eyelid. The MFD and MCD are important measurements for cosmetic symmetry of the eyelids. LE is the pivotal value in determining which surgical approach would best suit the patient (▶ Table 28.1).

The amount of lagophthalmos (LAG) present in gentle closure should also be estimated along with the movement and position of the globe at the time of eyelid closure (Bell's phenom-

enon). Marked LAG and poor corneal coverage necessitate a more conservative surgical approach to protect the ocular surface. Observations of chronic corneal exposure should prompt preoperative lubrication and management prior to surgery.

28.4.2 The Eye Examination

At the time when ptosis is first noted, a comprehensive eye examination is undertaken. Visual acuity is evaluated in each eye with a solid, adhesive patch placed over the contralateral eye. A young child will take every opportunity to "cheat" and "peak" around any occlusive method with moveable edges. A full sensorimotor examination should be performed to evaluate for underlying strabismus, as misalignment may need to be addressed prior to eyelid repositioning. Motility examination will aid in diagnosis of ptosis related to systemic disorders or syndromes such as DRS, myasthenia gravis, or thyroid-related ophthalmopathy. Inspection of the anterior and posterior segments is performed to detect other abnormalities such as cataracts or colobomas, which may hinder visual potential despite efforts to elevate the ptotic eyelid. Observed craniofacial or orbital dysmorphism may require the comanagement with plastic surgery, otolaryngology, or craniofacial surgeons.

Cycloplegic refraction is important. Even if the ptotic eyelid clears the pupillary margin, cycloplegic refraction may reveal anisometropic astigmatism associated with eyelid malposition. Anisometric amblyopia can be treated with refractive correction and patching, but this finding may also hasten the recommendation for surgical correction.

28.5 Management

Management in static myopathic ptosis is dictated by visual function, degree of ptosis, LE, and corneal protective mechanisms (degree of LAG, presence of Bell's phenomenon, and dry eye status).

28.5.1 Observation

Not all static congenital ptosis requires immediate surgery. If there is no frank occlusion of the pupil and the visual function of the two eyes is symmetric, serial examination may continue until there is a cause for surgical intervention. Appropriate visual development, maintained alignment, symmetric refraction, and the absence of adaptive head positioning allow the surgeon and patient to continue to observe the ptosis, and timing of the surgery remains elective. This allows tissues to grow, the child to mature, eyelid measurements to become reproducible, and neonatal anesthesia risks to minimize.

28.5.2 Timing of Surgical Intervention

There are some advantages to operating earlier in childhood: less disruption of daily routine, rapid healing, and less formed memory of surgical stress. There are landmark time periods in pediatric development that may help point to the appropriate time for surgery: in pediatric hospitals, anesthesia risks drop to normal levels at 12 months of age.[28] At 12 months of age, children move from prone to vertical navigation, and ptosis may become more disruptive to the vision. At age 4 or 5, physical

Table 28.1 Determination of surgical intervention based on the amount of levator excursion (LE)

Levator excursion	Surgical intervention
<4 mm	Frontalis suspension
4–8 mm	Frontalis suspension or levator resection
6–12 mm	Levator resection
>12 mm	Levator resection/levator aponeurosis advancement

awareness of differences intrudes on social development. As children approach the teenage years, ptosis surgery under local anesthetic becomes a possibility, and aesthetic concerns impact decision-making.

If the ptosis is amblyogenic, surgery is performed promptly. If the ptosis is moderate but not amblyogenic, 12 months of age may be appropriate for intervention. If the ptosis is mild and has minimal, if any, impact on the visual field, the family participates in the decision on when to proceed with surgery. The summer prior to kindergarten is a benchmark for optimizing the height of the eyelids to minimize social impacts of the congenital ptosis. As the patient matures, better cooperation for more accurate examination measurement as well as the ability to tolerate the procedure with local anesthesia may increase the chances of symmetric outcome.

28.5.3 The Surgical Approach

The goals of surgery are unobstructed and safe visual development, cosmetic symmetry, and ocular surface protection. The method of surgical repair is based on the degree of ptosis and LE (▶ Table 28.1). In the unusual case where the LE is normal (>12 mm), a levator aponeurosis advancement may be attempted but will likely need to be advanced further as compared to the adult patient with aponeurotic ptosis. In cases where the LE is < 4 mm, a frontalis sling is used to overcome the limitations of the existing levator muscle. In patients with LE between 8 and 12 mm, the most likely choice of surgical technique is levator resection. For the pediatric patient with levator function between 4 and 8 mm, other features of the examination help guide surgical decision-making; associated motility disorder, larger degree of preoperative LAG, pre-existing corneal epithelial irregularity, good frontalis function, and ocular dominance on the side of the ptotic lid would be features that point the surgeon toward frontalis suspension.

Levator resection surgery is challenging. The goal is to achieve an excellent eyelid height and contour while protecting the ocular surface. Numerous algorithms have been developed to determine the amount of surgery to be performed. If one perfect technique existed, it is unlikely that there would be so many choices. LE and the degree of ptosis remain at the center of each of these algorithms.

In the 1960s, Berke published a series that describes ideal intraoperative eyelid height at the conclusion of surgery based on a range of LEs, summarized in ▶ Table 28.2.[29,30,31] However, there are intraoperative issues that complicate the use of this guideline such as a change in the eyelid height due to anesthetic, hematoma, or change in position of gaze. That said, even when using other more formulaic techniques for ptosis repair, Berke's intraoperative observations remain useful for intraoperative assessment of lid position.

In the 1970s, Beard provided an algorithm for a specific amount of levator aponeurosis to resect based on preoperative LE and eyelid height, summarized in ▶ Table 28.3.[32] This algorithm eliminates the use of intraoperative measurements as in Berke's technique. This nomogram is still used today by many oculofacial surgeons.

In 1985, Putterman and Sarver developed another algorithm with the addition of the MLD as a determination of LE. This is the distance between the 6 o'clock inferior corneal limbus and the eyelid margin in upgaze when relaxing the ipsilateral frontalis muscle and raising the contralateral eyelid (▶ Fig. 28.9). The difference between the involved and the uninvolved eye represents the difference in LE. This value is multiplied by 3 and will be the amount of levator to be resected. The average normal MLD of 9 mm is the reference value subtracted from to obtain the aforementioned difference (▶ Table 28.4). This algorithm does not apply to patients with vertical strabismus. Putterman compared his measurements to Berke's algorithm, and, in cases with severe discrepancy, adjusted the amount of resection be closer to Berke's.[33]

There have since been further algorithms developed, such as a simple ratio of 4 mm of resection for every 1 mm of ptosis, mentioned in a recent review.[27] A familiarity with the application of several different algorithms is beneficial. Each surgeon finds the pattern that allows him or her to obtain the most predictable results.

Table 28.3 Amount of levator resection based on amount of ptosis and levator excursion by Beard[32]

Amount of ptosis	LE	Amount of resection
2 mm (mild)	0–5 mm (poor)	22–27 mm
	6–11 mm (fair)	16–21 mm
	12 or more (good)	10–15 mm
3 mm (moderate)	0–5 mm (poor)	30 mm (maximum)
	6–11 mm (fair)	22–27 mm
	12 or more (good)	16–21 mm
4 mm or more (severe)	0–5 mm (poor)	30 mm (maximum)
	6–11 mm (fair)	25–30 mm
	12 or more (good)	25–30 mm

Table 28.2 Final intraoperative eyelid height based on levator excursion by Berke[29,30,31]

Levator excursion	Upper eyelid position on cornea
> 10 mm	3–4 mm below limbus; eyelid should rise 2–3 mm postoperatively
8–9 mm	3 mm below the limbus; eyelid should rise 1–2 mm postoperatively
6–7 mm	2 mm below limbus; no change in position
5–6 mm	1 mm below limbus; eyelid may drop 1–2 mm postoperatively

Table 28.4 Amount of levator resection to perform based on Putterman's MLD formula[33]

Unilateral blepharoptosis	(MLD normal eyelid − MLD ptotic eyelid) × 3 = amount of levator resection
Bilateral blepharoptosis	(Average normal MLD of 9 − MLD ptotic eyelid) × 3 = amount of levator resection

Abbreviation: MLD, margin limbal distance.
Note: If the patient has vertical strabismus, this measurement tool is invalid.

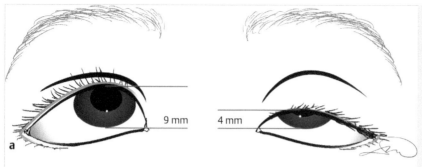

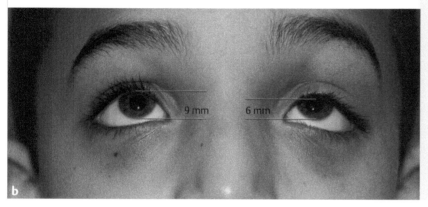

Fig. 28.9 **(a)** Illustration of MLD measurements in unilateral ptosis. The difference of 5 is multiplied by 3 indicating 15 mm of levator resection to correct the left upper eyelid ptosis. **(b)** Photograph with MLD measurements of unilateral ptosis. The difference of 3 is multiplied by 3 indicating 9 mm of levator resection to correct the left upper ptosis.

28.6 Conclusions

Diagnosing static myopathic ptosis is based on a thorough patient history, including family history, and physical examination. Management is based on the disruption of vision, degree of ptosis, LE, and assessment of corneal protective mechanisms. Surgical success is a result of a wise surgical procedure choice, excellent technical execution of the procedure, and a well-informed patient and family.

References

[1] Baldwin HC, Manners RM. Congenital blepharoptosis: a literature review of the histology of levator palpebrae superioris muscle. Ophthal Plast Reconstr Surg. 2002; 18(4):301–307

[2] Griepentrog GJ, Diehl NN, Mohney BG. Incidence and demographics of childhood ptosis. Ophthalmology. 2011; 118(6):1180–1183

[3] McMullan TF, Collins AR, Tyers AG, Robinson DO. A novel X-linked dominant condition: X-linked congenital isolated ptosis. Am J Hum Genet. 2000; 66(4): 1455–1460

[4] Pavone P, Barbagallo M, Parano E, Pavone L, Souayah N, Trifiletti RR. Clinical heterogeneity in familial congenital ptosis: analysis of fourteen cases in one family over five generations. Pediatr Neurol. 2005; 33(4): 251–254

[5] Genetics Home Reference. Blepharophimosis, ptosis, and epicanthus inversus syndrome. Available at: https://ghr.nlm.nih.gov/condition/blepharophimosis-ptosis-and-epicanthus-inversus-syndrome

[6] Whitman M, Hunter DG, Engle EC. Congenital fibrosis of the extraocular muscles. In: Adam MP, Ardinger HH, Pagon RA, Wallace SE, Bean LJH, Stephens K, Amemiya A, eds. GeneReviews®. Seattle, WA: University of Washington, Seattle; 2016

[7] Engle EC. Genetic basis of congenital strabismus. Arch Ophthalmol. 2007; 125 (2):189–195

[8] Tischfield MA, Baris HN, Wu C, et al. Human TUBB3 mutations perturb microtubule dynamics, kinesin interactions, and axon guidance. Cell. 2010; 140(1): 74–87

[9] Heidary G, Engle EC, Hunter DG. Congenital fibrosis of the extraocular muscles. Semin Ophthalmol. 2008; 23(1):3–8

[10] Genetics Home Reference. Congenital fibrosis of the extraocular muscles. Available at: https://ghr.nlm.nih.gov/condition/congenital-fibrosis-of-the-extraocular-muscles

[11] White JW. Paralysis of the superior rectus and inferior oblique muscles of the same eye. Arch Ophthalmol. 1942; 27:366–371

[12] Dunlop EA. Vertical displacement of horizontal recti. In: Symposium on Strabismus Transactions of the New Orleans Academy of Ophthalmology. St Louis, MO: Mosby; 1971:307–329

[13] Bagheri A, Sahebghalam R, Abrishami M. Double elevator palsy, subtypes and outcomes of surgery. J Ophthalmic Vis Res. 2008; 3(2):108–113

[14] Callahan MA. Surgically mismanaged ptosis associated with double elevator palsy. Arch Ophthalmol. 1981; 99(1):108–112

[15] Yurdakul NS, Ugurlu S, Maden A. Surgical treatment in patients with double elevator palsy. Eur J Ophthalmol. 2009; 19(5):697–701

[16] Gunn RM. Congenital ptosis with peculiar associated movements of the affected lid. Trans Ophthalmol Soc U K. 1883; 3:283–287

[17] Demirci H, Frueh BR, Nelson CC. Marcus Gunn jaw-winking synkinesis: clinical features and management. Ophthalmology. 2010; 117(7):1447–1452

[18] Dillman DB, Anderson RL. Levator myectomy in synkinetic ptosis. Arch Ophthalmol. 1984; 102(3):422–423

[19] Duane A. Congenital deficiency of abduction, associated with impairment of adduction, retraction movements, contraction of the palpebral fissure and oblique movements of the eye. 1905. Arch Ophthalmol. 1996; 114(10):1255–1256, discussion 1257

[20] Kekunnaya R, Negalur M. Duane retraction syndrome: causes, effects and management strategies. Clin Ophthalmol. 2017; 11:1917–1930

[21] Gutowski NJ, Ellard S. The congenital cranial dysinnervation disorders (CCDDs). Adv Clin Neurosci Rehabil. 2005; 5:8–10

[22] Isenberg S, Urist MJ. Clinical observations in 101 consecutive patients with Duane's retraction syndrome. Am J Ophthalmol. 1977; 84(3):419–425

[23] Kekunnaya R, Moharana R, Tibrewal S, Chhablani PP, Sachdeva V. A simple and novel grading method for retraction and overshoot in Duane retraction syndrome. Br J Ophthalmol. 2016; 100(11):1451–1454

[24] Mehendale RA, Dagi LR, Wu C, Ledoux D, Johnston S, Hunter DG. Superior rectus transposition and medial rectus recession for Duane syndrome and sixth nerve palsy. Arch Ophthalmol. 2012; 130(2):195–201

[25] Shauly Y, Weissman A, Meyer E. Ocular and systemic characteristics of Duane syndrome. J Pediatr Ophthalmol Strabismus. 1993; 30(3):178–183

[26] Morax S, Baudoin F, Hurbli T. [Surgery of post-traumatic ptosis]. Ann Chir Plast Esthet. 1995; 40(6):691–705

[27] Jubbal KT, Kania K, Braun TL, Katowitz WR, Marx DP. Pediatric blepharoptosis. Semin Plast Surg. 2017; 31(1):58–64

[28] Meyer HM, Thomas J, Wilson GS, de Kock M. Anesthesia-related and perioperative mortality: An audit of 8493 cases at a tertiary pediatric teaching hospital in South Africa. Paediatr Anaesth. 2017; 27(10):1021–1027

[29] Berke RN. Ophthalmic Plastic Surgery: A Manual. San Francisco, CA: American Academy of Ophthalmology and Otolaryngology; 1964:137

[30] Berke RN. Resection of the levator muscle through the external approach for congenital ptosis. Trans Pac Coast Otoophthalmol Soc Annu Meet 1964;45:207–214

[31] Berke RN. Results of resection of the levator muscle through a skin incision in congenital ptosis. AMA Arch Opthalmol. 1959; 61(2):177–201

[32] Beard C. Newer ptosis procedures. In: Ptosis. 2nd ed. St. Louis, MO: Mosby; 1976

[33] Sarver BL, Putterman AM. Margin limbal distance to determine amount of levator resection. Arch Ophthalmol. 1985; 103(3):354–356

29 Surgical Management of Levator Function Less Than 4 mm

Peter J. Dolman

Abstract

Frontalis slings are used to treat congenital or acquired ptosis with a levator palpebrae superioris excursion of less than 4 mm. Many patterns for sling placement and different materials have been reported over the past few decades. This chapter describes a simplified triangular pattern using silicone rods. The procedure is simple to perform with fewer incisions than other methods. The most common complications are undercorrection and late slippage. Fixation of the sling material to the tarsal plate using a nonabsorbable suture through an upper lid crease is preferable to stab incisions and no fixation, as the former has a better chance of creating a symmetric skin crease and avoiding upper lid lash ptosis, and it reduces the risk of recurrent ptosis from late sling slippage.

Keywords: frontalis sling, brow suspension, congenital ptosis, acquired ptosis, silicone rod, triangular pattern

29.1 Introduction

The surgical procedure commonly performed for congenital or acquired ptosis with a levator excursion of less than 4 mm is the frontalis sling, also termed "brow suspension," in which the upper eyelid is elevated by linking the tarsal plate to the frontalis muscle using a sling or an advancement flap from the frontalis muscle.[1,2] Levator resection in these cases typically is inadequate to correct the ptosis.

29.2 History of Frontalis Sling

Many variations of frontalis sling patterns, sling materials, and fixation methods have been performed through the years. A brief discussion of each follows.

29.2.1 Patterns of Sling

One of the first patterns for sling placement was the triple triangle, popularized by Jack Crawford (▶ Fig. 29.1).[3] Over the years, less elaborate patterns have been described eliminating the need for an incision in the mid-forehead region, including the double triangle, the rhomboid, and the square (▶ Fig. 29.2).[4,5] This chapter describes a simplified technique using a single triangle pattern (▶ Fig. 29.2).

29.2.2 Sling Materials

Autogenous, homologous, and alloplastic materials have been used as sling materials.[4,6,7]

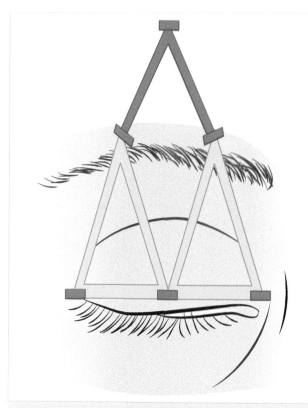

Fig. 29.1 Original three-triangle pattern with autogenous fascia lata described by Dr. Jack Crawford (*green and blue triangles*) and simplified two-triangle pattern (*green triangles*).

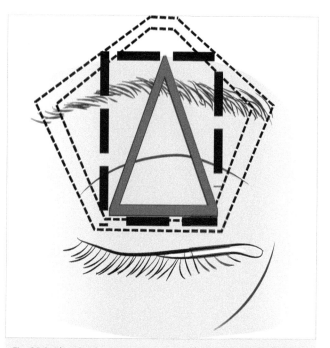

Fig. 29.2 Rhomboid pattern (*dotted outline*), square pattern (*black dashed line*), and simplified triangle technique (*red triangle*).

Autogenous tissues can be harvested from the leg (tensor fascia lata), arm (palmaris longus), and temple (temporalis fascia).[2,8,9] These are well tolerated, integrate well, and have low ptosis recurrence rates but require additional operative sites, special surgical equipment and time, and occasionally can have donor site morbidity.[7,10]

Homologous banked fascia lata avoids the need to harvest tissue but requires a tissue bank and may be less durable than autogenous choices. In addition, the risk of transmissible infections such as prion disease must be considered.

Popular alloplastic materials for frontalis slings include Mersilene polyester mesh,[11] expanded polytetrafluoroethylene (ePTFE)[12] or Gore-Tex, polypropylene (Prolene suture), supramid (polyfilament), and silicone rods.[13] These all have the benefit of avoiding extra surgical time and donor site morbidity from harvesting autogenous tissue. They are more likely to slip over time, and all of them may become exposed or cause foreign body granulomas.[11-13] Silicone rods have the benefit of inherent elasticity, which may allow better eyelid closure. A Cochrane systematic review is currently being conducted to compare different materials for frontalis slings.[14]

29.2.3 Fixation of Sling to Eyelid Tarsus

There are two common methods to fixate the distal loops of the sling material close to the eyelid margin. The first choice places small stab incisions through skin down to the tarsal surface, and the suspensory material is then drawn through the subcutaneous space using a Wright fascia needle that is threaded from one stab incision to the other (▶ Fig. 29.3a). This approach limits surgical dissection but does not allow creation of a defined lid crease. While fascia may be well integrated through this approach and limit slippage, several studies have shown a higher incidence of late slippage and recurrent ptosis in alloplastic sling cases.[1,15] In addition, upper lid lash ptosis (epiblepharon) is a common complication resulting from disruption by the sling.[16]

In the second approach, an upper lid crease incision symmetric with the opposite side is created through skin and orbicularis muscle, and the pretarsal plateau is exposed centrally approximately halfway down its width. The loops of the sling material are attached to the tarsus using nonabsorbable suture placed partial thickness (▶ Fig. 29.3b). Late slippage and secondary eyelash ptosis are less frequent with this approach. The skin is closed with two to three deep bites to the leading edge of the levator muscle without nicking the sling material, thus avoiding eyelash ptosis.[16]

29.3 Indications

- Frontalis sling is used in any form of congenital or acquired ptosis with poor levator excursion (less than or equal to 4 mm).
- Elevate the eyelid to prevent childhood amblyopia.
- Improve stereopsis in children and adults.
- Improve superior field of vision.
- Create aesthetic symmetry and so improve self-esteem.

29.4 Consequences

- Lagophthalmos at night on gentle eyelid closure.
- Reduced closure with blinking.
- Increased palpebral fissure (eyelid retraction) on downgaze, particularly noticeable in unilateral cases.
- Exacerbation of dry eye with associated discomfort or visual blurring.

29.5 Unique Considerations in Frontalis Suspension

29.5.1 Congenital Cases

A special consideration for children aged less than 8 years is the risk of deprivation amblyopia from the lid obscuring the visual axis. Young infants may require urgent surgery within a week to reduce the risk of amblyopia (▶ Fig. 29.4). The presentation of congenital ptosis with poor levator excursion may be unilateral or bilateral, and isolated or associated with a syndrome such as

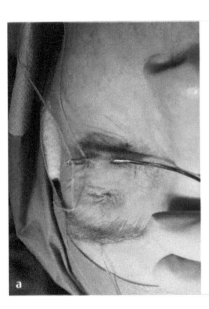
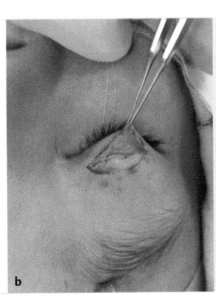

Fig. 29.3 (a) Sling passed across stab incisions close to lash line using Wright fascia needle. (b) Sling sutured in two places to tarsal plate through an upper lid skin crease incision.

Marcus Gunn jaw-wink, monocular elevation palsy, or blepharophimosis ptosis epicanthus inversus syndrome.

Marcus Gunn Jaw-Winking Ptosis

A pronounced jaw-wink may be treated by transecting the levator muscle close to Whitnall's suspensory ligament. In milder cases, the levator may be left alone as the patient often learns through practice how to avoid jaw muscle movements that precipitate the levator stimulation. Some surgeons advocate severing the opposite normal levator muscle and then placing slings in both lids, while others recommend bilateral slings without dividing the contralateral levator.[17] I leave the normal eyelid untouched but warn the patient that some asymmetry will be present, particularly with fatigue of the frontalis muscle.

Blepharophimosis Ptosis Epicanthus Inversus Syndrome

The levator slings are usually performed after the telecanthus and epicanthal folds are repaired, although recent literature has focused on one-stage surgery (▶ Fig. 29.5).[18]

29.5.2 Acquired Cases

Acquired myopathic ptoses with poor levator excursion may be a result of trauma, of a third nerve palsy, or of a heritable genetic disorder.

Genetically Inherited Myopathic Ptoses

Causes of acquired ptosis with poor levator excursion include myogenic ptosis in which the levator muscle is severely impaired from *mitochondrial myopathies, oculopharyngeal dystrophy, myotonic dystrophy,* or *other progressive myopathies* described in Chapter 31 (▶ Fig. 29.6).[19] In early mitochondrial myopathy, the levator function may be sufficiently strong (between 5 and 10 mm) to allow levator resection as repair. However, the natural history is for the disease to progress and recurrent ptosis is inevitable. Rather than subjecting the patients to repeat levator resections, many surgeons would recommend frontalis sling after the first recurrence.

Traumatic Injury

A second common category relates to poor levator function from *accidental or surgical trauma* to the muscle, its tendinous

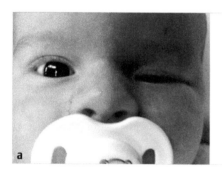
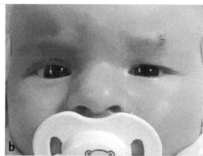

Fig. 29.4 (a) Congenital ptosis with risk of deprivation amblyopia. (b) Same patient following frontalis sling using triangle pattern; this case was complicated by an erosion of the silicone free ends through the left brow incision that required subsequent repair.

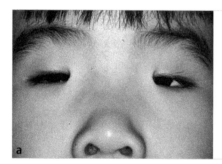
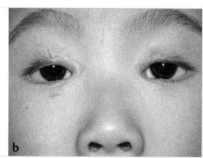

Fig. 29.5 (a) Blepharophimosis ptosis epicanthus inversus syndrome. (b) Epicanthal folds were repaired first followed by ptosis repair using a simplified frontalis sling triangle.

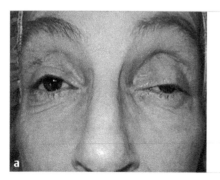
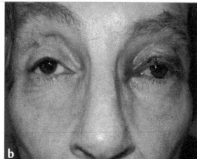

Fig. 29.6 (a) Mitochondrial myopathy with previous right frontalis triangular sling lifted just enough to clear the pupil. (b) Same patient following left frontalis sling. Each eye is performed separately to avoid bilateral corneal exposure complications.

insertion, or its innervation. Usually, a 6-month delay is recommended to allow for spontaneous improvement before selecting the procedure.

Third Nerve Palsy

Oculomotor nerve palsy may be caused by trauma, a Berry aneurysm, or a microvascular occlusion. Imaging is often necessary (*especially if the pupil is dilated*) to rule out an aneurysm. Surgery is usually delayed for 6 months to allow for spontaneous recovery of nerve function. The strabismus should be rectified as best as possible prior to planning ptosis repair.[20] A trial of taping up the affected lid allows the patient to determine if persistent diplopia will be too bothersome. Often, no surgery is performed due to intractable diplopia in all fields of gaze and poor corneal protective mechanisms.

Corneal Protective Mechanisms

Protective mechanisms such as eyelid closure, Bell's phenomenon, and tear function should be carefully assessed in acquired myogenic ptosis, as these may be suboptimal in mitochondrial myopathies and third nerve palsies. For this reason, unilateral surgery (even in cases of bilateral disease) is recommended to avoid simultaneous bilateral corneal breakdown.

29.6 Risks of the Procedure

- Undercorrection.
- Overcorrection.
- Eyelid contour abnormalities.
- Eyelash ptosis/epiblepharon.
- Penetrating ocular injury.
- Postoperative lagophthalmos.
- Postoperative exposure keratopathy.
- Worsening dry eye.
- Bradycardia or asystole from stimulating the oculocardiac reflex during the procedure, most commonly in anxious young adults.
- Sling slippage over time.

29.7 Benefits of the Procedure

- Improved visual acuity in deprivational cases.
- Improved stereopsis and restored fusion.
- Improved superior field of vision.
- Improved cosmesis and self-confidence.

29.8 Relative Contraindications

- Discontinue anticoagulants or platelet inhibitors prior to surgery upon approval of their internist, hematologist, or primary physician.
- In progressive myopathies like chronic progressive external ophthalmoplegia (CPEO), simultaneous bilateral frontalis sling surgery should be avoided because of the increased risk of corneal exposure and breakdown with the absence of a Bell's protective phenomenon in these cases.

- In patients with a third nerve palsy, the surgeon should assess whether the patient might have diplopia concerns prior to elevating the affected eyelid.

29.9 Informed Consent

Adult patients or parents of affected children must be fully informed about the benefits of the surgical procedure along with its intraoperative risks, postoperative consequences of the ptosis repair, and postoperative complications.

29.10 The Procedure

29.10.1 Surgical Supplies and Equipment

Sutures

- The 6–0 or 5–0 Prolene is used for suturing the silicone sling to the tarsus and for a lid margin retraction suture.
- The 6–0 Vicryl Rapide is used to close both the upper lid and brow cutaneous incisions in children.
- The 6–0 Prolene may be used for cutaneous closure in adults.

Cautery

Bipolar cautery and/or battery disposable hot wire cautery.

Sling Material

Silicone rods with a Watzke coupling sleeve.

Instruments

- Castroviejo needle holder.
- Straight hemostat.
- The #15 blade on Bard-Parker handle.
- Sharp Westcott scissors.
- A 0.5 toothed forceps.
- Wright fascia needle.

29.10.2 Preoperative Checklist

- Review procedure and complications with patient and with the family in children.
- Confirm and mark correct eyelid(s) for surgery.
- Ensure availability of equipment and surgical supplies, including the sling material.

29.10.3 Operative Technique

- The upper lid crease is marked in symmetry with the opposite eyelid. A 3- to 5-mm suprabrow incision is marked immediately temporal to the supraorbital notch (▶ Fig. 29.7**a**).
- Lidocaine 2% with epinephrine 1/100,000 is infiltrated subcutaneously along the upper lid crease and near the brow incision and in the region of the sling placement.
- A retraction suture is placed in the upper lid margin and held with a hemostat at the surgical drape.
- The #15 blade is used to incise the upper lid crease and dissection carried in the suborbicularis plane halfway down

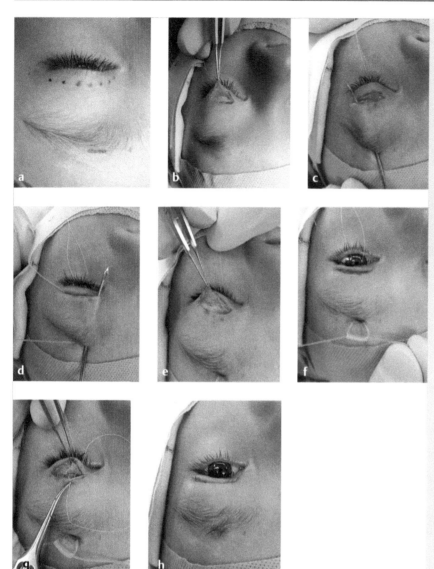

Fig. 29.7 (a) Surgical markings, including upper lid crease symmetric with opposite eyelid and brow incision just temporal to supraorbital notch. (b) Pretarsal pocket cleared to allow room for silicone sling loop. (c) Wright fascia needle passed from temporal aspect of brow wound in a postseptal plane and exiting at temporal margin of lid crease incision. (d) Needle withdrawn from the nasal aspect of the wound. (e) Polypropylene suture secures silicone rod at nasal and temporal limbus with the loop resting in a recess created in the pretarsal space. (f) Silicone at triangular apex is pulled at brow incision to ensure a pleasing contour of the eyelid. (g) A rapidly dissolving suture is used to close the upper lid crease with deep bites to the levator placed at the nasal and temporal limbus and through the silicone loop. (h) Eyelid is open at the end of the surgery but will close well when the patient is awake and after the anesthetic has worn off.

the height of the tarsus plate. Sufficient space is created centrally to accommodate the frontalis sling loop to avoid a flattened upper eyelid contour (▶ Fig. 29.7**b**).

- The suprabrow incision is created with a superior slant parallel to the hair shafts to avoid damage to the eyebrow follicles. Westcott sutures are used to create a subcutaneous pocket superior to this incision to bury the silicone coupling sleeve. Bipolar cautery controls bleeding.
- The Wright fascia needle is then passed from the temporal base of the brow wound inferiorly aiming for the lateral corneal limbus, erupting posterior to the septum through the lid crease opening (▶ Fig. 29.7**c**). The silicone rod is then passed through the eye of the fascia needle, which is withdrawn superiorly pulling the silicone rod along with it. The needle is then passed from the nasal base of the brow incision towards the nasal limbus in the postseptal plane and the other end of the silicone rod drawn up to the brow wound (▶ Fig. 29.7**d**).
- A 5–0 Prolene suture is then used to secure the silicone rod in the upper third of the tarsal plate at both the nasal and temporal limbus with the loop centrally curved inferiorly in a suborbicularis pocket (▶ Fig. 29.7**e**).

- The two ends of the silicone rods are pulled superiorly at the brow to ensure the lid opens with a pleasing contour. The two free ends of the rod are passed in opposing directions through the Watzke silicone sleeve but are not tightened yet to allow easier closure of the upper lid crease (▶ Fig. 29.7**f**).
- The crease incision is closed with three interrupted sutures, taking deep bites around the sling into the levator aponeurosis to recreate a crease line (▶ Fig. 29.7**g**). A running suture using 6–0 Prolene in adults and 6–0 Vicryl Rapide in children is used to close the eyelid crease wound (▶ Fig. 29.7**h**).
- The silicone rods are tightened symmetrically to achieve the right contour and margin fold, symmetric with the opposite side. The lid should be lifted to close to the desired height to be symmetric but should be easily closed with gentle traction. The free ends of the silicone are trimmed with approximately 4-mm tails to allow slackening of the silicone rod if overcorrected.
- The Watzke sleeve and barbs of silicone rod are buried in the pocket above the brow incision. A box suture is placed

subcutaneously at the brow and two interrupted sutures are placed. A small Steri-Strip is used to cover the brow incision. Antibiotic ointment is placed on the ocular surface and on the upper lid crease.

- A shield is used to protect the eye and its lids.

29.11 Expert Tips/Pearls/Suggestions

- A corneal protector can be used to prevent ocular penetration while passing the Wright needle.
- Care must be taken to avoid handling the silicone rod with toothed forceps or touching it with the needle as this will weaken it and possibly break it.
- Although needles are provided with the silicone rods, they are very flexible and not as consistent as the stiff Wright fascia needle in accurate placement of the silicone rod.
- A single silicone rod can be used for both sides, but only one Watzke sleeve is provided; therefore, another form of tightening would be necessary for the other lid or the Watzke sleeve may be divided in two and used on both sides.
- A suture tied around the silicone sleeve is not necessary nor is suturing of the sleeve to the underlying frontalis muscle.
- If the contour is not symmetric, the sutures holding the rod to the tarsal plates can be removed and shifted horizontally or vertically to improve the contour.
- In cases of suspected mitochondrial myopathy, a segment of orbicularis muscle can be resected without cautery and sent for mitochondrial deoxyribonucleic acid sequencing to look for large segment deletions (sporadic) or known microdeletions.[21]

29.12 Postoperative Care Checklist

- A broad-spectrum oral antibiotic (such as cephalexin).
- Tobramycin–dexamethasone ointment may be prescribed for a week to avoid infection from the implants.

- A Fox shield can be used at nighttime.
- For adults, especially with mitochondrial myopathies where the Bell's phenomenon is absent, an intentional undercorrection is preferred, and the cornea is monitored carefully and treated with frequent lubrication to avoid epithelial breakdown. Children tolerate lagophthalmos well and exposure keratopathy is seldom a complaint.

29.13 Complications and Their Management

Complications may be broken down into early and late. Their management is important.

29.13.1 Early Complications

Under- and Overcorrection

In a series review of over 75 frontalis slings using this technique performed by the author, 6% of eyelids were undercorrected, but none were overcorrected (▶ Fig. 29.8). Sling tightening may be performed through the eyebrow incision.

Exposure Keratopathy

Exposure changes arose in 15% of adult myogenic ptosis associated with mitochondrial myopathies or oculomotor palsy, largely due to concurrent lack of Bell's phenomenon from the CPEO and occasionally weak orbicularis tone.[22] No cases of corneal exposure were seen in pediatric cases, although pediatric frontalis slings may result in exposure later in adult life.[23] In these cases, more frequent lubrication is necessary. If insufficient, sling loosening may be performed.

Asymmetry and Contour Abnormalities

Approximately 86% of cases ultimately were within 1 mm of the height of the other eyelid (whether the second eyelid had been operated or not). Approximately 97% of patients or their parents were satisfied with the upper lid contour following this surgery (▶ Fig. 29.8, ▶ Fig. 29.9). In asymmetry, the sling can be

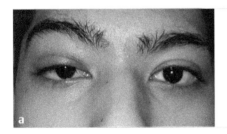
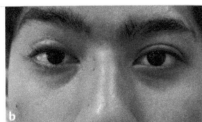

Fig. 29.8 (a) Right upper lid undercorrected by frontalis sling. (b) Sling advanced on the tarsal plate to improve height and contour.

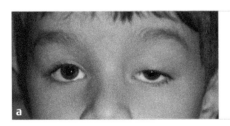
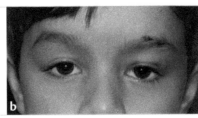

Fig. 29.9 (a) Sporadic left congenital ptosis. (b) Pleasing contour and well-defined lid crease 1 week following triangular frontalis sling.

tightened through the eyebrow and the contour can be altered through the eyelid skin crease incision.

Lash Epiblepharon

Approximately 5% of unilateral cases had a persistent lack of eyelid crease. This could be avoided by placing a deep bite from the skin to the leading edge of the levator in three places, nasal and temporal to the sling loop, and in the middle of the sling loop (▶ Fig. 29.8g).[24]

Prominent Forehead Scar

The eyelid incisions generally heal well but the thicker skin of the forehead is more prone to scarring.[4,6] The simplified triangle technique reduces the number of forehead incisions to a single 3- to 5-mm incision near the upper nasal brow margin, reducing its visibility.

Infected Sling

Infected slings need removal.

29.13.2 Late Complications

Exposure or Infection to Implant Material

While synthetic materials such as polyester mesh or ePTFE may erode through the forehead incision and occasionally form foreign body granulomas, this was rarely seen in our series using silicone rod.[4,6] This usually consisted of one or both free ends of the silicone rod protruding through the wound, and could be avoided by tucking the silicone barbs under the sleeve, and repaired by freshening the wound, trimming and repositioning the free ends, and closing the wound in layers (▶ Fig. 29.7). One child in the series had a contact sensitivity to the material requiring sling removal.

Nonresolving Corneal Exposure Keratopathy

The sling may be loosened, particularly in adult progressive myopathic ptoses. In severe myopathic ptoses, where the Bell's is limited and ptosis severe, a supramaximal blepharoplasty may be performed.[25]

Sling Slippage

Slippage of the frontalis sling occurred in 7% of the eyelids in the case series, most commonly in children rather than adults. In every case, this resulted from loss of fixation at the tarsal plate suture, rather than from loosening of the sleeve at the brow. The situation is best corrected by opening the lid crease, identifying the sling loop and its disinsertion from the tarsal plate, and advancing it back onto the tarsal plate with nonabsorbable sutures placed deeper into the tarsus.

References

[1] Takahashi Y, Leibovitch I, Kakizaki H. Frontalis suspension surgery in upper eyelid blepharoptosis. Open Ophthalmol J. 2010; 4:91–97

[2] Revere K, Katowitz WR, Nazemzadeh M, Katowitz JA. Eyelid developmental disorders. In: Fay A, Dolman PJ, eds. Diseases and Disorders of the Orbit and Ocular Adnexa. Edinburgh: Elsevier; 2017:149–152

[3] Crawford JS. Repair of ptosis using frontalis muscle and fascia lata. Trans Am Acad Ophthalmol Otolaryngol. 1956; 60(5):672–678

[4] Ben Simon GJ, Macedo AA, Schwarcz RM, Wang DY, McCann JD, Goldberg RA. Frontalis suspension for upper eyelid ptosis: evaluation of different surgical designs and suture material. Am J Ophthalmol. 2005; 140(5):877–885

[5] McCord CD, Codner MA. Frontalis suspension. In: McCord CD, Codner MA, eds. Eyelid and Periorbital Surgery. St Louis, MO: Quality Medical Publishing; 2008:439–448

[6] Pacella E, Mipatrini D, Pacella F, et al. Suspensory materials for surgery of blepharoptosis: A systematic review of observational studies. PLoS One. 2016; 11(9):e0160827

[7] Betharia SM. Frontalis sling: a modified simple technique. Br J Ophthalmol. 1985; 69(6):443–445

[8] Derby GS. Correction of ptosis by fascia lata hammock. Am. J. Ophth.. 1928; 11:352

[9] Wright WW. The use of living sutures in the treatment of ptosis. Arch. Ophth.. 1922; 51:99

[10] Bleyen I, Hardy I, Codère F. Muscle prolapse after harvesting autogenous fascia lata used for frontalis suspension in children. Ophthal Plast Reconstr Surg. 2009; 25(5):359–360

[11] Mehta P, Patel P, Olver JM. Functional results and complications of Mersilene mesh use for frontalis suspension ptosis surgery. Br J Ophthalmol. 2004; 88(3):361–364

[12] Elsamkary MA, Roshdy MMS. Clinical trial comparing autogenous fascia lata sling and Gore-Tex suspension in bilateral congenital ptosis. Clin Ophthalmol. 2016; 10:405–409

[13] Lee MJ, Oh JY, Choung HK, Kim NJ, Sung MS, Khwarg SI. Frontalis sling operation using silicone rod compared with preserved fascia lata for congenital ptosis a three-year follow-up study. Ophthalmology. 2009; 116(1):123–129

[14] Andersen J, Barmettler A, Rosenberg JB. Types of materials for frontalis sling surgery for congenital ptosis. Cochrane Database Syst Rev. 2017(7):CD012725

[15] Kim CY, Son BJ, Son J, Hong J, Lee SY. Analysis of the causes of recurrence after frontalis suspension using silicone rods for congenital ptosis. PLoS One. 2017; 12(2):e0171769

[16] Yagci A, Egrilmez S. Comparison of cosmetic results in frontalis sling operations: the eyelid crease incision versus the supralash stab incision. J Pediatr Ophthalmol Strabismus. 2003; 40(4):213–216

[17] Lee J-H, Kim Y-D. Surgical treatment of unilateral severe simple congenital ptosis. Taiwan J Ophthalmol. 2018; 8(1):3–8

[18] Bhattacharjee K, Bhattacharjee H, Kuri G, Shah ZT, Deori N. Single stage surgery for Blepharophimosis syndrome. Indian J Ophthalmol. 2012; 60(3):195–201

[19] Wong VA, Beckingsale PS, Oley CA, Sullivan TJ. Management of myogenic ptosis. Ophthalmology. 2002; 109(5):1023–1031

[20] Bagheri A, Borhani M, Salehirad S, Yazdani S, Tavakoli M. Blepharoptosis Associated With Third Cranial Nerve Palsy. Ophthal Plast Reconstr Surg. 2015; 31(5):357–360

[21] Roefs AM, Waters PJ, Moore GR, Dolman PJ. Orbicularis oculi muscle biopsies for mitochondrial DNA analysis in suspected mitochondrial myopathy. Br J Ophthalmol. 2012; 96(10):1296–1299

[22] Lelli GJ, Jr, Musch DC, Frueh BR, Nelson CC. Outcomes in silicone rod frontalis suspension surgery for high-risk noncongenital blepharoptosis. Ophthal Plast Reconstr Surg. 2009; 25(5):361–365

[23] Dollin M, Oestreicher JH. Adult-onset exposure keratitis after childhood ptosis repair with frontalis sling procedure. Can J Ophthalmol. 2009; 44(4):412–416

[24] Allen RC, Hong ES, Zimmerman MB, Morrison LA, Nerad JA, Carter KD. Factors affecting eyelid crease formation before and after silicone frontalis suspension for adult-onset myogenic ptosis. Ophthal Plast Reconstr Surg. 2015; 31(3):227–232

[25] Burnstine MA, Putterman AM. Upper blepharoplasty: a novel approach to improving progressive myopathic blepharoptosis. Ophthalmology. 1999; 106(11):2098–2100

30 Surgical Management of Static Congenital Ptosis with Levator Function between 4 and 10 mm

Jeremy Tan, Jill A. Foster

Abstract

Levator resection is an appropriate intervention for a patient with static congenital ptosis with moderate levator excursion (usually > 4 mm but < 10 mm). The foundational algorithms were presented in Chapter 28, and a working knowledge of each algorithm is useful until the surgeon gains experience to determine a best fit for the surgical technique. A challenge of these nomograms is finding consistent ways to measure the levator resection when the anatomy, elasticity, local anesthesia effects, and intraoperative bleeding create variability in individual cases. The authors favor Berke's intraoperative eyelid height as their primary guide in determining the desired eyelid position outcome. This chapter will address relevant anatomy, preoperative evaluation, surgical technique, and common complications in the postoperative period.

Keywords: moderate levator function, levator resection

30.1 Introduction

Levator resection is employed in patients with static congenital ptosis with levator excursion between 4 and 10 mm. The immediate goal of surgery in the pediatric patient is to provide an unobstructed visual axis for optimization of the child's developing vision. Surgery should be performed as soon as it is convenient and more rapidly in the child at risk for amblyopia. When there is no evidence of amblyopia, obstructed pupillary axis in primary gaze, asymmetric astigmatism, or significant chin-up posture, the surgery is less urgent and may be performed according to family and physician preferences. Advantages of early, nonurgent surgery include less disruption of the child's schedule, fast wound healing, and less patient/parent anxiety. Advantages of later surgery include more accurate lid measurements and better ability to assess and modify eyelid crease and eyelid fold for improved cosmesis. The algorithms reviewed in Chapter 28 allow the surgeon to determine the appropriate amount of levator resection. Individually customized modifications to the suggested algorithms will develop with surgeon experience.

30.2 The Anatomy of the Eyelid Crease

In normal eyelids, the levator aponeurosis divides into anterior and posterior portions prior to its insertion. The anterior portion is composed of fine leaflets of aponeurosis that insert into the septa between the pretarsal orbicularis muscle and the skin, forming the normal upper eyelid crease.[1,2] In congenital ptosis, there is a spectrum of lid crease formation from relatively normal to absent.[3] The surgeon may surgically create aponeurotic attachments to the pretarsal tissues to create a more prominent crease during ptosis surgery or in a staged approach. The goal is to create symmetry in the margin crease distance (MCD) and margin fold distance (MFD) in primary gaze.

30.3 Preoperative Assessment

The accuracy of the eyelid evaluation in pediatric patients requires patient cooperation and is challenging; repetition, patience, and skill to encourage patient cooperation are necessary. Important preoperative measurements include palpebral fissure, palpebral fissure on downgaze, margin reflex distance 1, MCD, MFD, lagophthalmos amount, Bell's phenomenon, and levator excursion. The preoperative encounter is the final opportunity to refine the surgical plan.

30.3.1 Indications

- Ptosis of the eyelid with fair to moderate levator excursion. The ideal candidate for this procedure is one with myopathic ptosis, levator excursion between 4 and 10 mm, good Bell's phenomenon, and no dry eye. The procedure may be performed in children and adults.
- The goals include eyelid elevation to prevent childhood amblyopia, improvement of superior field of vision, and better aesthetic symmetry between the eyelids in primary gaze.

30.3.2 Consequences of Levator Resection

- Increased palpebral fissure on downgaze, particularly noticeable in unilateral cases.
- Possible new onset or increase of lagophthalmos at night and on gentle eyelid closure.
- Alteration of blink mechanics.
- Exacerbation of dry eye, which may be associated with symptoms of conjunctival redness, blurred vision, and eye discomfort.

30.3.3 Risks of the Procedure

- Penetrating ocular injury.
- Undercorrection.
- Overcorrection.
- Postoperative lagophthalmos with resultant corneal exposure keratopathy.
- Worsening dry eye.
- Eyelid contour abnormalities with margin crease and margin fold asymmetries between sides.
- Bleeding.
- Infection.
- Scarring.
- Need for additional surgery.

- Double vision.
- Anesthesia reactions.
- Blindness.
- Death.

30.3.4 Benefits of the Procedure

- Reduction of visual obstruction and risk for deprivational amblyopia.
- Clearance of the visual axis and improved eyelid symmetry in primary gaze.
- Improved superior visual field.
- Improved symmetry of the lid position in primary gaze.

30.3.5 Relative Contraindications

- Patients with poor Bell's phenomenon, limited extraocular motility, or poor corneal sensation have greater risks for postoperative ocular surface exposure. In these cases, a more conservative elevation of the eyelid may be considered.
- Preexisting corneal surface exposure limits the options to lift the eyelid.

30.3.6 Alternatives

- If no amblyopia exists, the surgeon can observe with close follow-up to ensure no visual delay develops as time progresses.
- If amblyopia develops, the surgeon must ensure the patient has appropriate refraction and occlusion therapy.
  - If vision stabilizes, the surgeon may continue to observe the patient.
  - If vision does not improve or deteriorates, surgery to lift the affected eye is recommended.
- Frontalis suspension may be performed to preserve the levator aponeurosis.

30.4 Informed Consent

Adult patients or parents of affected children must be informed of the benefits, risks, and alternatives of the surgical procedure, including the intraoperative risks, postoperative consequences of levator resection, and postoperative complications.

30.5 Instrumentation

- Local anesthetic on 3-mL syringe with 30-gauge needle:
  - Marcaine 0.025% with 1:200,000 epinephrine for infants.
  - Lidocaine 1% or 2% and 0.75% bupivacaine (50/50 mix) with 1:200,000 epinephrine for older children and adults.
- Marking pen.
- Protective scleral shell.
- A 0.3 toothed forceps.
- A #15 blade.
- Westcott scissors.
- Straight iris scissors.
- Ptosis clamp.
- Monopolar needle-tip cautery.
- Castroviejo needle drivers.

- Desmarres retractor.
- Serafin clamps.
- Suture:
  - Three double-armed 5–0 or 6–0 Vicryl on spatulated needles per side.
  - The 6–0 plain absorbing gut.
  - The 6–0 polypropylene on a P-1 needle for older children or adults.

30.6 The Levator Resection Procedure

- The eyelid crease is marked prior to local infiltration (before sedation in the adult and after in the child).
  - In unilateral cases, the contralateral eyelid crease is used for comparison.
  - In bilateral surgery, the more natural eyelid crease height is used.
  - If neither eyelid presents a distinct crease, gentle digital upward lift of the margin will often delineate the most natural fold and crease.
- Inject local anesthetic with epinephrine to improve postoperative comfort, provide hemostasis, and delineate tissue planes.
  - Pediatric patients may reach toxic level of local anesthetic.
    - Lidocaine maximum dosage of 4.5 mg/kg (7 mg/kg is allowable with use of lidocaine with epinephrine).
    - Bupivacaine maximum dosage of 3 mg/kg.
- A protective scleral contact lens may be used for ocular surface protection.
- Incise the eyelid crease at the previously made skin marking with a #15 blade.
- Sharply dissect through orbicularis and septum with Westcott scissors.
  - Septum and fat are teased away from the levator aponeurosis and muscle and pushed superiorly to reveal Whitnall's ligament.
- Decide if degree of levator resection requires some removal of conjunctiva to prevent conjunctival prolapse.
  - The larger the resection, the more likely one will wish to prophylactically remove 2 to 5 mm of conjunctiva to prevent conjunctival prolapse postoperatively.
  - Large resection:
    - Perform a full-thickness punch incision nasally and temporally (performed with sharp iris scissors above the tarsus starting at the anterior surface and exiting through the conjunctiva) (▶ Fig. 30.1a). The lid is everted so that the exit sites above the tarsus are directly visualized as the scissor tip is advanced (▶ Fig. 30.1b).
    - Cut full thickness above the tarsal plate to unite the punch incisions (▶ Fig. 30.1c).
    - Place the ptosis clamp on the tissue above the incision, incorporating conjunctiva, Müller's muscle, and levator aponeurosis. If further separation of the septum and fat from the eyelid elevators is desired, it is easier to do with the ptosis clamp in position to act as a retractor (▶ Fig. 30.1d).
    - Use the straight iris scissors to bluntly separate the conjunctiva from Müller's muscle. Müller's muscle is

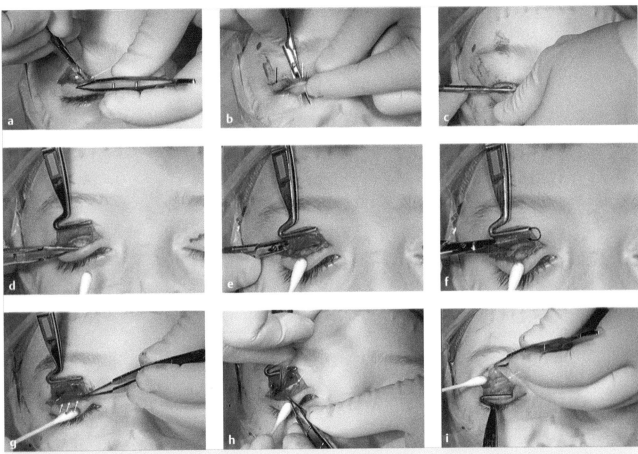

Fig. 30.1 Illustrated is a large levator resection with need of conjunctival resection. For smaller levator resections, conjunctiva may be left intact as described in the text below. **(a)** Full-thickness buttonhole superior to the tarsus after initial skin–muscle incision. *White arrow*: superior border of tarsus. **(b)** Eyelid eversion denoting full-thickness buttonhole with iris scissors. Note the eyelid eversion to avoid globe penetration and ensure superior tarsal border stab incision placement. *White arrow*: active nasal stab incision. *Black arrow*: area of the site of temporal stab incision. **(c)** Full-thickness transection from temporal to nasal stab incision. **(d)** Retractor complex placement in ptosis clamp. **(e)** Dissection of conjunctiva from Müller's muscle with iris scissors. **(f)** Scissors prepared for transection of mobilized conjunctiva. Amount to be resected delineated between *black arrows*. This technique is used to avoid postoperative conjunctival prolapse in large levator resections. **(g)** Gut suture placement of conjunctiva to the superior tarsal border edge when conjunctiva is resected in the setting of large levator resections. *White arrows* at the anastomosed end of transected conjunctiva to superior tarsus. **(h)** Posterior separation of Müller's muscle from conjunctiva up to the posterior aspect of Whitnall's ligament is performed (*white arrow*). **(i)** Dissection is performed, separating levator aponeurosis from orbital fat and septum. Blunt anterior dissection carried superiorly past Whitnall's ligament (*white arrow*). *(Continued)*

firmly adherent to conjunctiva. The tip of the scissors is inserted about 3 mm above the clamp between the conjunctiva and Müller's muscle, spread, and then pulled out without closing the scissor, bluntly dissecting with slow horizontal movement across the backside of the eyelid (► Fig. 30.1**e**). Once the entire horizontal breadth of the conjunctiva is lifted away from the Müller's muscle, the conjunctiva is horizontally transected at a level above the clamp that leaves the excess conjunctiva in the clamp (► Fig. 30.1**f**).

– After the conjunctival transection, additional superior separation of the conjunctiva from the Müller's muscle and aponeurosis is accomplished with the Westcott scissors. The height of the separation extends to just above the desired placement of the fixation sutures. The incised conjunctival edge is sutured to the superior border of the tarsus with 6–0 gut suture (► Fig. 30.1**g**).

○ Smaller resections do not require conjunctival disinsertion.

– While applying downward traction on the eyelid margin, make a central snip incision to open the levator aponeurosis and Müller's muscle just above the tarsal plate. Undermine medially and laterally with Westcott scissors to raise up the edge of the lid retractors from the conjunctiva across the horizontal breadth of the eyelid.

– Dissect in a preconjunctival plane just enough to elevate the upper lid retractor complex.

– Place the ptosis clamp on the edge of Müller's muscle and levator aponeurosis.

• Dissect conjunctiva from Müller's muscle. With the clamp rotated towards the surgeon sitting at the head of the bed, sharply dissect Müller's muscle off the conjunctiva with a blunt Westcott scissors and continue dissection up past the origin of Müller's muscle (► Fig. 30.1**h**).

• Dissect the orbital septum from the levator. With the clamp then rotated downward towards the eyelid margin, elevate

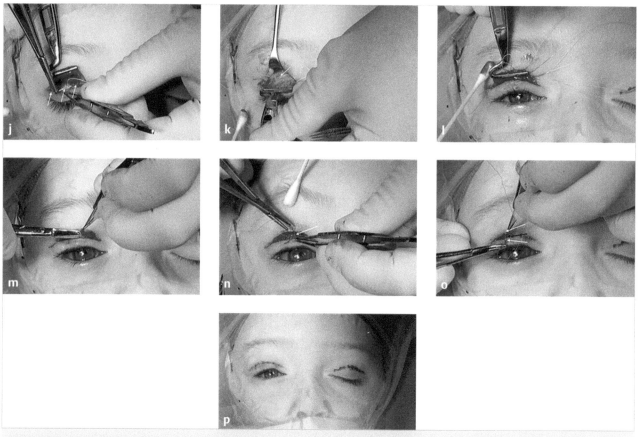

Fig. 30.1 (*Continued*) (**j**) Placement of three partial-thickness tarsal double-armed sutures at *white arrows* for levator resection. (**k**) Full-thickness placement of suture through the retractor complex for levator resection. Arrow points at needle emerging from posterior to anterior side of complex. Note that the ptosis clamp is pulled inferiorly to place the sutures. (**l**) Removal of scleral shell to assess intraoperative eyelid height and contour. Sutures are held with slipknots for ease of adjustments. (**m**) Resection of excess retractor complex after sutures are tied in square knots. (**n**) Crease-forming sutures are placed. Deep lid crease reformation with buried interrupted sutures from pretarsal orbicularis to advanced levator stump (*white arrow*) to pretarsal orbicularis (*black arrow*). (**o**) Further crease-forming suture placement with skin (*white arrow*) to levator stump (*black arrow*) to skin (*white arrow*) with interrupted sutures. (**p**) Final closure completed with intervening simple interrupted sutures.

the septum and fat off the levator complex anteriorly. Attempt to leave the fat with the septum. Elevate the septum and fat to above the desired level for placement of the sutures (▶ Fig. 30.1**i**).

- Perform the resection.
  - Place three double-armed 5–0 or 6–0 polyglactin suture partial thickness through the tarsus nasally, centrally, and temporally (▶ Fig. 30.1**j**).
  - Measure the amount of levator retractor complex to be resected and place the double-armed sutures through the clamped material (▶ Fig. 30.1**k**).
  - Tie sutures in slipknots.
  - Remove scleral shell for assessment of intraoperative eyelid height and contour (▶ Fig. 30.1**l**).
  - Adjust sutures as necessary to provide the desired eyelid gap and contour.
  - When satisfied, convert to square knots.
  - Remove excess retractors distal to suture placement (▶ Fig. 30.1**m**).
- Consider conservative skin/orbicularis excision.
  - Once the eyelid has been elevated, there may be skin and/or orbicularis redundancy along the incision. Drape the upper tissue above the incision over the line of the

resection to assess how much skin overlap is present. One to two millimeters of overlap is appropriate. A small skin–muscle ellipse may be removed while assessing to ensure that the anterior lamellar length will not limit eyelid closure.

- Close incision with eyelid crease formation sutures.
  - Orbicularis to advanced levator stump to orbicularis in an interrupted buried fashion (▶ Fig. 30.1**n**).
  - Skin to advanced levator stump to skin (▶ Fig. 30.1**o**).
  - A simple interrupted dissolvable suture is used to close the remaining wound (▶ Fig. 30.1**p**).
- A typical pre- and postoperative result is noted in ▶ Fig. 30.2.

30.7 Expert Tips/Pearls/ Suggestions

- Corneal protectors may be used to protect the eye during surgery.
- Dissection to expose the levator aponeurosis and muscle:
  - Gentle retropulsion on the globe can help identify the orbital fat bulge posterior to the septum to provide anatomic orientation.

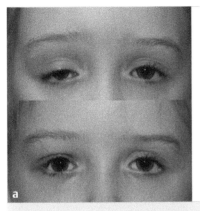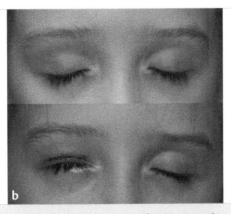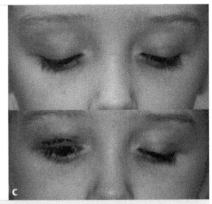

Fig. 30.2 **(a)** Pre- and postoperative lid position in primary gaze in a patient with static myopathic ptosis with levator function of 8 mm. **(b)** Pre- and postoperative eyelid position with gentle closure in the same patient in ▶ Fig. 30.2a at 1 week after external levator resection. **(c)** Pre- and postoperative eyelid position in downgaze with nearly equivalent postoperative vertical palpebral fissures (▶ Fig. 30.2a). Note the postoperative increased palpebral fissure on downgaze, which should be discussed during preoperative evaluation.

○ Attempt to keep fat pads behind septum.
- If the fat is protruding, light cautery can shrink it back out of the way.
- Avoid fat removal in children.
○ If dissection proceeds too deeply, the surgeon may lose the levator edge.
- Remember, the preaponeurotic fat pad lies anterior to the levator aponeurosis.
- Grasping and pulling the superior tissues inferiorly at the deepest identifiable edge will aid in the identification of the layers.
○ Avoid septum in your levator resection suture passes as these may cause cicatricial changes, which result in lagophthalmos.
- Hematomas distort the tissue and surgical measurements.
○ Intraoperative digital pressure and massage may help to spread out the collection of blood and flatten tissues, but the distortion diminishes the predictability of the procedure.
- Full-thickness passes of the suture through the tarsus may occur, especially in the relatively smaller tissues of the pediatric patient. Use scleral shell to protect the globe to avoid ocular penetration and evert the eyelid to check for full-thickness passes, which may result in corneal abrasions.
○ If unsure whether a full-thickness pass has occurred, pinpoint bleeding is a good clue, and repassing the tarsal bite is prudent.
- Organize your free suture ends with Serafin clamps. Loose suture is frustrating.

30.8 Postoperative Care

- Keep ocular surface liberally lubricated during the first week. Maxitrol is preferred.
○ Assess degree of lagophthalmos and eyelid excursion at first postoperative visit to determine tapering schedule of the lubrication.
○ The eyes of children are often able to adapt the tear film for successful protection even with large levator resections with resultant lagophthalmos.

- It is difficult to apply ice or restrictions in the pediatric population. Be flexible with this instruction.
- Give parents signs and symptoms of orbital hemorrhage or infection.
- Tylenol may be used for pain management.
- Maintain any ongoing amblyopia regimen.

30.9 Complications and Their Management

- Undercorrection:
○ If the eyelid is out of the visual axis and not causing astigmatism, it can be observed.
○ Follow-up regularly to ensure no visual delay from intermittent obstruction.
○ Reoperate when appropriate.
- Overcorrection may lead to exposure keratopathy, corneal desiccation, scarring, and permanent vision loss.
○ Observe for signs of ocular surface decompensation.
○ Lubricate with artificial tears and ointments.
○ If the ocular surface decompensates with adequate medical management, proceed with surgical lysis of sutures and adhesions to allow closure of the palpebral aperture.
- In some cases, even with the lid at an appropriate height, the eye will develop problems with ocular surface exposure. In these cases, a temporary serpentine tarsorrhaphy may be used to protect the cornea until the edema from surgery resolves and the lid function improves.
- If this is unsuccessful, the lid may be lowered as above.
- Orbital hemorrhage:
○ Dissection planes are deep to the orbital septum and hematoma collection may cause compartment syndrome.
- When identified, immediate surgical evacuation should be performed.

– If orbital hemorrhage is severe, canthotomy and cantholysis may be necessary.
- Infection:
  ○ Infection limited to the skin or preseptal tissues:
    – Oral antibiotics.
    – Signs and symptoms of worsening should be discussed, including worsening pain, double vision, fevers, and discharge.
    – Close follow-up.
  ○ Infection involving deeper orbital structures:
    – Admit to the hospital for intravenous antibiotics, orbital imaging, and patient monitoring.
    – Orbitotomy for drainage as necessary.
    – Close follow-up.

30.10 Conclusion

Levator resection is an excellent technique to treat static myopathic ptosis with levator excursion between 4 and 10 mm.

Thoughtful patient management with clear communication of postoperative expectations and careful attention to surgical technique yield excellent patient results.

References

[1] Pandit S, Ahuja MS. Gross and microscopic study of insertion of levator palpebrae superioris and its anatomical correlation in superior palpebral crease formation and its clinical relevance. Med J Armed Forces India. 2015; 71(4): 330–336

[2] Kakizaki H, Madge SN, Selva D. Insertion of the levator aponeurosis and Müller's muscle on the tarsus: a cadaveric study in Caucasians. Clin Exp Ophthalmol. 2010; 38(6):635–637

[3] Guercio JR, Martyn LJ. Congenital malformations of the eye and orbit. Otolaryngol Clin North Am. 2007; 40(1):113–140, vii

31 Progressive Myogenic Ptosis: Evaluation and Management

Liat Attas-Fox, François Codère

Abstract

This chapter introduces the approach to and management of different forms of progressive myogenic ptosis. In this ptosis category, there is usually localized or diffuse intrinsic muscular disease that results in poor levator excursion. These ptoses are rare, usually inherited, and bilateral, and may have associated ocular or systemic abnormalities. There may be poor extraocular motility and orbicularis muscle function. The amount of levator function indicates the extent of the disease and helps inform the surgeon's choice for corrective surgery.

Keywords: oculopharyngeal muscular dystrophy, chronic progressive ophthalmoplegia, Kearns–Sayre, myotonic dystrophies, congenital progressive ptoses

31.1 Introduction

Progressive myogenic ptoses consist mostly of genetic diseases that are intrinsic to the levator muscle. The levator, orbicularis, and extraocular muscles are often affected. Understanding the common presentations and physical findings observed in this ptosis group makes diagnosis and treatment straightforward.[1] When suspected, it is important to obtain a thorough family history even though variable penetrance may obscure a hereditary pattern or mutations may be sporadic.

Management of progressive myopathic ptosis depends upon the degree of upper eyelid ptosis, measurement of levator excursion, and intactness of corneal protective mechanisms (lagophthalmos, intact Bell's phenomenon, and extent of dry eye).

31.2 Causes of Progressive Myopathic Ptosis

Progressive myopathic ptosis may occur in children and adults. Those seen in children are rare, frequently fatal, and discussed in Chapter 32. Below, we discuss the most common disorders seen in adulthood. Appropriate workup may include referral to other specialists and systemic testing to evaluate potentially life-threatening issues.

31.2.1 Oculopharyngeal Muscular Dystrophy

Oculopharyngeal muscular dystrophy (OPMD) is an autosomal dominant muscle disorder, usually of late onset.[2] Patients become symptomatic by the fifth and sixth decades. It is characterized by progressive bilateral ptosis of the eyelids, dysphagia, and proximal muscle weakness (▶ Fig. 31.1). Although other extraocular muscles may become gradually involved, complete external ophthalmoplegia is rare and intrinsic eye muscles are not affected. The ptosis is progressive and symmetrical as a result of levator weakness. Patients have good orbicularis function and Bell's phenomenon. There are different phenotypes. In early onset disease, there is usually rapid progression of symptoms and severe disease. In late onset disease, there is slower progression and milder disease. OPMD occurs because of a stable mutation causing an expansion in the *PABPN1* gene located on chromosome 14. Filamentous intranuclear inclusions in muscle fibers of OPMD patients are the pathological hallmark of the disease.[3]

OPMD has a worldwide distribution with the largest cluster in Quebec followed by Bukhara Jews in Israel.[4] Also, an unexpected large OPMD population of Hispanic offspring living in New Mexico have been revealed.[5] To confirm the diagnosis in patients clinically suspected of having OPMD, molecular genetic testing is performed. The most common ptosis treatment options include levator resection and advancement in mild or moderate cases and frontalis suspension of the eyelids in more advanced cases.[6]

31.2.2 Chronic Progressive External Ophthalmoplegia

Chronic progressive external ophthalmoplegia (CPEO) is a progressive myopathy affecting the external eye muscles bilaterally

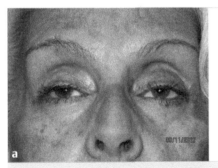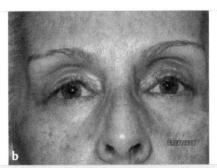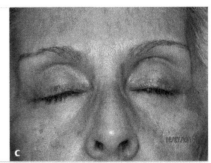

Fig. 31.1 A 71-year-old female with progressive eyelid ptosis, positive family history for OPMD with trouble swallowing meat, diminished extraocular motility, and LE of 6 mm OD and 7 mm OS **(a)**. She underwent bilateral levator resections (19 mm OU) **(b)**. Note the postoperative lagophthalmos **(c)**. The ptosis will recur over time. (The images are provided courtesy of Michael A. Burnstine, MD, and Eyesthetica.)

and usually occurs sporadically (▶ Fig. 31.2). CPEO usually results from genetic defects that affect mitochondrial function. It is the most common manifestation of mitochondrial myopathy. Patients usually present in young adulthood. Progressive paralysis of the extraocular muscles is seen. The phenotype is varied due to the number of mitochondria involved. The ptosis develops and is associated with an extreme loss of ocular motility, to the point of no motility of lids and eyebrows.[7] The orbicularis is usually weak as well and therefore there is poor eyelid closure. Pupillary muscle fibers are spared and the ptosis may precede the motility problem.

Kearns–Sayre syndrome is a variant of CPEO, often called CPEO Plus.[8] It is associated with other tissue changes including heart block, pigmentary retinopathy, and sometimes peripheral muscle weakness. These patients should have a neurologic

workup.[9] In both CPEO and Kearns–Sayre syndrome, hearing loss and diabetes mellitus can precede the onset of muscle involvement by years.[10]

Ptosis associated with CPEO is one of the most difficult to manage. Due to weakness of the orbicularis oculi muscles and poor eyelid closure, the lids should not be raised in excess. Conservative frontalis sling procedures are useful to elevate the lids.[11,12] Due to poor Bell's phenomenon, incomplete blink and lack of eye movements, exposure keratopathy can be common postoperatively. Additional procedures are often required to minimize the dryness.

31.2.3 Myotonic Dystrophies

Myotonic dystrophy is a disease that affects muscles and other body systems, characterized by progressive muscle loss and weakness (▶ Fig. 31.3). It is the most common form of adult-onset muscular dystrophy. Myotonic dystrophy is inherited in an autosomal dominant pattern.[13] It is characterized by unstable mutations. The mutations occur when a piece of DNA is abnormally repeated a number of times, which makes the gene unstable. The phenotype varies depending on variation of the genotype.

Unlike OPMD, myotonic dystrophy is associated with abnormalities in other organ systems. Almost any other tissue or organ can be involved including the crystalline lenses (Christmas tree cataract), the brain, testicles, and hair.[13]

The ptosis can be mild to severe and is known to progress slowly. Unlike CPEO, motility loss is usually mild. Severity of disease pattern varies based on the genotype. Ultimately, a conservative frontalis sling is required to elevate the lids. The repair can be complicated by facial weakness.

31.2.4 The Masquerader of Progressive Myopathic Ptosis

Juvenile myasthenia gravis (MG) can masquerade as simple congenital ptosis.[14] The chance of misdiagnosis increases in bilateral cases.[15] MG is an autoimmune disorder that affects the neuromuscular junction rather than an intrinsic levator muscle disorder (▶ Fig. 31.4). Although adult MG is an acquired autoimmune disease, congenital MG is a rare, nonimmune inheritable disorder. It is termed ocular myasthenia gravis (OMG) when weakness is limited exclusively to the eyelids and extraocular muscles.[16]

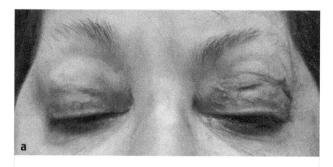
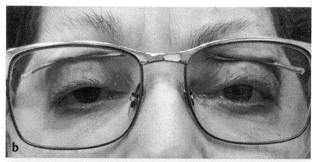

Fig. 31.2 A 65-year-old female with history of CPEO suffering systemic manifestation of muscle weakness in shoulders, hands, and legs, and diminished extraocular motility. Levator excursion of 0 mm bilaterally and MRD1 of –2 bilaterally (a). Using glasses that have a "ptosis crutch" to lift the upper eyelids (b). (The images are provided courtesy of Prof. Arik Y. Nemet, Meir Medical Center, Israel.)

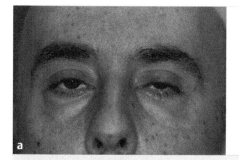
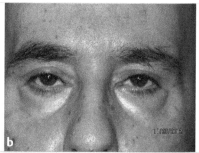
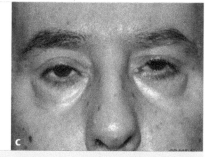

Fig. 31.3 A 43-year-old man with myotonic dystrophy and profound ptosis, facial wasting, and diminished Bell's phenomenon with levator excursion of 10 mm (a). He underwent bilateral conservative levator repair (b). Five years later, the ptosis has recurred (c). He will likely need frontalis suspension. (The images are provided courtesy of Michael A. Burnstine, MD, and Eyesthetica.)

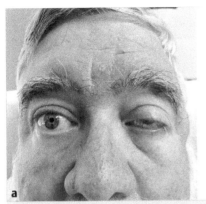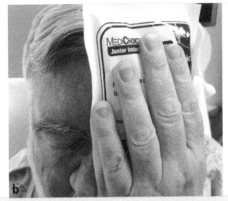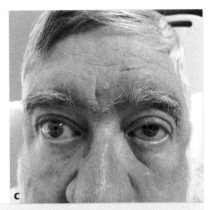

Fig. 31.4 A 68-year-old man presented with unilateral ptosis and no other symptoms. The neurologic examination revealed ptosis of the left eye after sustained upgaze (**a**). Extraocular motility was normal. Myasthenia gravis was suspected, and the ice test was performed with a cold pack placed over the left eye (**b**). After 2 minutes, the ptosis was improved, indicating a positive test (**c**). The diagnosis was supported by the presence of serum anti-acetylcholine receptor antibodies and by electrodiagnostic testing, which showed a decremental response to repetitive nerve stimulation. The ice pack test can be a useful tool to distinguish MG from other causes of ptosis or ophthalmoparesis. The inhibition of acetylcholinesterase activity at a reduced muscle temperature is thought to underlie the observed clinical improvement. The patient was treated with pyridostigmine, and the ptosis was diminished. (Image courtesy of Liu and Chen and the New England Journal of Medicine (NEJM) 2016;375:e39.)

Medical therapy includes acetylcholinesterase inhibitors, pyridostigmine (Mestinon), oral corticosteroids, and immunomodulators. These drugs have no effect on the underlying disease process; they are purely to help manage symptoms.[17] Meticulous examination is the key to the correct diagnosis.

31.3 History and Physical Examination

Progressive myogenic ptosis types are rare. When suspected, a proper history and examination are the key to the correct diagnosis.[1] It is our goal to identify the ptosis and to formulate a treatment plan. Factors suggesting an uncommon type of ptosis are positive family history and other associated ocular, muscular, or systemic problems.

31.3.1 The History

Obtaining a thorough history of present illness and family history of ptosis are critical to making the progressive myopathic ptosis diagnosis.

History of Present Illness

Most patients will report that their eyelids have dropped over time and eyelid height does not vary throughout the day. They will deny double vision and will occasionally report decreased extraocular motility.

Second, a thorough review of systems is important: whether there are swallowing problems as seen in OPMD or heart problems, facial weakness, hearing loss, and ataxia as seen in CPEO and myotonic dystrophy variants.

Family History of Ptosis

A family history of ptosis may be gleaned from the patient or by review of older family photographs. A history of parents,

grandparents, siblings, and cousins should be acquired if a heritable etiology is entertained in the differential diagnosis.

31.3.2 Physical Examination

In addition to a thorough history, a complete physical examination should be performed, paying particular attention to the basic eye examination. Visual acuity, extraocular motility, dilated fundus examination, and eyelid measurements are important data points.

Eye Examination

Measuring visual acuity and assessing a dilated fundus for pigmentary changes may aid in the diagnosis of some progressive myopathies such as Kearns–Sayre syndrome. Evaluating diminished extraocular motility may also aid in the diagnosis.

Facial Weakness

Facial atrophy and wasting is important to note in myotonic dystrophies and OPMD.

Eyelid Measurements

Standard periocular measurements for ptosis are important and include palpebral fissure (PF), margin reflex distance 1 (MRD1), margin crease distance (MCD), and margin fold distances (MFD). Levator excursion (LE) is measured in isolation of frontalis muscle use. Typically, patients with myopathic ptoses have a decreased PF, MRD1 with increased MCD and MFD. LE varies based on the disease and extent of the myopathy. Orbicularis function and lagophthalmos on gentle eyelid closure should also be assessed.

Corneal Protective Mechanisms

In myopathic ptosis, it is critical to assess orbicularis function, dry eye status, lagophthalmos with gentle eyelid closure and

Bell's phenomenon. It is common to have diminished orbicularis tone and a decreased or absent Bell's phenomenon from progressive disease, which affects the orbicularis and extraocular skeletal muscles. When the eye is at risk from diminished corneal protection, conservative management of the ptosis becomes critical.

31.4 Management of Progressive Myopathic Ptosis

Surgical repair of progressive myogenic ptosis is guided by degree of ptosis, ability to protect the cornea and LE. Advancement or shortening procedures work less as the levator function decreases.[18] With intact corneal protective mechanisms, patients with LE between 0 and 4 mm receive frontalis suspension, between 4 and 10 mm receive levator resection, and greater than 10 mm receive levator advancement. For those patients with weakened orbicularis oculi function with a poor Bell's phenomenon that places the patient at risk for lagophthalmos and corneal keratopathy/breakdown (i.e., CPEO and myotonic dystrophy type 1), nonsurgical correction with ptosis crutches on spectacles, a vaulted PROSE lens (both discussed in Chapter 37) or skin-only blepharoplasty may be used.[12,19] Adjunctive techniques such as raising the lower eyelids to mitigate the effects of lagophthalmos have also been promoted to minimize corneal exposure.[20]

31.4.1 Timing of Repair

Repair is considered when the ptosis is affecting the patient's ability to function. Difficulties driving and reading are frequent complaints.

31.4.2 Our Workhorse Procedure

The levator function and pathophysiology of the disease are the most important factors in choosing the type of ptosis correction. In progressive myogenic ptosis in which the patients will progress over the years, a simple upper blepharoplasty or levator resection yield large rates of ptosis recurrence. In such cases, frontalis suspension should be advocated early in the disease process.[2]

Frontalis suspension surgery is based on connecting the tarsal plate to the eyebrow. The sling utilizes the power of the frontalis muscle to elevate the poorly functioning eyelid (see Chapter 29).[20] Various techniques and materials can be used. Fascia lata can be harvested as sling material which is more complicated as compared to using synthetic materials. Our suspensory material of choice is Prolene because this material is readily available and easily adjustable. It was reported that the "box-shaped" technique (▶ Fig. 31.5) is simpler to perform and yields similar outcomes to the "modified Crawford" technique (▶ Fig. 31.6) in patients with ptosis due to OPMD.[6] In the box technique, two supraciliary incisions are placed (medially and laterally) 2 mm above the cilia measuring 2 mm in length. Medial and lateral incisions are placed just above the brow. The Prolene suture is passed to the brow in a suborbicularis plane with a lid protector in the eye and tied at the medial incision in the brow. This operation can also cause lagophthalmos, made worse by a diminished Bell's phenomenon.[6] Patients must be educated about lubricating the eye postsurgery to avoid exposure keratopathy.[18,19]

31.5 Conclusions

Progressive myopathic ptosis may be a difficult diagnosis to make. Usually, the ptosis is inherited, but it may be sporadic. Appropriate workup may include referral to other specialists and systemic testing to manage the other sequelae of the disease processes. Careful surgical decision-making is critical to improve the ptosis while maintaining eye protection.

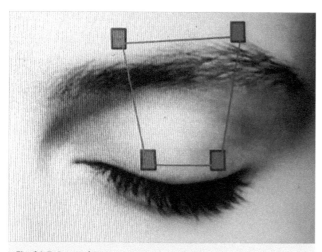

Fig. 31.5 Box technique.

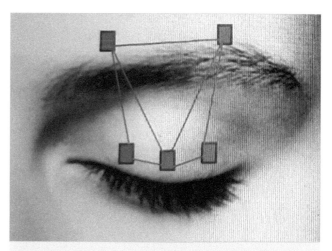

Fig. 31.6 Modified Crawford technique with interlocking triangles.

References

[1] Wong VA, Beckingsale PS, Oley CA, Sullivan TJ. Management of myogenic ptosis. Ophthalmology. 2002; 109(5):1023–1031

[2] Codère F, Brais B, Rouleau G, Lafontaine E. Oculopharyngeal muscular dystrophy: what's new? Orbit. 2001; 20(4):259–266

[3] Corbeil-Girard LP, Klein AF, Sasseville AM, et al. PABPN1 overexpression leads to upregulation of genes encoding nuclear proteins that are sequestered in oculopharyngeal muscular dystrophy nuclear inclusions. Neurobiol Dis. 2005; 18(3):551–567

[4] Blumen SC, Nisipeanu P, Sadeh M, et al. Epidemiology and inheritance of oculopharyngeal muscular dystrophy in Israel. Neuromuscul Disord. 1997; 7 Suppl 1:S38–S40

[5] Becher MW, Morrison L, Davis LE, et al. Oculopharyngeal muscular dystrophy in Hispanic New Mexicans. JAMA. 2001; 286(19):2437–2440

[6] Kalin-Hajdu E, Attas-Fox L, Huang X, Hardy I, Codère F. Comparison of two polypropylene frontalis suspension techniques in 92 patients with oculopharyngeal muscular dystrophy. Ophthal Plast Reconstr Surg. 2017; 33(1):57–60

[7] Bau V, Zierz S. Update on chronic progressive external ophthalmoplegia. Strabismus. 2005; 13(3):133–142

[8] Shemesh A, Margolin E. Kearns Sayre syndrome. In: StatPearls [Internet]. Treasure Island, FL: StatPearls Publishing; 2018

[9] Sharma AK, Jain N, Kharwar RB, Narain VS. Classical triad of Kearns-Sayre syndrome. BMJ Case Rep. 2016; 2016:2016

[10] Ho J, Pacaud D, Khan A. Kearns-Sayre syndrome is a rare cause of diabetes. Can J Diabetes. 2016; 40(2):110–111

[11] Shah KP, Mukherjee B. Efficacy of frontalis suspension with silicone rods in ptosis patients with poor Bell's phenomenon. Taiwan J Ophthalmol. 2017; 7(3):143–148

[12] Burnstine MA, Putterman AM. Upper blepharoplasty: a novel approach to improving progressive myopathic blepharoptosis. Ophthalmology. 1999; 106(11):2098–2100

[13] Bird TD. Myotonic dystrophy type 1. In: Adam MP, Ardinger HH, Pagon RA, Wallace SE, Bean LJH, Stephens K, Amemiya A, eds. GeneReviews®[Internet]. Seattle, WA: University of Washington, Seattle; 1993–2019

[14] Peragallo JH. Pediatric myasthenia gravis. Semin Pediatr Neurol. 2017; 24(2):116–121

[15] Alam MS, Devi Nivean P. Early onset bilateral juvenile myasthenia gravis masquerading as simple congenital ptosis. GMS Ophthalmol Cases. 2017; 7:Doc07

[16] Cornblath WT. Treatment of ocular myasthenia gravis. Asia Pac J Ophthalmol (Phila). 2018; 7(4):257–259

[17] Farmakidis C, Pasnoor M, Barohn RJ, Dimachkie MM. Congenital myasthenic syndromes: a clinical and treatment approach. Curr Treat Options Neurol. 2018; 20(9):36

[18] Shields M, Putterman A. Blepharoptosis correction. Curr Opin Otolaryngol Head Neck Surg. 2003; 11(4):261–266

[19] Lapid O, Lapid-Gortzak R, Barr J, Rosenberg L. Eyelid crutches for ptosis: a forgotten solution. Plast Reconstr Surg. 2000; 106(5):1213–1214

[20] Doherty M, Winterton R, Griffiths PG. Eyelid surgery in ocular myopathies. Orbit. 2013; 32(1):12–15

32 Syndromic Blepharoptoses

Christine Greer, Michael A. Burnstine, Diana K. Lee, Jonathan W. Kim

Abstract

Syndromic blepharoptosis refers to patients who present with ptosis and other ocular and systemic findings. This differs from static maldevelopment ptosis which is present from birth (i.e., classic congenital ptosis). The syndromic forms of ptosis covered in this chapter are aberrant innervation syndromes, static myopathic ptoses involving other extraocular muscles, and myopathic ptoses that affect the levator muscle in children and adulthood.

Keywords: congenital ptosis, syndromes with ptosis, myopathic ptosisMarcus Gunn jaw-winking syndrome, blepharophimosis-ptosis-epicanthus inversus-syndrome (BPES), congenital myopathies, muscular dystrophies

32.1 Introduction

Syndromic blepharoptoses refers to a category of eyelid ptoses associated with other ocular and systemic findings. This is distinct from the classic congenital ptosis described in Chapter 28. Frequently, in patients with syndromes there is an underlying genetic basis for the phenotypic presentation. In some cases, the associated phenotypic manifestations may be fatal.

To date, syndromic ptosis has never been categorized and presented in a comprehensive, effective manner. For clarity, the syndromic forms of ptoses covered in this chapter have been subdivided into sections: aberrant innervation syndromes, static myopathic ptoses involving the extraocular muscles, myopathic ptoses that affect the levator muscle and other muscle groups presenting in childhood, and progressive myopathic ptoses seen in adulthood (▶ Table 32.1).

32.2 Aberrant Innervation Syndromes

The presentation of an aberrant innervation syndrome depends on the nerves involved and can range from syndromes isolated to the levator muscle (i.e., Marcus Gunn jaw-winking syndrome) to more severe forms accompanied by ophthalmoparesis and possibly strabismus (i.e., Duane's syndrome). Age of onset, symptoms, progression, inheritance, genetics, and treatments for these disorders are summarized in the ▶ Table 32.1.

32.3 Static Myopathic Ptoses Involving the Extraocular Muscles

Blepharophimosis-ptosis-epicanthus inversus syndrome (BPES) is a well-characterized syndrome affecting eyelid development, which presents with the classic constellation of severe bilateral blepharoptosis, blepharophimosis, epicanthus inversus, and telecanthus (see Chapter 28). The levator palpebrae superioris muscle has markedly decreased function due to fibrosis,[52] and

the tarsal plates can be hypoplastic. Fibrosis of the extraocular muscles and the levator is also seen in congenital fibrosis of the extraocular muscles (CFEOM) and monocular elevation deficiency. Age of onset, symptoms, progression, inheritance, genetics, and treatments are summarized in the ▶ Table 32.1.

32.4 Progressive Myopathic Ptoses that Affect the Levator and Other Muscle Groups Presenting in Childhood

Congenital myopathies (CMs) are a heterogenous inherited group of disorders that can cause blepharoptosis and should be considered when an infant or young child presents with generalized hypotonia, facial nerve weakness, ophthalmoparesis, and blepharoptosis. They differ from congenital muscular dystrophies (CMDs) in their histochemical and electron microscopy findings.[38] In such cases, a muscle biopsy confirms the diagnosis. Other congenital syndromes that have myopathic ptosis are listed in the ▶ Table 32.1.

32.5 Progressive Myopathic Ptoses Seen in Adulthood

Many of the conditions discussed herein are muscular dystrophies. The muscular dystrophies are a heterogeneous group of disorders characterized by progressive weakness and characterized by their clinical, genetic, and biochemical features.[28] These include: myotonic dystrophy (type I and II) and oculopharyngeal muscular dystrophy. Limb girdle muscular dystrophy is categorized under myopathic ptoses that affect the levator in childhood, given its onset early in life. Other muscular dystrophies, including Duchenne–Becker, facioscapulohumeral distal, and the congenital muscular dystrophies classically present with minimal or no eye findings and will not be discussed in this chapter.

Other inherited conditions presenting with ptosis in adulthood include chronic progressive external ophthalmoplegia (CPEO) and desmin (myofibrillary) myopathy. Age of onset, symptoms, progression, inheritance, genetics, and treatments are summarized in the ▶ Table 32.1.

32.6 Management and Conclusions

Syndromic blepharoptoses include many disorders. Subdividing the disorders into aberrant innervation syndromes, static myopathic ptosis involving the extraocular muscles, myopathic ptoses that affect the levator muscle and other muscle groups in childhood (progressive or non-progressive), and progressive myopathic ptoses seen in adulthood can aid in patient management. The latter two categories may require established care with necessary interdisciplinary teams to manage the systemic

Table 32.1 Summary of syndromic progressive myopathic ptoses

Disease	Age of onset	Symptoms	Progressive/nonprogressive	Inheritance	Gene	Treatment
Aberrant innervation syndromes						
Duane's syndrome[1]	Birth	Patients have deficiency of abduction and/or adduction with associated co-contraction of the medial and lateral recti causing globe retraction and narrowing of the palpebral aperture on lateral gaze. Symptoms occur secondary to a cranial nerve III-VI synkinesis. Blepharoptosis can occur secondarily.	Nonprogressive	Majority sporadic 5–10% inherited AD Rarely AR	Sporadic mutations involve *CHN1* gene (chimerin 1, GTP-ase-activating protein)	Surgical correction of strabismus and blepharoptosis where indicated
Marcus Gunn jaw-winking syndrome[2–5,6]	Birth	Patients typically present with congenital blepharoptosis with an upper eyelid that elevates with opening of the mouth or moving the jaw. Symptoms are secondary to cranial nerve III-V synkinesis.	Nonprogressive	Nonhereditary	N/A	For patients with mild blepharoptosis, observation. For patients with severe ptosis, levator aponeurosis disinsertion, and frontalis suspension
Marin-Amat syndrome, "Inverted Marcus Gunn phenomenon"[7]	Typically acquired after facial nerve palsy, rarely congenital	Synkinesis of cranial nerves V and VII, whereby jaw opening leads to eyelid closure	Nonprogressive	Can be acquired or inherited (rare); unknown genetics	Unknown	Facial neuromuscular retraining and in select cases, botulinum toxin
Static myopathic ptoses involving the extraocular muscles						
Blepharophimosis-ptosis-epicanthus inversus syndrome[8,9]	Birth	Classically, patients have severe bilateral blepharoptosis, blepharophimosis, epicanthus inversus, and telecanthus. Other periorbital findings include lower lid ectropion, hypertelorism, superior orbital rim hypoplasia, and lacrimal system abnormalities, present in varying degrees. Type I is associated with ovarian insufficiency	Nonprogressive, possible improvement of telecanthus with growth	AD	*FOXL2* (forehead box protein 2) is responsible for types I and II	Surgical correction of blepharoptosis and phimosis
Congenital fibrosis of the extraocular muscles syndrome (CFEOM)[10,11]	Birth	Bilateral blepharoptosis and external ophthalmoplegia involving vertical gaze, and to a variable degree horizontal gaze. Patients have hypotropia in the affected eye with chin up head posture.	Nonprogressive	CFEOM1 AD CFEOM2 AR CFEOM3 AD Tukel AR	1: *KIF21A* (kinesin family member 7)/ *TUBB3* (tubulin beta 3 class III) 2: *PHOX2A* (paired like homeobox 2a) 3: *KIF21A*/*TUBB3* Tukel: Unknown	Surgical correction of strabismus and blepharoptosis where indicated
Monocular elevation deficiency, formerly "double elevator palsy"[12–14]	Present at birth, or acquired	Unilateral syndrome, in which the eye is not able to supraduct in all fields of gaze. Hypotropia is present in primary position. Can be associated with blepharoptosis	Nonprogressive	Sporadic	N/A	Surgical correction of strabismus, followed by surgical correction of blepharoptosis

(*Continued*)

Table 32.1 (*Continued*) Summary of syndromic progressive myopathic ptoses

Disease	Age of onset	Symptoms	Progressive/nonprogressive	Inheritance	Gene	Treatment
Progressive myopathic ptoses affecting the levator muscle and other muscle groups that present in childhood						
Autosomal dominant optic atrophy plus syndrome (Treft Sanborn Carey syndrome)[15]	Childhood	Bilateral optic atrophy, sensorineural hearing loss, myopathy leading to ophthalmoplegia, blepharoptosis, ataxia, and peripheral neuropathy	Progressive	AD	OPA1 (OPA1 protein, a mitochondrial dynamin like GTPase)	Supportive measures. Surgical correction of strabismus and blepharoptosis where indicated
Central core myopathy (Shy-Magee Syndrome), muscle core disease, central fibrillary myopathy[16,17]	Birth	Hypotonia, limb weakness, blepharoptosis	Nonprogressive or progressive	AD	RYR1 gene (skeletal muscle ryanodine receptor, calcium channel in the sarcoplasmic reticulum)	**Supportive care. Salbutamol may help with weakness.** Surgical correction of blepharoptosis
Centronuclear myopathy, X-linked myotubular myopathy (XLMM)[a,18,19]	Infancy, early childhood	Facial and neck muscle weakness, including ocular (blepharoptosis, ophthalmoparesis), limb weakness, diaphragmatic weakness	Often progressive	XLR, AD, or AR	More common: DNM2 gene (dynamin 2), BIN1 (bridging integrator 1), TTN (Titin). Less common: CCDC78 gene (coiled-coil domain containing 78), SPEG (A member of the myosin light chain kinase family, required for myocyte cytoskeletal development), RYR1 (skeletal muscle ryanodine receptor, calcium channel in the sarcoplasmic reticulum). XLMM: MTM1 (myotubularin)	Supportive care. Surgical correction of strabismus and ptosis where indicated
Chromosome 3p-syndrome[20,21]	Birth	Poor growth, developmental delay, intellectual disability, microcephaly, autism spectrum disorder, hypotonia, blepharoptosis	Nonprogressive	Nonhereditary	Chromosomal: Secondary to a deletion of a segment of the short arm of chromosome 3	Supportive care. Surgical correction of blepharoptosis in indicated cases
Congenital fiber-type disproportion[a,22–25]	Birth	Floppiness, limb and facial weakness; ptosis, ophthalmoplegia, bulbar weakness and diaphragmatic weakness	Usually non-progressive or may show improvement over time	AD, AR, or XLR	ACTA1 (skeletal muscle actin), SEPN1 (Selenoprotein N), TPM3 (Tropomyosin 3)	Supportive care. Surgical correction of strabismus and blepharoptosis where indicated
Gillum-Anderson syndrome[26]	Congenital	Ectopia lentis, myopia, blepharoptosis with reduction in strength of the levator aponeurosis, findings likely secondary to connective tissue abnormalities	Non-progressive	AD	Unknown	Definitive treatment for ectopia lentis and blepharoptosis is surgical

(*Continued*)

Table 32.1 (Continued) Summary of syndromic progressive myopathic ptoses

Disease	Age of onset	Symptoms	Progressive/nonprogressive	Inheritance	Gene	Treatment
Kugelberg-Welander syndrome[a,27]	After 1 year	Hypotonia and weakness proximal > distal. 50% have scoliosis and restrictive lung disease. Diaphragmatic weakness may occur late in the disease. May have blepharoptosis.	Progressive	AR	SMN (survival motor neuron protein), NAIP (neuronal apoptosis inhibitory protein)	Supportive care Surgical correction of blepharoptosis
Limb girdle muscular dystrophy[b,28,29,30]	Early childhood	Progressive weakness the shoulder and hip girdle muscles with sparing of the facial muscles (type I and type II based on inheritance). Subtype LGMD1C presents with proximal muscle weakness, ophthalmoplegia, exophthalmos, and blepharoptosis. GMPPB subtype with mental retardation, microcephaly, epilepsy, cataract, strabismus, nystagmus, and blepharoptosis.	Progressive	AR (type 2 90%), AD (type 1)	1B: *LMNA* (Lamins A and C are intermediate filaments which are components of the nuclear envelope) 1C: *Caveolin 3* gene (caveolin 3, plays a role in the formation of muscle fibers) 2A: *CAPN3* (calpain-3) 2B: *DYSF* (dysferlin) 2C-2F: SGCA (sarcoglycan protein complex) 2J: *TTN* (Titin) 2L: *ANO5* (anoctamin-5) 2I, 2K, 2M-N: GMPPB gene/protein POMGNT1 gene/protein	Supportive care Surgical correction of strabismus and blepharoptosis in indicated cases
Lymphedema-distichiasis-syndrome[31–33]	Variable	Lymphedema, distichiasis, blepharoptosis in 30% of patients. Possible systemic associations include cardiac defects, cleft palate, spinal cord cysts, and scoliosis	Lymphedema develops by age 40, distichiasis occurs in 94%, presentation of blepharoptosis is variable	AD; 25% sporadic	FOXC3 gene (forkhead box C2, a transcription factor)	Treatment of lymphedema and distichiasis by conventional methods. Surgical correction of blepharoptosis
Mitochondrial neurogastrointestinal encephalopathy syndrome (MNGIE)[34]	Variable (infancy to adulthood)	Gastrointestinal dysmotility, cachexia, peripheral neuropathy, leukoencephalopathy, blepharoptosis	Progressive	AR	TYMP (thymidine phosphorylase)	Supportive care Surgical correction of blepharoptosis in indicated cases
Multiminicore myopathy[a,17,35,36]	Birth, infancy	Hypotonia, generalized muscle weakness (predominately axial), facial weakness, blepharoptosis, ophthalmoplegia	Static or progressive	AR	RYR1 gene in atypical cases (skeletal muscle ryanodine receptor, Calcium channel in the sarcoplasmic reticulum), *SELENON* gene in classic cases (Selenoprotein N)	Supportive care Surgical correction of strabismus and blepharoptosis

(*Continued*)

199

Table 32.1 (*Continued*) Summary of syndromic progressive myopathic ptoses

Disease	Age of onset	Symptoms	Progressive/nonprogressive	Inheritance	Gene	Treatment
Myotonia congenita[37]	Variable	Intermittent episodes of myotonia, may include ocular muscles, relieved with repeated contractions; Thomsen disease is more mild, Becker disease more common. Symptoms may improve later in life	Nonprogressive	AD (Thomsen), AR (Becker)	CLCN1 gene, (chloride voltage gated channel 1)	Treatment of muscle stiffness.
Myotubular myopathy[a,17]	Birth to childhood	Severe weakness, hypotonia, facial weakness, bulbar weakness, diaphragmatic weakness	Frequently fatal in childhood	XLR (most severe form), AD (least severe and does not affect eyes), AR	MTM1 gene (myotubularin)	Supportive care Surgical correction of blepharoptosis where indicated
Nemaline myopathy[17,38,39]	Childhood	Generalized hypotonia and diaphragmatic weakness. Distal weakness of lower extremities, severe facial and bulbar weakness.	Nonprogressive	AD, AR, or sporadic	ACTA1 TPM2 TPM3 NEB TNNT1 KBTBD CFL2 Genes encode protein components of the muscle thin filament, most commonly nebulin protein (NEB) or alpha actin.	Supportive care Surgical correction of blepharoptosis
Noonan syndrome[40]	Birth	Distinct facies notable for hypertelorism, epicanthal folds, blepharoptosis, micrognathia, webbed neck, low posterior hairline, pectus carinatum, short stature, kyphosis/scoliosis, cardiac anomalies, platelet deficiency, cryptorchidism	Nonprogressive	AD	PTPN11 (50%) SOS 1 (10–13%) RAF1 (5%) RIT1 (these genes encode proteins important in the RAS/MAPK cell signaling pathway important for cell division, growth, differentiation and migraine) KRAS (<5%) Less frequent: NRAS BRAF MEK2 RRAS RASA2 A2ML1 SOS2 LZTR1	Surgical correction of blepharoptosis in indicated cases

(*Continued*)

Table 32.1 (*Continued*) Summary of syndromic progressive myopathic ptoses

Disease	Age of onset	Symptoms	Progressive/nonprogressive	Inheritance	Gene	Treatment
Parry Romberg syndrome[41]	Late childhood/early adulthood	Hemifacial atrophy initially affecting the maxilla and between the nasolabial folds. The tongue and soft palate may be involved. Ocular manifestations include enophthalmos, blepharoptosis, uveitis	Progressive	Nonhereditary	N/A	Reconstructive or microvascular surgery where indicated
Sensory ataxic neuropathy, dysarthria and ophthalmoplegia (SANDO)[42,43]	Variable (5–17 years of age)	Sensory ataxic neuropathy, dysarthria, ophthalmoparesis. Hearing loss, seizures, myopathy may occur and lead to blepharoptosis.	Progressive	AR (nuclear coded mitrochondrial DNA)	POLG (DNA polymerase gamma gene)	Supportive care Surgical correction of strabismus and blepharoptosis in indicated cases
Saethre-Chotezen syndrome (acrocephalosyndactyly)[44]	Birth	Craniosynostosis with midface hypoplasia, hypoplastic maxilla, blepharoptosis, hypertelorism	Nonprogressive	AD	TWIST1 (encodes TWIST 1 protein, a transcription factor)	Patients may require craniofacial reconstruction, including blepharoptosis repair
Vertebral fusion posterior lumbosacral blepharoptosis[45]	Birth	Congenital blepharoptosis, posterior fusion of lumbosacral vertebrae	Nonprogressive	AD	Unknown	Treatment of lumbosacral vertebral fusion by conventional methods; surgical correction of blepharoptosis
Progressive myopathic ptoses seen in adulthood						
Chronic progressive external ophthalmoplegia[17,46]	Early adulthood	Generalized weakness, blepharoptosis, ophthalmoplegia, facial weakness including orbicularis; Plus syndrome includes sensorineural hearing loss, ataxia, parkinsonism	Progressive	AR, AD, MM	Nuclear DNA (AD): POLG TWNK SLC25A4 Nuclear DNA (AR): POLG RRM2B Mutation in these genes leads to large deletions of mtDNA in muscle cells; mechanism unclear Mitochondrial DNA: MT-TL1 (disrupt tRNA function, thus interrupting production of proteins involved in oxidative phosphorylation)	Surgical correction of strabismus, followed by surgical correction of blepharoptosis where indicated

(*Continued*)

Table 32.1 (Continued) Summary of syndromic progressive myopathic ptoses

Disease	Age of onset	Symptoms	Progressive/nonprogressive	Inheritance	Gene	Treatment
Desmin (myofibrillary) myopathy[47,48]	Infancy to adulthood (more common)	Muscle weakness distally, progresses to proximal muscles, peripheral neuropathy, cardiomyopathy, blepharoptosis without ophthalmoparesis	Progressive	AD, AR, XLR, or sporadic	AD: DES (Desmin) TTN (Titin) DNAJB6 (Dnaj heat shock protein family (Hsp40) member B6) MYOT (Myotilin) LDB3 (LIM domain binding 3) FLNC (filamin C) BAG3 (BCL2 associated athanogene 3) XLR: FHL1 (four and a half LIM domains 1) AR: CRYAB (Crystallin alpha B)	Supportive care Treatment of blepharoptosis where indicated.
Myotonic dystrophy type I and I (DMI, DMII)[b,28,49]	Congenital, juvenile, and adult forms	Hypotonia, blepharoptosis, diaphragmatic weakness, atrophy, myotonia, cardiac conduction abnormalities. DMII is less severe.	Progressive	AD	DMI: DMPK DMII: CNBP Leads to expanded microsatellite sequences and intranuclear accumulation of mutated transcripts	Supportive care; surgical correction of blepharoptosis where indicated
Oculopharyngeal muscular dystrophy[b,17]	Adulthood (40–60 years of age)	Ophthalmoplegia and blepharoptosis, dysphagia, proximal weakness	Progressive	AD, AR	PABPN1 (polyadenylate binding protein nuclear 1)	Supportive care, surgical correction of strabismus and blepharoptosis in indicated cases
Oculopharyngodistal myopathy[28,50,51]	Adulthood	Blepharoptosis, external ophthalmoplegia, dysphagia, and distal weakness.	Progressive	AD, AR	Unknown	Supportive care Surgical correction of strabismus and blepharoptosis in indicated cases

Abbreviations: AD, autosomal dominant; AR, autosomal recessive; MM, maternal mitochondrial; N/A, not applicable; XLR, X-linked recessive,
[a]Denotes fatal genetic mutation over time due to respiratory failure and pneumonia.
[b]Denotes muscular dystrophy.

sequelae of the genetic abnormalities. A thorough medical and family history should be taken to document the congenital timeline, other systemic problems, and to determine if the blepharoptosis defect is isolated and sporadic. Making the syndromic diagnosis early will maximize patient outcomes by recruiting other subspecialists to care for patients with these challenging conditions.

References

[1] Isolated duane retraction syndrome. Available at: ghr.nml.nih.gov. Updated 2018. Accessed June 10, 2018

[2] Yin X, Pu CQ, Wang Q, Liu JX, Mao YL. Clinical and pathological features of patients with nemaline myopathy. Mol Med Rep. 2014; 10(1):175–182

[3] Demirci H, Frueh BR, Nelson CC. Marcus Gunn jaw-winking synkinesis: clinical features and management. Ophthalmology. 2010; 117(7):1447–1452

[4] Khwarg SI, Tarbet KJ, Dortzbach RK, Lucarelli MJ. Management of moderate-to-severe Marcus-Gunn jaw-winking ptosis. Ophthalmology. 1999; 106(6):1191–1196

[5] Pearce FC, McNab AA, Hardy TG. Marcus Gunn jaw-winking syndrome: a comprehensive review and report of four novel cases. Ophthalmic Plast Reconstr Surg. 2017;33(5):325–328

[6] Pratt SG, Beyer CK, Johnson CC. The Marcus Gunn phenomenon. A review of 71 cases. Ophthalmology. 1984; 91(1):27–30

[7] Rana PVS, Wadia RS. The Marin-Amat syndrome: an unusual facial synkinesia. J Neurol Neurosurg Psychiatry. 1985; 48(9):939–941

[8] Allen CE, Rubin PA. Blepharophimosis-ptosis-epicanthus inversus syndrome (BPES): clinical manifestation and treatment. Int Ophthalmol Clin. 2008; 48(2):15–23

[9] Fang J, Dagenais SL, Erickson RP, et al. Mutations in FOXC2 (MFH-1), a forkhead family transcription factor, are responsible for the hereditary lymphedema-distichiasis syndrome. Am J Hum Genet. 2000; 67(6):1382–1388

[10] Doherty E, Macy M, Sener SW. CFEOM3: a new extra ocular congenital fibrosis syndrome that maps to 16q24.2–24.3. Invest Ophthalmol Vis Sci. 1999; 40:1687–1694

[11] Engle EC, Kunkel LM, Specht LA, Beggs AH. Mapping a gene for congenital fibrosis of the extraocular muscles to the centromeric region of chromosome 12. Nat Genet. 1994; 7(1):69–73

[12] Bagheri A, Sahebghalam R, Abrishami M. Double elevator palsy, subtypes and outcomes of surgery. J Ophthalmic Vis Res. 2008; 3(2):108–113

[13] Jampel RS, Fells P. Monocular elevation paresis caused by a central nervous system lesion. Arch Ophthalmol. 1968; 80(1):45–57

[14] Scott WE, Jackson OB. Double elevator palsy: the significance of inferior rectus restriction. Am Orthopt J. 1977; 27:5–10

[15] Miller NR, Subramanian P, Patel V. Walsh & Hoyt's Clinical Neuro-ophthalmology: The Essentials. 3rd ed. Philadelphia, PA: Wolters Kluwer Health; 2015

[16] Central core disease of muscle, MIM number: 117000. In: Online mendelian inheritance in man, OMIM. Baltimore, MD: Johns Hopkins University; Updated 2015. Available at https://www.omim.org/entry/117000. Accessed May 1, 2018

[17] Kahn ND, Weinberg DA. Myogenic ptosis. In: Cohen AJ, Weinberg DA, eds. Evaluation and Management of Blepharoptosis. Springer Science and Business Media; 2011

[18] Myopathy C. X-linked, MIM number: 310400; In: Online mendelian inheritance in man, OMIM. Baltimore, MD: Johns Hopkins University. Updated 2016. Available at https://www.omim.org/entry/310400. Accessed May 1, 2018

[19] Centronuclear myopathy 1, MIM number: 160150. In: Online mendelian inheritance in man, OMIM. Baltimore, MD: Johns Hopkins University; Updated 2015. Available at https://www.omim.org/entry/160150. Accessed May 1, 2018

[20] Chromosome 3p deletion: Genetic and rare diseases information center, national center for advancing translational sciences. Available at https://rarediseases.info.nih.gov/diseases/37/chromosome-3p-deletion. Updated 2015. Accessed May 16, 2018

[21] 3p deletion syndrome: National library of medicine (US). Genetics home reference. Available at https://ghr.nlm.nih.gov/condition/3p-deletion-syndrome#sourcesforpage. Updated 2018

[22] Clarke NF. Congenital fiber-type disproportion. Semin Pediatr Neurol. 2011; 18(4):264–271

[23] Tropomyosin 3; TPM3, MIM number: 191030; In: Online mendelian inheritance in man, OMIM. Baltimore, MD: Johns Hopkins University; Updated 2016. Available at https://www.omim.org/entry/191030. Accessed May 1, 2018

[24] Myopathy, congenital, with fiber type disproportion, MIM number: 255310; In: Online mendelian inheritance in man, OMIM. Baltimore, MD: Johns Hopkins University; Updated 2014. Available at https://www.omim.org/entry/255310. Accessed May 1, 2018

[25] Selenoprotein N. selenon, MIM number: 606210. In: Online mendelian inheritance in man, OMIM. Baltimore, MD: Johns Hopkins University; Updated 2016. Available at https://www.omim.org/entry/606210. Accessed May 1, 2018

[26] Winter RM, Baraitser M. Gillum Anderson syndrome. In: Multiple congenital anomalies: A diagnostic compendium. Springer-Science; 2013:1430

[27] National Organization for Rare Disorders. Russman BS. Kugelberg Welander syndrome. Available at https://rarediseases.org/rare-diseases/kugelberg-welander-syndrome/. Updated 2012. Accessed June 10, 2018

[28] Evliyaoglu F, Burakgazi AZ. Ocular findings in muscular dystrophies. Journal of Medicine and Medical Sciences. 2015; 6(9):234–242

[29] Muscular dystrophy, limb girdle, type 2A, MIM number: 253600. In: Online mendelian inheritance in man, OMIM. Baltimore, MD: Johns Hopkins University; Updated 2010. Available at https://www.omim.org/entry/253600. Accessed May 1, 2018

[30] Lamin A. CAPN3; TITIN; CAV3; ANO5; DYSF. In: Online mendelian inheritance in man, OMIM. Baltimore, MD: Johns Hopkins University. Available at https://www.omim.org. Accessed May 1, 2018

[31] Brice G, Mansour S, Bell R, et al. Analysis of the phenotypic abnormalities in lymphoedema-distichiasis syndrome in 74 patients with FOXC2 mutations or linkage to 16q24. J Med Genet. 2002; 39(7):478–483

[32] Rosbotham JL, Brice GW, Child AH, Nunan TO, Mortimer PS, Burnand KG. Distichiasis-lymphoedema: clinical features, venous function and lymphoscintigraphy. Br J Dermatol. 2000; 142(1):148–152

[33] McDermott S, Lahiff C. Lymphedema-distichiasis syndrome. CMAJ. 2016; 188(2):E44

[34] Mitochondrial DNA depletion syndrome 1 (MNGIE TYPE), MIM number: 603041; In: Online mendelian inheritance in man, OMIM. Baltimore, MD: Johns Hopkins University; Updated 2018. Available at https://www.omim.org/entry/603041. Accessed May 1, 2018

[35] Ferreiro A, Estournet B, Chateau D, et al. Multi-minicore disease–searching for boundaries: phenotype analysis of 38 cases. Ann Neurol. 2000; 48(5):745–757

[36] Ferreiro A, Fardeau M. 80th ENMC international workshop on multi-minicore disease: 1st international MmD workshop 12–13th may, 2000, Soestduinen, The Netherlands. Neuromuscul Disord. 2002; 12(1):60–68

[37] Myotonia congenita, autosomal dominant, MIM number: 160800. In: Online mendelian inheritance in man, OMIM. Baltimore, MD: Johns Hopkins University; Updated 2016. Available at https://www.omim.org/entry/160800. Accessed May 1, 2018

[38] Gilbreath HR, Castro D, Iannaccone ST. Congenital myopathies and muscular dystrophies. Neurol Clin. 2014; 32(3):689–703, viii

[39] Wallgren-Pettersson C, Sewry CA, Nowak KJ, Laing NG. Nemaline myopathies. Semin Pediatr Neurol. 2011; 18(4):230–238

[40] Noonan syndrome 1, MIM number 163950. In: Online mendelian inheritance in man, OMIM. Baltimore, MD: Johns Hopkins University. Updated 2017. Available at https://www.omim.org/entry/163950. Accessed May 1, 2018

[41] Stone J. Parry Romberg syndrome. In: National organization for rare disorders (NORD). 2016. Available at https://rarediseases.org/rare-diseases/parry-romberg-syndrome/. Accessed June 10, 2018

[42] Polymerase DNA. Gamma; POLG, MIM number: 174763; In: Online mendelian inheritance in man, OMIM. Baltimore, MD: Johns Hopkins University; Updated 2016. Available at https://www.omim.org/entry/174763. Accessed May 1, 2018

[43] Sensory ataxic neuropathy, dysarthria and ophthalmoparesis; SANDO, MIM number: 607459; In: Online mendelian inheritance in man, OMIM. Baltimore, MD: Johns Hopkins University; Updated 2016. Available at https://www.omim.org/entry/607459. Accessed May 1, 2018

[44] Saethre-Chotzen syndrome with eyelid anomalies, MIM number 101400. In: Online mendelian inheritance in man, OMIM. Baltimore, MD: Johns Hopkins University; Updated 2017. Available at https://www.omim.org/entry/101400. Accessed May 1, 2018

[45] Fusion V. posterior lumbrosacral with blepharoptosis, MIM number: 192800; In: Online mendelian inheritance in man, OMIM. Baltimore, MD: Johns Hopkins University; Updated 1995. Available at https://www.omim.org/entry/192800. Accessed May 1, 2018

[46] Progressive external ophthalmoplegia with mitochondrial DNA deletions, Autosomal dominant 5, OMIM number: 613077; In: Online mendelian inheritance in man, OMIM. Baltimore, MD: Johns Hopkins University; Updated 2012. Available at https://www.omim.org/entry/613077. Accessed May 1, 2018

[47] Myofibrillar myopathy; Desmin; Myotilin; Filamin; DNAJB6. In: Online mendelian inheritance in man, OMIM. Baltimore, MD: Johns Hopkins University. Available at https://www.omim.org. Accessed May 1, 2018

[48] Myofibrillar myopathy: Genetic and rare diseases information center, national center for advancing translational sciences; Available at https://rarediseases.info.nih.gov/diseases/10529/myofibrillar-myopathy. Updated 2015. Accessed 5/9/2018

[49] Bird TD. Myotonic dystrophy. NORD (National Organization for Rare Disorders) web site. Available at https://rarediseases.org/rare-diseases/dystrophy-myotonic/. Updated 2017. Accessed 5/1/2018

[50] Durmus H, Laval SH, Deymeer F, et al. Oculopharyngodistal myopathy is a distinct entity: clinical and genetic features of 47 patients. Neurology. 2011; 76 (3):227–235

[51] Oculopharyngodistal myopathy, MIM number: 164310. In: Online mendelian inheritance in man, OMIM. Baltimore, MD: Johns Hopkins University; Updated 2016. Available at https://www.omim.org/entry/164310. Accessed May 1, 2018

[52] Kohn R, Romano PE. Blepharoptosis, blepharophimosis, epicanthus inversus, and telecanthus–a syndrome with no name. Am J Ophthalmol. 1971; 72(3): 625–632

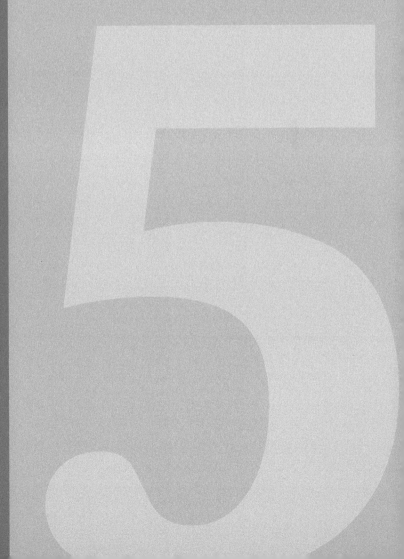

Section V Neurogenic Ptosis

33 Neurogenic Ptosis: Evaluation and Management

Kimberly K. Gokoffski, Vivek R. Patel

Abstract

In this chapter, we discuss neurogenic ptosis using an anatomical approach. Neurogenic forms of ptosis are important to recognize; in fact, in some cases ptosis is a key sign leading to the diagnosis of a life-threatening condition. The neuroanatomical circuitry is well characterized; however, following damage, interesting and complex reorganization can take place. Accurate diagnosis and appropriate intervention depends on a solid understanding of the underlying pathophysiology of these aberrant regeneration syndromes. We will cover the most common of these entities here, with representative examples throughout.

Keywords: neurogenic ptosis, Horner's syndrome, myasthenia gravis, third nerve palsy, aberrant innervation

33.1 Introduction

Most cases of blepharoptosis seen in clinical practice are due to aponeurotic or myopathic causes. While relatively rare, neurogenic blepharoptosis is important to recognize due to potential life-threatening concerns in some cases. Frequently, there are associated oculomotor and/or pupillary findings as well as other neurologic findings. Most cases of neurogenic ptosis seen in clinical practice are due to lesions of the oculomotor nerve (cranial nerve [CN] III) or disruption of the oculosympathetic pathway (Horner's syndrome). Rarely, cortical pathology may lead to neurogenic ptosis. In this chapter, we discuss neurogenic ptosis through a neuroanatomical lens, further differentiating patients who present with congenital versus acquired ptosis.

33.2 Neuroanatomic Considerations

Understanding neural pathways is critical to understanding the pathophysiology behind neurogenic ptosis. The important neurocircuitry discussed in this chapter includes cortical and supranuclear pathways, the oculomotor nerve nucleus and pathway, oculosympathetic projections, and the neuromuscular junction.

33.2.1 Cortical and Supranuclear Pathways

Ptosis produced by cerebral hemisphere dysfunction has been reported to be bilateral or unilateral.[1-4] Apraxia of eyelid opening, an inability to initiate voluntary eyelid opening in the presence of spontaneous lid elevation, hemispheric stroke, degenerative conditions, and blepharospasm fall under this rubric.

33.2.2 Oculomotor Nerve

Damage to the third nerve anywhere in its course from its nucleus in the dorsal mesencephalon, its fascicles in the brainstem parenchyma, the nerve root in the subarachnoid space, or in the cavernous sinus or posterior orbit can cause ptosis (▶ Fig. 33.1). Visual acuity is typically unaffected. The affected eye position is usually down and out (exotropic and hypotropic position) in cases with complete involvement. Limitation of eye elevation, depression, and adduction are noted due to innervation deficits to the superior rectus, inferior rectus, and medial rectus muscles, respectively. The pupil may be dilated and not light-responsive, reactive with normal response to light, or partially dilated and slightly responsive to light.

33.2.3 Oculosympathetic Pathway

A patient with a Horner's syndrome may present with ptosis, reverse ptosis of the lower eyelid, miosis in dim illumination, dilation lag, anhidrosis, lower intraocular pressure, and enhanced accommodation. In congenital cases, decreased iris

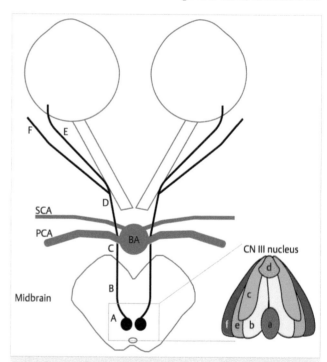

Fig. 33.1 Schematic of cranial nerve III pathway. A: CN III nucleus; B: fascicle of CN III; C: interpeduncular CN III; D: intercavernous CN III; E: superior branch of CN III; F: inferior branch CN III; a: central caudal nucleus; b: superior rectus nucleus; c: inferior rectus nucleus; d: Edinger–Westphal nuclei; e: inferior oblique nucleus; f: medial rectus nucleus; PCA: posterior cerebral artery; SCA: superior cerebellar artery; BA: basilar artery. A single central caudal nucleus controls both levator palpebrae muscles. The inferior oblique and medial rectus nuclei lie inferior to the nuclei of the superior rectus.

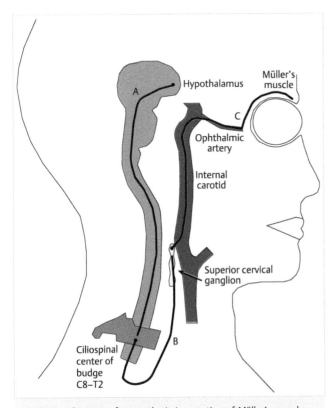

Fig. 33.2 Schematic of sympathetic innervation of Müller's muscle. A: the first-order neuron in the sympathetic chain originates in the hypothalamus and travels paramedian down the brainstem to synapse with second order neurons whose nuclei lie in the ciliospinal center of Budge. B: second-order neurons travel superiorly to synapse at the superior cervical ganglion. C: third-order neurons travel with the internal carotid, following the ophthalmic artery branch, through the optic canal, to synapse with Müllers muscle.

pigmentation is often seen. A Horner syndrome can result from a lesion or pathology anywhere along the three neuron adrenergic (sympathetic) pathway (▶ Fig. 33.2). The first-order neuron descends caudally from the hypothalamus to the first synapse at the lower cervical spinal cord (C8–T2; ciliospinal center of Budge). The second-order neuron travels from the sympathetic trunk through the brachial plexus, to the lung apex, and then ascends to the superior cervical ganglion located near the angle of the mandible and common carotid bifurcation. The third-order neuron then ascends adjacent to the internal carotid artery, through the cavernous sinus in close proximity to CN VI. The oculosympathetic pathway then joins the fifth CN (V1; ophthalmic division) to proceed to innervate the iris dilator muscle, Müller's muscle of the upper eyelid, and tarsal muscle of the lower eyelid. Postganglionic sympathetic fibers that are responsible for sweating follow the external carotid artery to the facial sweat glands.

33.2.4 Neuromuscular Junction

Autoantibodies at the neuromuscular junction acetylcholine (Ach) nicotinic postsynaptic receptors can cause variable ptosis, as seen in myasthenia gravis (MG) (▶ Fig. 33.3). A reduction in

the number of active Ach receptors results in the characteristic pattern of progressively diminished muscle strength with repeated use (fatigue) and recovery with rest. Other ocular findings may include double vision and a weakening of eyelid closure. The pupil is typically spared.

33.3 Localization

33.3.1 Supranuclear/Cortical Localization

Pathology above the third nerve nucleus and sympathetic pathways can lead to ptosis. Lesions in the hemispheres, brainstem, and degenerative conditions can all cause neurogenic ptosis.

Cerebral Hemorrhage

Large nondominant hemispheric strokes can lead to bilateral cortical ptosis. This ptosis, which is usually transient, lasting days to months, can be asymmetric and accompanied by gaze palsies with the eyes being deviated toward the nondominant, involved hemisphere.[5] Interestingly, a small prospective series of patients with large hemispheric strokes found complete bilateral or asymmetric ptosis to be the first sign of imminent herniation, preceding pupillary dilation and ophthalmoplegia. Cases of cortical ptosis resulting from bilateral frontal lobe infarcts have also been reported.[6]

Degenerative Conditions

Degeneration of the extrapyramidal tracts in the midbrain has been associated with eyelid apraxia. Eyelid apraxia is characterized by bilateral transient (on the order of 30 seconds) inability to open the eyelids after initiation of the blink reflex. Generally seen in patients with Parkinson's disease and progressive supranuclear palsy,[7,8] eyelid apraxia has also been described in Creutzfeldt–Jakob disease, amyotrophic lateral sclerosis, and Huntington's disease.[9,10] Electromyographic (EMG) studies divide patients with eyelid apraxia into three groups: (1) patients with intermittent inhibition of levator contraction without orbicularis oculi contraction, (2) patients with transient pretarsal orbicularis oculi contraction (atypical blepharospasm), and (3) patients who are unable to relax transient pretarsal contraction after blinking. This may explain variable responses to Botox injections. In addition to Botox, reports suggest some benefit from several drugs including L-dopa, desipramine, olanzapine, and riluzole. Blepharoplasty with orbicularis muscle extirpation should be considered in patients with dermatochalasis in conjunction with eyelid apraxia to alleviate any associated mechanical ptosis.

33.3.2 Brainstem Localization

Central First-Order Neuron Horner's Syndrome

Sympathetic innervation to Müller's muscle originates in the hypothalamus and travels paramedian down the entire length of the brainstem before synapsing in the ciliospinal center of Budge, located between C8–T2. Given the long, nondecussating,

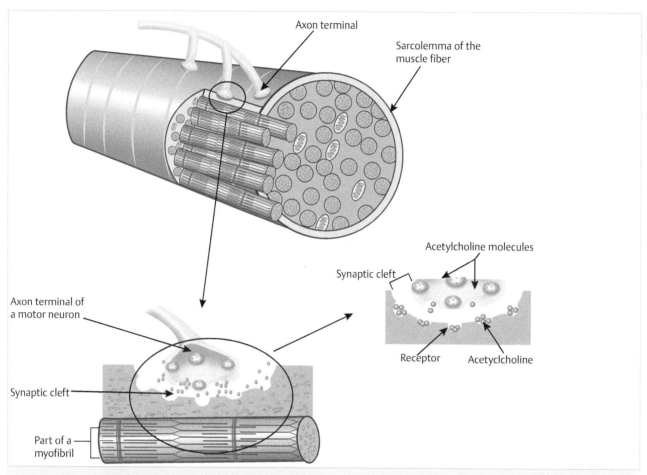

Fig. 33.3 Neuromuscular junction.

course of the central first-order sympathetic neuron, it is no wonder that brainstem lesions such as hemorrhage, ischemia, demyelination, and metastatic disease can cause ipsilateral Horner's syndrome with resulting ptosis. Patients with a first-order Horner syndrome will demonstrate the typical triad of ptosis, miosis, and facial anhidrosis due to involvement of ipsilateral facial sudomotor fibers. Given that Müller's muscle accounts for approximately 2 mm of upper lid elevation, ptosis is mild in Horner's syndrome relative to CN III palsies (discussed in Section 33.3.5). As sympathetic fibers also innervate the inferior lid retractors, inverse ptosis of the lower eyelids can also be observed (▶ Fig. 33.4).

Central/first-order Horner's syndrome can usually be distinguished from lower order syndromes involving the second- or third-order sympathetic fibers by involvement of other localizing clinical signs. For example, in Wallenberg's syndrome, damage to the lateral medulla results in ipsilateral Horner's syndrome, ataxia, ipsilateral face with contralateral body pain and temperature hypoesthesia, and lateropulsion (deviating to the side of the lesion) secondary to co-disruption of the descending oculosympathetics, ipsilateral spinal trigeminal tract, ascending decussated spinothalamic tract fibers, and vestibular nuclei, respectively. Infarction of the anterior inferior cerebellar artery can result in Foville's syndrome, which is characterized by ipsilateral Horner's syndrome and CN V, VI, VII, and sometimes even VIII palsy, with contralateral hemiparesis.

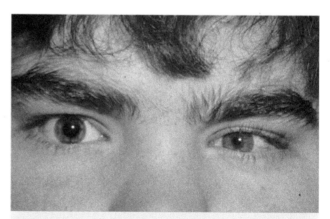

Fig. 33.4 Left Horner's syndrome: 21-year-old man with left eye upper and lower lid (inverse) ptosis, with pupillary miosis. Note the lateral conjunctival injection due to loss of vasoconstrictive tone to ocular surface vascular smooth muscle. The mild esotropia suggests third-order neuron localization due to the co-localization of the sympathetic fibers with the intracavernous portion of the abducens nerve.

If a first-order Horner syndrome is suspected, a magnetic resonance imaging (MRI) of the brain with and without contrast is the investigation of choice.

Potent direct sympathomimetic agents such as phenylephrine will demonstrate mild improvement in ptosis in patients with Horner's syndrome. Instillation of apraclonidine, a weak alpha-1 adrenergic agent, can result in reversal (or significant reduction of) anisocoria, due to denervation supersensitivity, which can develop within 48 hours of damage to the sympathetic chain in acute cases. Cocaine (4% or 10%) drops may still be useful in the most acute of presentations (blocks reuptake of noradrenaline, hence development of supersensitivity is not required); however, apraclonidine testing has all but replaced use of cocaine drops in all other settings. Neither drop helps differentiate between pre- and post-ganglionic presentations, but can be very helpful to confirm diagnostic suspicion of a Horner's syndrome.

Thalamic Hemorrhage

Similar to cases of cortical ptosis, transient bilateral ptosis after thalamic hemorrhage has been reported in the literature.[11] Ptosis is thought to result from concurrent involvement of either the rostral interstitial medial longitudinal fasciculus (which lies caudal to the thalamus) or the posterior limb of the internal capsule (which lies temporal to the thalamus), leading to disruption of supranuclear cortical control of the central caudal nucleus of CN III.

Dorsal Midbrain (Parinaud's) Syndrome

Classically, dorsal midbrain syndrome leads to eyelid retraction (Collier's sign, ▶ Fig. 33.5) from release of inhibition on the central caudal nucleus of CN III by inhibitory neurons of the posterior commissure. However, when damage to the dorsal midbrain is severe and results in concurrent damage to the central caudal nucleus of CN III, patients can experience severe bilateral ptosis.

Familial Dysautonomia/Riley–Day Syndrome

Riley–Day syndrome is an inherited dysautonomia whose ophthalmic examination is characterized by corneal hypoesthesia, decreased lacrimation, exodeviations, retinal vasculature tortuosity, anisocoria, and ptosis.[12] Described most often in patients of Ashkenazy descent, ptosis in this inherited dysautonomia is thought to result from sympathetic denervation and

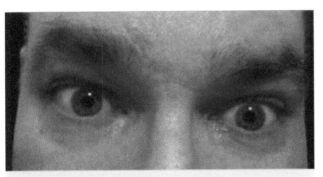

Fig. 33.5 Bilateral symmetric upper eyelid retraction in Parinaud's (dorsal midbrain) syndrome (Collier's sign). This finding is often associated with inability to elevate the eyes, convergence-retraction nystagmus on attempted upgaze, and light-near dissociation of the pupillary response.

has been found to improve with instillation of dilute sympathomimetics.[13]

33.3.3 Spinal Cord and Paravertebral Ganglia Localization

Second-Order Neuron Horner's Syndrome

Second-order sympathetic nerve originates in the ciliospinal center of Budge and travels superiorly over the apex of the lung, under the subclavian artery, up the common carotid to synapse on the superior cervical ganglion which sits near the bifurcation of the common carotid into the external and internal carotid arteries. Because sudomotor fibers that innervate the sweat glands of the face branch off at this point, anhidrosis of the ipsilateral face can be a localizing sign of first- or second-order sympathetic neuron damage. Given its trajectory, the differential diagnosis for second-order Horner's syndrome includes tumors of the apex of the lung, thyroid, or carotid sheath, and iatrogenic causes (central line placement). The diagnostic studies of choice here are magnetic resonance angiogram (MRA) or computed tomography angiogram (CTA) of the neck and soft tissue views (CT or MRI) of the upper chest and neck.

33.3.4 Carotid Artery and Cavernous Sinus Localization

Third-Order Neuron Horner's Syndrome

Third-order sympathetic neuron originates in the superior cervical ganglion, traveling up the internal carotid artery until it enters the cavernous sinus, at which point the sympathetic fibers briefly join CN VI before transitioning to the nasociliary branch of CN V. However, nerves bound for the eyelid continue with the internal carotid, then ophthalmic artery, through the optic canal to innervate Müller's muscle and its lower eyelid counterpart. Pharmacological testing with hydroxyamphetamine can be used to distinguish third-order Horner's syndrome from preganglionic etiologies: after confirmation of Horner's syndrome with cocaine or apraclonidine eye drops, instillation of hydroxyamphetamine will lead to pupillary dilation if the third-order sympathetic neuron is intact (i.e., the lesion is preganglionic). At least 48 hours should separate hydroxyamphetamine from either cocaine or apraclonidine testing.

Although the differential diagnosis for a third-order Horner's syndrome is broad, by far the most feared etiology is a carotid artery dissection. It is widely recommended that patients presenting with isolated, painful Horner's syndrome undergo urgent angiography to rule out carotid artery dissection. Other etiologies to consider include cavernous sinus syndromes, which typically have concurrent involvement of CNs IV, V, or VI, as well as orbital apex syndromes.

33.3.5 Nuclear Localization

Brainstem: Central Caudal Nucleus of CN III

The central caudal nucleus of CN III provides bilateral equal innervation to the levator muscles. As such, lesions to the midbrain generally result in bilateral, symmetric, and severe ptosis.

Generally, mesencephalic causes of ptosis are associated with other localizing signs (e.g., ophthalmoplegia, Horner's); however, rarely they can occur in isolation. Acquired etiologies include ischemia, hemorrhage, infection, demyelinating, and malignancy.

Ophthalmoplegic Migraine

In young patients with a history of migraine, recurrent ptosis, ophthalmoplegia, and mydriasis lasting a few days (but up to 6–8 weeks) can sometimes be attributed to ophthalmoplegic migraines. The International Classification of Headache Disorders classifies ophthalmoplegic migraines as at least two attacks of migraine-like headache followed by CNs III, IV, or VI palsy within 4 days, without evidence of compressive lesion, infarction, infection, or thrombosis on imaging, that resolves over the course of weeks. The etiology of ophthalmoplegic migraines is unknown. Some propose cranial neuropathy to result from intermittent vascular compression by dilated carotid or basilar arteries while others suggest an ischemic neuropathy as the underlying etiology.[14] Some patients have been documented to have enhancement of CN III, leading others to propose recurrent demyelination as the etiology of ophthalmoplegic migraines.[15]

Cyclic Oculomotor Paresis Syndrome

Cyclic oculomotor paresis syndrome is a rare condition in which partial or complete CN III palsy is interspersed, about every 2 minutes, with spastic episodes of CN III hyperfunction (lid elevation, globe adduction, miosis, and increased accommodation) lasting about 10 to 30 seconds.[16] Likened to ocular neuromyotonia, cyclic oculomotor paresis syndrome is generally diagnosed early in life and manifests throughout life. These patients can have concurrent deprivational amblyopia in the involved eye although normal vision has been reported as well.

33.3.6 Infranuclear Localization

Fascicular CN III Palsy

Unlike nuclear CN III palsies, damage to CN III fascicle leads to unilateral ptosis. Damage to the CN III fascicle is generally associated with involvement of the other extraocular muscles controlled by CN III, including superior rectus, medial rectus, inferior rectus, and inferior oblique, and may or may not involve the pupil. Depending on the extent of damage and involvement of surrounding nuclei, fascicular damage to CN III may be associated with a contralateral rubral tremor (Benedikt's syndrome or paramedian midbrain syndrome from concurrent red nucleus involvement), contralateral hemiparesis (Weber's syndrome from concurrent cerebral peduncle involvement), and ipsilateral cerebellar ataxia (Nothnagel's syndrome from concurrent superior cerebellar peduncle involvement). Causes of fascicular CN III damage include intrinsic etiologies (ischemia, hemorrhage, infection, demyelination) and extrinsic etiologies (tumor).

Peripheral CN III Palsy

CN III fascicle turns into CN III peripheral nerve when it exits the midbrain ventrally. CN III peripheral nerve then traverses between the posterior cerebral artery and superior cerebellar artery to enter the interpeduncular space, lateral to the posterior communicating artery, before piercing the dura to enter the cavernous sinus where it divides into superior and inferior branches. Similar to fascicular CN III damage, peripheral CN III palsy is unilateral, usually accompanied by involvement of the other extraocular muscles subserved by CN III, and may or may not involve the pupil (▶ Fig. 33.6). Rarely, ptosis may proceed involvement of extraocular muscles or pupil.

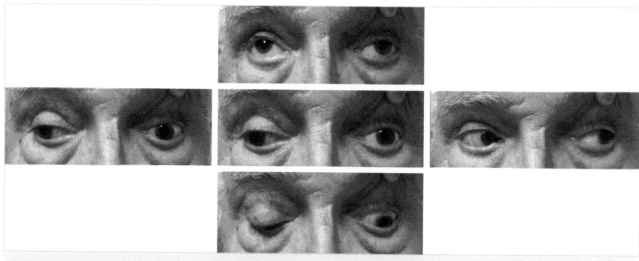

Fig. 33.6 A 76-year-old man with a near-complete left oculomotor nerve palsy. The eyelid is being manually elevated to demonstrate the limitations of adduction, elevation, and partial depression deficit. The pupils are pharmacologically dilated. Note the appearance of a large right exotropia in primary position, potentially resulting in the erroneous initial assumption that the right eye is the source of the misalignment. Rather, the patient is attempting to fixate with the paretic left eye, resulting in a large exotropia of the right eye, explained by Hering's law of reciprocal innervation.

Pupil Involving

The most dreaded etiology of a peripheral CN III palsy is compression by a posterior communicating artery aneurysm (PCOMM). Aneurysms greater than 3 mm in maximal dimension are more likely to be symptomatic; if rupture occurs, a roughly 50% mortality rate remains, despite recent advances (▶ Fig. 33.7).

Superior Divisional

Isolated involvement of the superior vision alone results in ptosis along with an elevation deficit of the same eye (superior rectus dysfunction). Damage can occur anywhere between the anterior-most portion of the cavernous sinus to the posterior orbit (▶ Fig. 33.8).

33.4 Aberrant Innervation Syndromes

33.4.1 Compressive/Trauma

When compressive or traumatic injury to CN III leads to disruption of the perineurial sheath, peripheral nerve bundles can make miswired connections during the regenerative phase. Aberrant connections can occur between the extraocular muscles, pupillary sphincter muscle, and levator palpebrae superioris. The most common aberrant connection occurs between fibers of the medial or inferior rectus with levator palpebrae, leading to eyelid elevation during adduction or infraduction, respectively. Although ptosis is often the first clinical deficit to improve postcompressive or traumatic CN III injury,

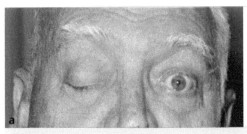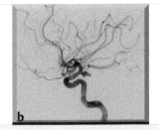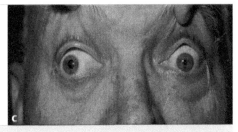

Fig. 33.7 (a–c) A 66-year-old man with right eyelid ptosis progressing to complete occlusion over 6 days, associated with periorbital pain. Manual elevation of the eyelid reveals a large relative unreactive pupil and an exotropic and mildly hypotropic right eye. Roughly 95% of compressive CN III palsies will produce some degree of pupillary dysfunction, and can present with partial or complete EOM limitation with the oculomotor nerve territory.

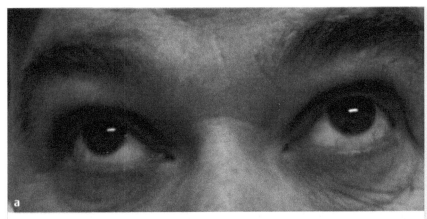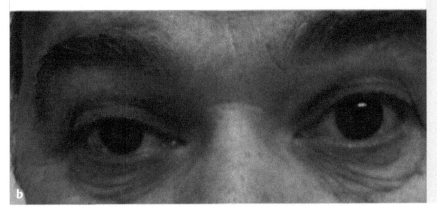

Fig. 33.8 (a, b) Right superior divisional CN III palsy. Subtle right upper eyelid ptosis in primary position, noted in **(b)**. In **(a)**, the patient is looking upwards, revealing the mild deficit of elevation of the right eye, due to mild right superior rectus dysfunction.

the improvement is more commonly from aberrancy than from true peripheral nerve regeneration. Importantly, aberrant regeneration *never* occurs following microvascular ischemic injury. Evidence of aberrant regeneration on initial presentation of the CN III palsy (primary aberrancy) or development of aberrancy weeks to months after the initial presentation (secondary aberrant regeneration), warrants immediate neuroimaging—preferably an MRI with and without contrast, or a CTA if a vascular lesion is highest on the differential (▶ Fig. 33.9).

33.4.2 Marin-Amat's Syndrome

Ptosis associated with opening of the mouth is often referred to as reverse or inverse jaw winking Marcus Gunn jaw-wink phenomenon. This terminology may be misleading, as it erroneously suggests that Marin-Amat's syndrome is a congenital disorder. Although an EMG study has shown that activation of the external pterygoid muscle when the jaw is thrusted to the opposite side leads to inhibition of the levator without activation of the orbicularis,[17] this reported case is of congenital origin, and likely not analogous to the more common form of Marin-Amat, which is an acquired disorder seen after traumatic damage to the facial nerve. The case reported by Lubkin is likely a true inverse jaw-winking case, whereas in Marin-Amat's syndrome the aberrancy lies at the level of the CN VII. The facial nerve carries the proprioceptive impulses generated by wide opening of the mouth. When the facial nerve is damaged, aberrant regeneration between these proprioceptive fibers and orbicularis oculi (both are branches of CN VII) could trigger eyelid closure by orbicularis oculi stimulation (▶ Fig. 33.10). Indeed EMG confirmation in these cases shows contraction of the orbicularis in response to full mouth opening without associated change in levator palpebrae superioris firing.[18] Given this ambiguity we concur that the term inverse jaw-winking should be reserved for congenital cases (between trigeminal and oculomotor innervated groups), and Marin-Amat's syndrome be used to describe eyelid closure following acquired CN VII damage.

33.4.3 Synkinesis

Synkinesis is aberrant innervation between different muscle groups that develop during gestation and can lead to transient ptosis.

Supranuclear Oculopalpebral Synkinesis

Supranuclear oculopalpebral synkinesis is characterized by ptosis in eccentric fields of gaze. On primary gaze, the palpebral fissure is typically of normal caliber. Ptosis arises on adduction (occasionally abduction) secondary to concurrent supranuclear inhibition of levator palpebrae.

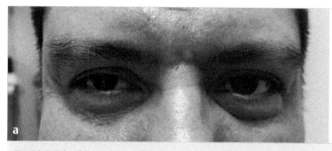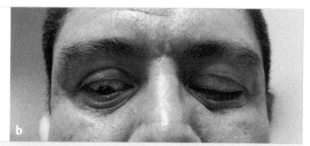

Fig. 33.9 (a) Mild right upper eyelid ptosis in primary position secondary to a right CN III palsy. (b) Note the right upper eyelid retraction on attempted downgaze, resulting from aberrant miswiring of branches of the damaged oculomotor nerve (pseudo-Von Graefe's sign). Here, branches innervating the right inferior rectus have made aberrant connections to the levator palpebrae superioris.

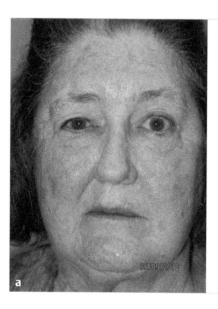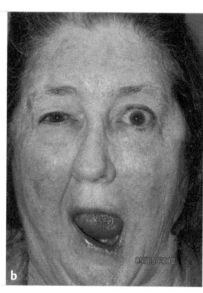

Fig. 33.10 (a) Patient with a history of right facial trauma 3 years ago, initially resulting in a right seventh nerve paresis. At time of current presentation, features of aberrant re-innervation are present, including relative deepening of the right nasolabial fold, and narrowing of the right palpebral fissure. (b) Marin-Amat's syndrome: accentuation of right eye palpebral fissure narrowing due to aberrant stimulation of the orbicularis oculi, elicited by wide opening of the mouth (cranial nerve V–VII aberrancy). (These images are provided courtesy of Dr. Michael A. Burnstine, MD, and Eyesthetica.)

Duane's Syndrome

Positional ptosis can also be seen in Duane's syndrome, a condition in which CN VI nucleus and nerve fail to develop properly. These patients develop synkinesis between CN III and CN VI. Patients with Duane's syndrome typically manifest ptosis on adduction secondary to globe retraction from co-contraction of both medial and lateral recti.

Marcus Gunn Jaw-Winking

Marcus Gunn jaw-winking phenomenon is characterized by ptosis and elevation of the eyelid with jaw movement. This phenomenon results from synkinesis between levator palpebrae and one of the pterygoid muscles of the jaw, more commonly the external rather than internal pterygoid. At rest, the eyelid is usually ptotic. Activation of the pterygoid muscles, such as with thrusting of the mandible to the contralateral side (ipsilateral external pterygoid contraction), forward thrusting of the jaw (bilateral external pterygoid contraction), or opening of the mouth widely, will lead to elevation of the upper eyelid. Patients are usually diagnosed in infancy after parents note eyelid movement during sucking. This condition can be associated with anisometropia, strabismus, and nystagmus and can lead to amblyopia. When indicated, surgical treatment usually consists of weakening of the levator palpebrae combined with a lid suspension procedure.[20]

33.5 Diseases of the Neuromuscular Junction

33.5.1 Myasthenia Gravis

Myasthenia gravis (MG) is an autoimmune condition that leads to decreased signal transduction at the neuromuscular junction (postsynaptic localization). About 70% of patients with MG will have ocular findings at the time of initial presentation. Thus, it is not uncommon for the ophthalmologist to make the initial diagnosis. MG has a reported incidence of 4 to 5/100,000 with a bimodal distribution. Typical presentations include patients in their 30s with a second peak involving males in their 60s. Of patients with isolated ocular MG, rates of conversion to generalized have been reported between 35 and 50% within 2 years of presentation. Generalization rates decrease significantly after the 2-year mark.

Diagnosis of ocular MG is based on clinical examination findings. Ptosis can be an isolated finding in patients with MG but is more often associated with orbicularis weakness, strabismus, and normal pupillary and deep tendon reflexes. When ptosis is present, it can be unilateral or bilateral—when bilateral, it is often asymmetric. The palpebral fissure will narrow with the lid fatigue test (patient is asked to hold extreme upgaze for 1 minute) and improve with the ice pack test (ice held to lid for 2 minutes) (▶ Fig. 33.11). When strabismus is present, saccadic velocities are initially "lightning" fast (supranormal velocity) but fatigue (slowing and hypometria) is apparent with repetitive movement. The hallmark of ptosis associated with MG is that of *moment to moment fluctuation* (▶ Fig. 33.12). Analogously, a Cogan lid twitch can be elicited by asking the patient to first look up for 5 to 10 seconds, followed by sustained downgaze for 10 seconds. Then the patient is asked to redirect gaze up to the examiner's nose. The levator palpebrae will demonstrate a small amplitude, momentary overshoot when the eyes are brought to primary position followed by a depression. The "see-saw sign" (a manifestation of Hering's law of reciprocal innervation) is another helpful sign, wherein manual elevation of the more ptotic eyelid results in increased in ptosis of the contralateral eyelid.

A positive Tensilon test, where an injection of edrophonium chloride results in immediate improvement in ptosis or strabismus, is pathognomonic for MG (▶ Fig. 33.13). If Tensilon testing

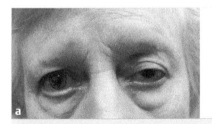 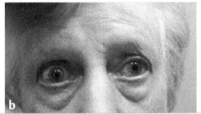 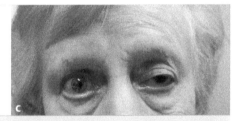

Fig. 33.11 Ice pack test for suspected ocular myasthenia gravis (MG). **(a)** A 74-year-old woman with left upper lid ptosis, before ice pack placement over the left upper eyelid. **(b)** Marked improvement in ptosis noted immediately after 2 minutes of ice pack application. **(c)** Return to baseline level of left upper eyelid ptosis, 5 minutes after completion of ice pack test.

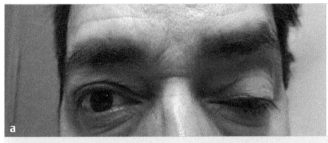 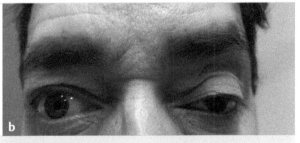

Fig. 33.12 Patient with ocular myasthenia gravis (MG) with profound left upper eyelid ptosis, exhibiting marked moment-to-moment fluctuation in lid height. **(a)** Photograph taken at moment of near-complete ptosis and **(b)** seconds later, noted to have a larger palpebral fissure, varying spontaneously.

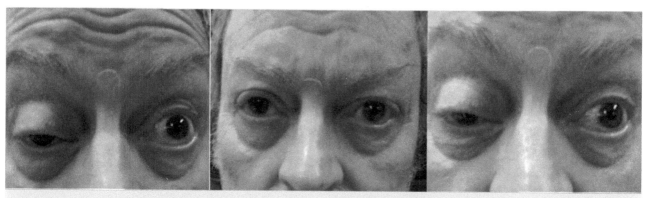

Fig. 33.13 A 71-year-old man was referred to with suspicion for right upper eyelid ptosis, and relative left eye proptosis. Rather, pseudoproptosis secondary to unequal palpebral fissures was considered, and ocular myasthenia gravis (MG) was suspected. Photo on the left shows marked right upper eyelid ptosis, left upper eyelid retraction and significant frontalis recruitment. The middle photo was taken 3 minutes after intravenous (IV) administration of 4 mg of edrophonium chloride. Note the relative normalization of the palpebral fissures and reduction in compensatory frontalis contraction. The right photos was taken just 10 minutes after the previous one, demonstrating findings nearly identical to baseline, underscoring the dramatic but short-lived effect of edrophonium chloride. This test should be administered with atropine 1 mg on hand in case of bradycardia, and performed under heart rate, blood pressure, and oxygen saturation monitoring.

cannot be performed, diagnosis of ocular MG can be facilitated with laboratory testing for anti-acetylcholine receptor binding, blocking, and modulating antibodies. Although up to 90% of patients with generalized MG can have positive serology, only 50% of patients with ocular-isolated MG will have positive antibodies. Of note, patients with ocular-isolated MG do not demonstrate positivity to anti-Musk antibody and thus we do not recommend this on routine testing. A retrospective study by Kupersmith et al[25] suggest that a short course of oral prednisone (slow titrated up to so as to prevent myasthenic crisis) in antibody-positive, ocular-isolated MG patients decreases the rate of conversion to generalized MG from 36 to 7%; thus, we routinely prescribe prednisone in antibody-positive patients. When MG serology is negative, a single-fiber electromyography (sf-EMG) can be obtained of the orbicularis oculi or frontalis muscles to assist with diagnosis. Sf-EMG will demonstrate increased jitter response in myasthenic patients. The authors recommend CT chest to evaluate for thymoma in patients with confirmed MG.

Pediatric Myasthenia Gravis

Pediatric MG can be grouped into three categories: transient neonatal myasthenia, congenital myasthenic syndrome, and juvenile myasthenia gravis (JMG). As suggested by the name, transient neonatal myasthenia is a transient condition that can occur in infants of mothers with active MG who pass their anti-acetylcholine receptor antibodies onto their infant during breast feeding. Muscle weakness resolves as the antibodies are cleared from the body.[22] In contrast, congenital myasthenic syndrome is a collection of inherited mutations of the motor endplate, most commonly of the acetylcholine receptor.[23] As such, the mainstay of treatment for patients with congenital myasthenic syndrome focuses on increasing acetylcholine signaling such as with receptor agonists. Although JMG is an autoimmune condition associated with variable ptosis and ophthalmoplegia, its clinical course differs from its adult counterpart.[24] JMG patients generally present before age 5, do well with pyridostigmine alone, and generalize at a much lower rate than adult MG. JMG patients

stabilize on average 37.9 months after presentation, with some even demonstrating complete resolution.

33.5.2 Lambert–Eaton Syndrome

Lambert–Eaton syndrome (LEMS) is a rare paraneoplastic syndrome most often associated with small cell lung cancer (SCLC), but also reported in association with non-small cell lung cancer (NSCLC), breast cancer, and lymphosarcoma. In contrast to MG, in LEMS the pathophysiological dysfunction occurs at the presynaptic membrane. Specifically, autoantibodies attack a specific population of voltage-gated calcium channels (VGCC), disrupting release of acetylcholine into the synaptic cleft. The clinical findings of ocular motor and levator palpebrae superioris dysfunction overlap with MG, but knowledge of some important differences can help the clinician differentiate between the two entities. Unlike MG, LEMS can affect the deep tendon reflexes, and autonomic dysfunction (labile blood pressure, dry eyes, dry mouth) are commonly seen. In LEMS, ocular findings do not present in isolation of the systemic afflictions. For patients presenting with findings suggestive of LEMS, a systemic workup including sending for a paraneoplastic antibody panel, chest/abdomen/pelvis imaging (CT or MRI), and referral to a neurologist is required, irrespective of whether the patient is known to have a malignancy.

33.6 Congenital Presentations

Both CN III and Horner's syndrome may present at birth.

33.6.1 Third Nerve Palsy

Isolated congenital CN III palsy is a rare condition.[25] In addition to ptosis, mydriasis, and ophthalmoplegia, congenital CN III palsies can be associated with aberrant regeneration, even in the absence of a history of birth trauma or forceps delivery. Patients with congenital CN III palsy can develop oculomotor paresis with cyclical spasm (see Section 33.3.5).

33.6.2 Congenital Horner's Syndrome

The most common etiology for congenital Horner's syndrome is delivery trauma from forceps use, vacuum extraction, fetal rotation, or central line placement.[26] A clinical sign that distinguishes congenital (or at least long-standing) Horner's from the acquired syndrome is the presence of heterochromia, with the abnormal iris being lighter in color. Decreased pigmentation results from decreased sympathetic stimulation of iris melanophores, which depend on norepinephrine for development. Heterochromia of the iris occurs irrespective of whether the Horner's is preganglionic or postganglionic as anterograde degeneration of the postganglionic neuron occurs in first- and second-order congenital Horner's. Patients with very blue irides do not manifest heterochromia. Of note, congenital Horner's can also result from congenital tumors and postviral infections. Thus, in the absence of obvious clinical history or physical evidence of delivery trauma (neck incision, shoulder dystocia), urgent imaging is recommended to rule out central causes of sympathetic dysinnervation.

33.7 Summary

Neurogenic ptosis should not be missed by the clinician because treatment is usually aimed at addressing the underlying anatomic pathology. A thorough understanding of the neurocircuitry is necessary to localize the disease and create a treatment plan.

References

[1] Caplan LR. Ptosis. J Neurol Neurosurg Psychiatry. 1974; 37(1):1–7
[2] Nutt JG. Lid abnormalities secondary to cerebral hemisphere lesions. Ann Neurol. 1977; 1(2):149–151
[3] Lepore FE. Bilateral cerebral ptosis. Neurology. 1987; 37(6):1043–1046
[4] Hamedani AG, Gold DR. Eyelid dysfunction in neurodegenenerative, neurogenetic, and neurometabolic disease. Front Neurol. 2017; 8:329–5
[5] Averbuch-Heller L, Leigh RJ, Mermelstein V, Zagalsky L, Streifler JY. Ptosis in patients with hemispheric strokes. Neurology. 2002; 58(4):620–624
[6] Krohel GB, Griffin JF. Cortical blepharoptosis. Am J Ophthalmol. 1978; 85(5 Pt 1):632–634
[7] Lee KC, Finley R, Miller B. Apraxia of lid opening: dose-dependent response to carbidopa-levodopa. Pharmacotherapy. 2004; 24(3):401–403
[8] Dehaene I. Apraxia of eyelid opening in progressive supranuclear palsy. Ann Neurol. 1984; 15(1):115–116
[9] Bonelli RM, Niederwieser G. Apraxia of eyelid closure in Huntington's disease. J Neural Transm (Vienna). 2002; 109(2):197–201
[10] Goldstein JE, Cogan DG. Apraxia of lid opening. Arch Ophthalmol. 1965; 73:155–159
[11] Lampl Y, Gilad R. Bilateral ptosis and changes in state of alertness in thalamic infarction. Clin Neurol Neurosurg. 1999; 101(1):49–52
[12] Goldberg MF, Payne JW, Brunt PW. Ophthalmologic studies of familial dysautonomia. The Riley-Day syndrome. Arch Ophthalmol. 1968; 80(6):732–743
[13] Liebman SD. Riley-Day syndrome: long-term ophthalmologic observations. Trans Am Ophthalmol Soc. 1968; 66:95–116
[14] Vijayan N. Ophthalmoplegic migraine: ischemic or compressive neuropathy? Headache. 1980; 20(6):300–304
[15] Gelfand AA, Gelfand JM, Prabakhar P, Goadsby PJ. Ophthalmoplegic "migraine" or recurrent ophthalmoplegic cranial neuropathy: new cases and a systematic review. J Child Neurol. 2012; 27(6):759–766
[16] Loewenfeld IE, Thompson HS. Oculomotor paresis with cyclic spasms. A critical review of the literature and a new case. Surv Ophthalmol. 1975; 20(2):81–124
[17] Lubkin V. The inverse Marcus Gunn phenomenon. An electromyographic contribution. Arch Neurol. 1978; 35(4):249
[18] Rana PV, Wadia RS. The Marin-Amat syndrome: an unusual facial synkinesia. J Neurol Neurosurg Psychiatry. 1985; 48(9):939–941
[19] Pratt SG, Beyer CK, Johnson CC. The Marcus Gunn phenomenon. A review of 71 cases. Ophthalmology. 1984; 91(1):27–30
[20] Bowyer JD, Sullivan TJ. Management of Marcus Gunn jaw winking synkinesis. Ophthal Plast Reconstr Surg. 2004; 20(2):92–98
[21] Kupersmith MJ, Latkany R, Homel P. Development of generalized disease at 2 years in patients with ocular myasthenia gravis. Arch Neurol. 2003;60(2):243–248
[22] Papazian O. Transient neonatal myasthenia gravis. J Child Neurol. 1992; 7(2):135–141
[23] Engel AG, Shen XM, Selcen D, Sine SM. Congenital myasthenic syndromes: pathogenesis, diagnosis, and treatment. Lancet Neurol. 2015; 14(5):461
[24] Ortiz S, Borchert M. Long-term outcomes of pediatric ocular myasthenia gravis. Ophthalmology. 2008; 115(7):1245–1248.e1
[25] Miller NR. Solitary oculomotor nerve palsy in childhood. Am J Ophthalmol. 1977; 83(1):106–111
[26] Jeffery AR, Ellis FJ, Repka MX, Buncic JR. Pediatric Horner syndrome. J AAPOS. 1998; 2(3):159–167

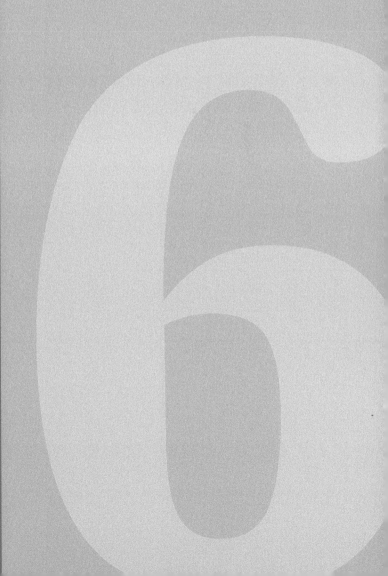

Section VI Pseudoptosis

34 Pseudoptosis: Evaluation and Management

Helen A. Merritt

Abstract

This chapter discusses the diseases and conditions that result in the perceived appearance of blepharoptosis without abnormality of the levator muscle. These periocular disorders result in manifestations mimicking ptosis including decreased vertical palpebral fissure height, deep superior sulcus, and elevated upper eyelid crease. The chapter discusses conditions causing pseudoptosis such as dermatochalasis, vertical strabismus, contralateral eyelid retraction, enophthalmos, ocular abnormalities, and protractor overaction.

Keywords: pseudoptosis, ptosis, superior sulcus, dermatochalasis, enophthalmos, silent sinus syndrome, anophthalmic socket, blepharospasm, hypotropia, orbital fracture

34.1 Introduction

Pseudoptosis describes a group of periocular disorders that resemble blepharoptosis but are not due to primary levator muscle abnormality. Pseudoptosis often results from underlying changes in the size or position of the eye and orbital contents, but can also include problems with the periocular muscles of protraction. This chapter will describe common conditions associated with pseudoptosis and explore factors important for evaluation and management.

The manifestations of true blepharoptosis due to abnormality or dehiscence of the levator muscle include decreased vertical palpebral fissure height, deep superior sulcus, and elevated upper eyelid crease. The entities that create pseudoptosis mimic these physical signs but have causes other than retractor muscle dysfunction. Most commonly, pseudoptosis is secondary to the perceived appearance of a decrease in palpebral fissure height while the margin reflex distance (MRD1) is normal. This phenomenon is often present bilaterally, as is seen with dermatochalasis causing excess skin to obscure the eyes. Additionally, a relative decrease in palpebral fissure height in comparison to the contralateral eye can create this effect. Pseudoptosis can also be present when there is presence of a deep superior sulcus or elevated upper eyelid crease. Pseudoptosis may also be secondary to overaction of the muscles of protraction as in hemifacial spasm or benign essential blepharospasm.

34.1.1 Dermatochalasis

Most commonly, pseudoptosis is secondary to the perception of a decrease in palpebral fissure height. The most frequently

encountered underlying abnormality is dermatochalasis. Excess upper eyelid skin obscures the palpebral fissure; giving the appearance of a decreased MRD1 while the underlying lid function is preserved. Lifting the eyelid skin reveals normal palpebral fissure height (▶ Fig. 34.1). Surgical management of dermatochalasis and mechanical ptosis has been extensively discussed in Section II.

34.1.2 Vertical Strabismus

Evaluation of ptosis should always include thorough assessment of the relative positions of the globes as well as extraocular muscle function. Misalignment of the eyes, as in vertical strabismus, may lead to a pseudoptosis due to close relationship between the upper eyelid and globe position. As the superior rectus muscle and levator muscle are closely linked, the upper eyelid can follow the malpositioned globe and create the appearance of ptosis. An ipsilateral hypotropia, where an eye is deviated downward in comparison to the fellow eye, can decrease the palpebral fissure height due to the lid following the globe inferiorly (▶ Fig. 34.2). This phenomenon, which is seen in conditions such as monocular elevation deficiency, can be assessed by occluding the fellow eye and observing a return of the pseudoptotic lid to normal position with fixation.[1] By a similar mechanism, the presence of a contralateral hypertropia can give the appearance of ptosis if the patient fixates with the hypertropic eye. Pseudoptosis resulting from such eye misalignment is often corrected by strabismus surgery.

34.1.3 Contralateral Eyelid Retraction

Patients presenting with unilateral or asymmetric eyelid retraction may be first thought to have ptosis of the contralateral eye (▶ Fig. 34.3). This phenomenon is due to the appearance of a relatively lower MRD1 in comparison to the retracted eyelid. Investigation of the etiology of eyelid retraction is important in these cases of pseudoptosis. The most common cause of eyelid retraction is thyroid eye disease, but other causes can include dorsal midbrain syndrome, aberrant regeneration of the facial nerve, and scarring or fibrotic changes of the upper eyelid. Treatment of pseudoptosis due to these conditions focuses on therapy for the underlying disorder and recession of the retracted eyelid.

Patients with thyroid eye disease may also exhibit overuse of the muscles of protraction in an attempt to improve symptoms of corneal exposure and discomfort associated with eyelid retraction.[2] This overaction of the corrugator and procerus

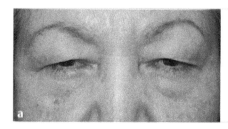
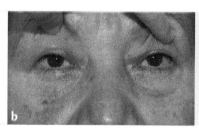

Fig. 34.1 **(a)** Dermatochalasis causing the appearance of ptosis due to skin overriding the lid margin. **(b)** Improved appearance of ptosis after skin elevation.

muscles can lead to glabellar rhytids, medial brow ptosis, altered brow contour, and further eyelid asymmetry.[3] In these cases, treatment with botulinum toxin chemodenervation of the glabellar muscles may improve brow position and eyelid symmetry.[3]

34.1.4 Enophthalmos

The increase in orbital volume or decrease in ocular volume creates the clinical appearance of ptosis by changes in the palpebral fissure height, deepening of the superior sulcus, and elevation of the eyelid crease. A variety of conditions can create this appearance, but enophthalmos is the most common. Enophthalmos, or posterior displacement of the globe within the orbit, can result from traumatic, degenerative, neoplastic, or involutional changes of the bony structures and contents of the

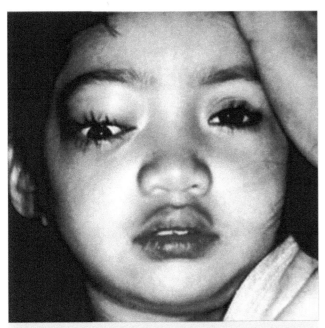

Fig. 34.2 Right pseudoptosis due to hypoglobus and hypotropia from orbital rhabdomyosarcoma.

orbit. Recognition and evaluation of these causes is important to treatment of both the periorbital manifestations and underlying disease. Evaluation of enophthalmos should include detailed history of trauma and systemic disease, full ophthalmic assessment, exophthalmometry, and radiographic imaging. It is important to distinguish true enophthalmos from relative asymmetry due to contralateral exophthalmos. Each specific mechanism of enophthalmos requires varied management and intervention.

Orbital Fracture

While blunt trauma can lead to ptosis from direct damage to the levator muscle or cranial nerve III, trauma can also lead to the development of pseudoptosis. Fractures of the orbital bones can increase the effective orbital volume causing posterior displacement of the globe, thereby leading to consequent changes of the upper eyelid position. Fractures of the medial wall and floor of the orbit are more likely to cause enophthalmos than the lateral wall or roof of the orbit.[4] Patients presenting with ptosis after trauma should have a tailored examination to investigate the orbital anatomy including assessment of motility and exophthalmometry, which is the measurement of the distance from the corneal apex to the lateral orbital rim. Radiographic imaging with orbital computed tomography (CT) is necessary to view the orbital bones and position of the globe (▶ Fig. 34.4). Enophthalmos is more likely in cases of large (> 50%) floor fractures or combined floor and medial wall fractures.[5–7] In cases of traumatic enophthalmos, the restoration of normal orbital volume by fracture repair and/or orbital volume augmentation can correct the position of the globe and resolve pseudoptosis. Orbital fractures should be repaired in cases of early manifest enophthalmos, symptomatic diplopia, or in cases of large orbital floor fractures causing significant latent enophthalmos or hypoglobus.[8]

Silent Sinus Syndrome

Silent sinus syndrome is a disease characterized by inferior displacement of the orbital floor secondary to chronic maxillary sinusitis and atelectasis. The abnormal sinus lacks aeration, and

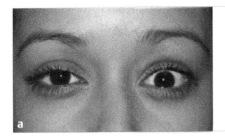
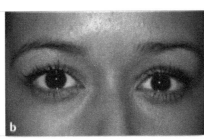

Fig. 34.3 (a) Right pseudoptosis due to contralateral eyelid retraction. (b) Resolution of right pseudoptosis after left upper eyelid retraction repair.

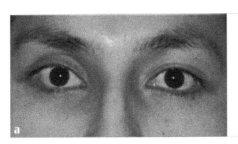
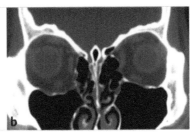

Fig. 34.4 (a) Right pseudoptosis after orbital fracture. (b) Computed tomography (CT) imaging revealing a right orbital floor and medial wall fracture.

this leads to negative pressure. Consequent collapse of the maxillary sinus and increase in orbital volume can lead to enophthalmos, hypoglobus, and pseudoptosis (▶ Fig. 34.5). As silent sinus syndrome can lead to varied levels of enophthalmos and hypoglobus, resultant eyelid malposition can range from pseudoretraction to pseudoptosis to a subtler hollowing of the superior sulcus. Pseudoretraction may be the more common associated eyelid finding, seen in 90% of cases in one large series, and explained by a relatively larger component of hypoglobus when compared to other spontaneous enophthalmos syndromes.[9] The most important measure in the treatment of silent sinus syndrome is restoration of maxillary sinus aeration via antrostomy. Treatment of the remaining orbital floor abnormality can be accomplished with an orbital floor implant. While many surgeons choose to address the orbital floor at the time of the initial antrostomy with aeration of the sinus, some argue that the floor repair should be staged to allow inflammation to subside and monitor for spontaneous improvement.[10]

Orbital Fat Atrophy

Orbital fat atrophy can also lead to pseudoptosis by deepening of the superior sulcus and elevation of the eyelid crease. While age-related factors and traumatic mechanisms of injury and previous surgery are classically associated with fat atrophy, the rising use of prostaglandin analogues for glaucoma treatment has become a common factor. Prostaglandin-associated periorbitopathy (PAP) can lead to enophthalmos, superior sulcus deformity, high eyelid crease, and pseudoptosis or retraction.[11] Careful evaluation of eyelid position and levator function is important in patients on prostaglandin inhibitors, as true ptosis and levator muscle dysfunction have also been found to be associated with use.[12] Discontinuation of prostaglandin analogue therapy may reverse fat atrophy and may restore normal eyelid position (▶ Fig. 34.6).[13]

Other Causes of Enophthalmos

Pseudoptosis can also result from enophthalmos secondary to nontraumatic, degenerative, or fibrotic changes of the orbital contents and bones. Orbital malignancy and other fibrotic processes can lead to findings of deepened superior sulcus and elevated eyelid crease. Metastatic scirrhous breast carcinoma of the orbit can cause enophthalmos and pseudoptosis, and these findings may present prior to systemic diagnosis.[14] Other nonneoplastic atrophic and fibrotic disorders such as linear scleroderma, hemifacial atrophy, and changes related to previous radiotherapy can lead to similar periorbital changes and enophthalmos.[15] Additionally, a relative pseudoenophthalmos may be present due to contralateral exophthalmos.

In cases of enophthalmos or orbital asymmetry of unknown etiology, radiographic investigation with computed tomogra-

phy (CT) or magnetic resonance imaging (MRI) is important to assess anatomic changes. Therapy for eyelid malposition associated with these disorders should be targeted to treatment of the underlying condition.

34.1.5 Ocular Abnormalities

Reduced volume of the globe can lead to the appearance of enophthalmos without true axial displacement of the globe. As with true enophthalmos, this change in ocular volume may result in insufficient support of the upper eyelid by the globe and pseudoptosis.

The etiology of ocular volume abnormality can include congenital causes such as nanophthalmos, microphthalmos, and congenital anophthalmos. Acquired conditions include surgical or traumatic anophthalmos and phthisis bulbi, a process of atrophy and disorganization of the globe due to insult. Pseudoptosis in these patients results from deepening of the superior sulcus, elevation of the eyelid crease, and asymmetry in comparison to the contralateral healthy eye. The likely pathophysiologic basis behind these findings is a disruption in the normal orbital spatial architecture and disturbance of the relationships of the orbital soft tissue.[16] In cases of postsurgical or acquired ocular abnormality, fat atrophy, contracture, and cicatricial changes may also play a role.

Pseudoptosis may also occur due to limitation of levator function caused by an inappropriately sized prosthesis (▶ Fig. 34.7).

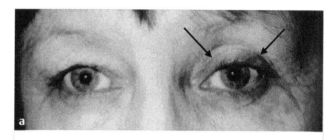

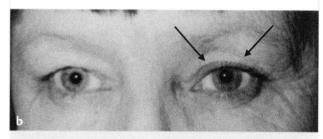

Fig. 34.6 (a) Left pseudoptosis due to unilateral prostaglandin associated periorbitopathy causing deepening of the superior sulcus. **(b)** Resolution of pseudoptosis after prostaglandin cessation. (The images are provided courtesy of Peplinski LS, Albiani Smith K. Deepening of lid sulcus from topical bimatoprost therapy. Optom Vis Sci 2004 Aug;81(8):574–577.)

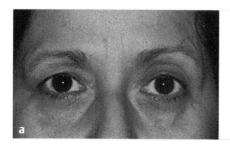

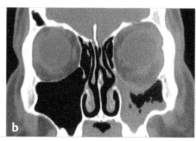

Fig. 34.5 (a) Left pseudoptosis due to silent sinus syndrome. **(b)** Computed tomography (CT) imaging demonstrating left maxillary sinus atelectasis.

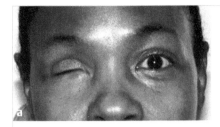
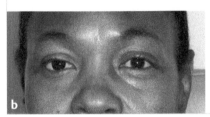
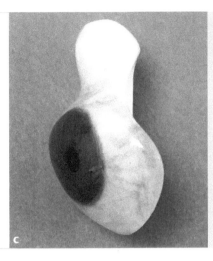

Fig. 34.7 **(a)** Right pseudoptosis in an anophthalmic patient. **(b)** Improvement in eyelid position after prosthesis adjustment. **(c)** Prosthesis with ptosis adjustment. (The images are provided courtesy of Stephen Haddad, BCO.)

Diminished levator function has been demonstrated in anophthalmic sockets in comparison to normal orbits, and this function is improved by a prosthesis of proper height.[17] Close collaboration with an ocularist regarding the shape and size of the prosthesis is therefore the first step in addressing pseudoptosis in this patient population.

Pseudoptosis in patients with blind microphthalmic, nanophthalmic, or phthisical eyes may be improved by a scleral shell to restore volume. Options for these patients with pseudoptosis due to volume loss and a deep superior sulcus include reshaping of the prosthesis, adding a scleral shell, orbital implant exchange, orbital dermis fat grafting, and orbital volume augmentation with subperiosteal implants. More recently described procedures include filler or dermis fat graft placement to the superior sulcus.[18]

34.1.6 Eyelid Protractor Overaction

Spasm or overaction of the orbicularis oculi muscle can also lead to pseudoptosis. Aberrant regeneration of the facial nerve can occur after trauma, surgery, Bell's palsy, and similar disorders leading to synkinesis of the orbicularis oculi and other facial muscles. This aberrant activation of the protractors can therefore cause the appearance of ptosis by narrowing the palpebral fissure. Similarly, conditions such as benign essential blepharospasm and hemifacial spasm also lead to pseudoptosis by involuntary contractions of the orbicularis. These patients usually demonstrate normal levator excursion, symmetric eyelid creases, and improved MRD1 after treatment of the orbicularis with paralytic agents.

While these etiologies do not involve abnormality of the levator muscle, the resultant pseudoptosis may still be visually significant. Described treatments of overaction, spasm, or aberrant innervation of the orbicularis muscle include botulinum toxin, biofeedback rehabilitation, and surgery.[19] Injection of botulinum toxin should be performed superficially in the pretarsal orbicularis with the lowest effective dose to avoid side effects such as true ptosis, diplopia, or lagophthalmos.[19,20]

References

[1] Ficker LA, Collin JR, Lee JP. Management of ipsilateral ptosis with hypotropia. Br J Ophthalmol. 1986; 70(10):732–736

[2] Saks ND, Burnstine MA, Putterman AM. Glabellar rhytids in thyroid-associated orbitopathy. Ophthal Plast Reconstr Surg. 2001; 17(2):91–95

[3] Olver JM. Botulinum toxin A treatment of overactive corrugator supercilii in thyroid eye disease. Br J Ophthalmol. 1998; 82(5):528–533

[4] Parsons GS, Mathog RH. Orbital wall and volume relationships. Arch Otolaryngol Head Neck Surg. 1988; 114(7):743–747

[5] Jin HR, Shin SO, Choo MJ, Choi YS. Relationship between the extent of fracture and the degree of enophthalmos in isolated blowout fractures of the medial orbital wall. J Oral Maxillofac Surg. 2000; 58(6):617–620, discussion 620–621

[6] Raskin EM, Millman AL, Lubkin V, della Rocca RC, Lisman RD, Maher EA. Prediction of late enophthalmos by volumetric analysis of orbital fractures. Ophthal Plast Reconstr Surg. 1998; 14(1):19–26

[7] Burm JS, Chung CH, Oh SJ. Pure orbital blowout fracture: new concepts and importance of medial orbital blowout fracture. Plast Reconstr Surg. 1999; 103 (7):1839–1849

[8] Burnstine MA. Clinical recommendations for repair of isolated orbital floor fractures: an evidence-based analysis. Ophthalmology. 2002; 109(7):1207–1210, discussion 1210–1211, quiz 1212–1213

[9] Soparkar CN, Patrinely JR, Davidson JK. Silent sinus syndrome-new perspectives? Ophthalmology. 2004; 111(2):414–415, author reply 415–416

[10] Numa WA, Desai U, Gold DR, Heher KL, Annino DJ. Silent sinus syndrome: a case presentation and comprehensive review of all 84 reported cases. Ann Otol Rhinol Laryngol. 2005; 114(9):688–694

[11] Rabinowitz MP, Katz LJ, Moster MR, et al. Unilateral prostaglandin-associated periorbitopathy: a syndrome involving upper eyelid retraction distinguishable from the aging sunken eyelid. Ophthal Plast Reconstr Surg. 2015; 31(5): 373–378

[12] Shah M, Lee G, Lefebvre DR, et al. A cross-sectional survey of the association between bilateral topical prostaglandin analogue use and ocular adnexal features. PLoS One. 2013; 8(5):e61638

[13] Custer PL, Kent TL. Observations on prostaglandin orbitopathy. Ophthal Plast Reconstr Surg. 2016; 32(2):102–105

[14] Mohadjer Y, Holds JB. Orbital metastasis as the initial finding of breast carcinoma: a ten-year survival. Ophthal Plast Reconstr Surg. 2005; 21(1):65–66

[15] Hamedani M, Pournaras JA, Goldblum D. Diagnosis and management of enophthalmos. Surv Ophthalmol. 2007; 52(5):457–473

[16] Kronish JW, Gonnering RS, Dortzbach RK, et al. The pathophysiology of the anophthalmic socket. Part II. Analysis of orbital fat. Ophthal Plast Reconstr Surg. 1990; 6(2):88–95

[17] Kim NJ, Khwarg SI. Decrease in levator function in the anophthalmic orbit. Ophthalmologica. 2008; 222(5):351–356

[18] Shah CT, Hughes MO, Kirzhner M. Anophthalmic syndrome: a review of management. Ophthal Plast Reconstr Surg. 2014; 30(5):361–365

[19] McElhinny ER, Reich I, Burt B, et al. Treatment of pseudoptosis secondary to aberrant regeneration of the facial nerve with botulinum toxin type A. Ophthal Plast Reconstr Surg. 2013; 29(3):175–178

[20] Lolekha P, Choolam A, Kulkantrakorn K. A comparative crossover study on the treatment of hemifacial spasm and blepharospasm: preseptal and pretarsal botulinum toxin injection techniques. Neurol Sci. 2017; 38(11): 2031–2036

Section VII Additional Considerations in Upper Facial Surgery

7

35 Eyelash Ptosis Management

Nicholas R. Mahoney

Abstract

Eyelash ptosis can occur in isolation or in the setting of floppy eyelid syndrome, blepharoptosis, trichomegaly, or a poorly formed lid crease. The supporting connecting tissue in the pretarsal eyelid margin might be lax and/or the levator aponeurosis can fail to provide adequate support. Correction of the primary underlying pathology is often adequate to treat eyelash ptosis but additional techniques can be used in combination or isolation to rotate the lashes.

Keywords: eyelash ptosis, lash ptosis, entropion, floppy eyelid syndrome

35.1 Introduction

Eyelash ptosis is an under-recognized finding that can both contribute to functional visual axis obstruction and be of aesthetic concern. It can occur in isolation or in the setting of blepharoptosis, of either acquired or congenital etiologies. Eyelash ptosis might be of more significance in patients with trichomegaly, hypertrichosis, or naturally long eyelashes.[1] Patients with less well-defined eyelid creases may have a more mechanical eyelash ptosis. Floppy eyelid syndrome with associated progressive degenerative changes to the eyelid micro-architecture can be thought of as a more involutional eyelash ptosis. Lastly, eyelash ptosis can be found in patients with frank upper eyelid cicatricial entropion. Here we review how eyelash ptosis presents and adds to the complexity of some already difficult to master entities and discuss the management from a variety of etiologies (▶ Fig. 35.1).

35.2 Anatomical Considerations

35.2.1 Eyelash Cilia

The normal eyelash follicles are located 1.5 to 2.5 mm deep to the lid margin epithelium either just anterior to the tarsal plate or, less commonly, embedded in the anterior surface.[2,3] There are approximately 100 eyelashes on the upper eyelid and each bulb measures just under 200 μm.[3] The orbicularis oculi is located anterior to the follicles and the muscle of Riolan is typically just posterior.[3] Eyelashes grow in a 4- to 9-month cycle and compared to other hairs in the body, the anagen phase is shorter (30 days) and the telogen phase is longer (3–8 months).[1,3] The normal lashes curve away from the globe in a parallel manner.[4] There is no arrectores pilorum to affect the eyelash position or curvature and lash position is entirely dependent on the surrounding sturctures.[4]

Trichiasis and entropion represent pathology wherein the eyelid margin or the eyelash follicle is abnormally directed toward the globe. For the purposes of this discussion, these entities differ from eyelash ptosis or downward pointing lashes without disruptive misdirection of the eyelash follicle or eyelid margin rotation.

Trichomegaly refers to an increase in length or thickness of lashes. It can be congenital (Oliver-McFarlane syndrome, Cornelia de Lange syndrome, familial trichomegaly, cone-rod dystrophy, Goldstein-Hutt syndrome), drug-related (epidermal growth factor receptor inhibitors, prostaglandin analogues, interferon, cyclosporin), or acquired (human immunodeficiency virus [HIV] infection).[1] The heaviness of the long, thick lashes can result in eyelash ptosis and disruption of the follicle support.

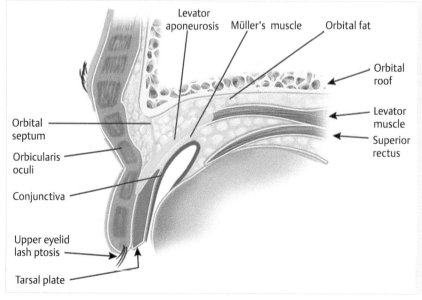

Fig. 35.1 Upper eyelid anatomy for a patient with eyelash ptosis.

Floppy eyelid syndrome is a condition characterized clinically by lax, easily evertable upper eyelids, and tarsal expansion.[5] In addition to the rubbery, loose tarsus and reactive changes on the posterior conjunctiva from mechanical irritation there is eyelash ptosis in the majority of patients.[4] There is upregulation of elastolytic enzymes and elastin degradation in the tarsal plate and the connective tissue around the eyelash roots and eyelash ptosis results.[5]

Other causes of cilia root disruption included ocular leprosy and congenital lamellar ichthyosis.[6]

35.2.2 Levator Aponeurosis and Eyelid Crease

A similar phenomenon of eyelash ptosis can be seen in patients with alterations in the levator aponeurosis. The normal levator aponeurosis is well described elsewhere. It inserts onto the anterior surface of the tarsal plate and into the pretarsal skin. There is a normal zone of fusion with the septum superior to the tarsal plate for several millimeters. The insertion through the orbicularis oculi fibers into the subdermal tissue and the strength of this entire apparatus results in the location and definition of the lid crease.

In studies of congenital ptosis, eyelash ptosis of some degree has been identified in more than 90% of patients.[6] It is theorized that this occurs from dysgenesis of these aponeurosis fibers and the resultant absence of their strengthening of the connecting tissue around the eyelash root.[6] It can also be found in cases of more significant acquired blepharoptosis, particularly with associated loss of lid crease definition.

As described elsewhere, the Asian eyelid has a variation in the location and extent of the lid crease and associated eyelid fold. This occurs because of variation in the zone of fusion between the septum and levator aponeurosis, often with little to no fusion and an insertion point well below the superior tarsal border.[7] Lash ptosis of a mild degree has been observed in the non-ptotic eyelid of Asian patients as well as with increasing frequency in patients with acquired blepharoptosis.[7] This is likely related to similar loss of support from a less robust levator aponeurosis insertion and indeed the degree of lash ptosis seems to be worse in patients without a history of a double eyelid fold.[7]

35.3 Goals of Intervention/ Indications

The main goal of eyelash ptosis repair is to elevate and rotate the downturned eyelashes out of the visual axis into a more normal position.

35.4 Risks of the Procedure

Risks are within the typical scope for eyelid surgery and include:
- Bleeding.
- Infection.
- Asymmetry.
- Need for further surgery or failure to achieve desired result.
- Focal madarosis.

35.5 Benefits of the Procedure

When successful, eyelash ptosis repair can:
- Clear the obstructing lashes from the visual axis.
- Improve aesthetics of the eyelid.
- Occasionally improve blepharitis in patients with anterior debris.

35.6 Informed Consent

- A thorough discussion of the risks and benefits of surgical repair.
- Given eyelash ptosis is also found in the setting of other eyelid malpositions, a discussion on the approaches of all problems is necessary with a discussion of alternative management strategies (i.e., there is more than one way to fix blepharoptosis but if eyelash ptosis is also being treated, an anterior incision is likely to be indicated).

35.7 Contraindications

There are no contraindications of surgical repair for eyelash ptosis.

35.8 Procedure

Eyelash ptosis as a secondary phenomenon in the setting of another primary eyelid malposition is likely to improve with treatment of the primary condition alone. Eyelash rotation can be performed in combination with these other techniques or it can be performed in isolation. (It should be noted that in this chapter the author is referring to methods to correct eyelash ptosis and rotate the eyelashes in an otherwise normal, nonentropic eyelid margin.) Primary condition correction is detailed elsewhere but briefly:
- In patients with mild to moderate floppy eyelid syndrome who require horizontal tightening, a wedge resection alone can result in improvement in their eyelash ptosis. This might be less predictable when patients undergo lateral tarsal strip as tightening procedure.
- In patients with congenital ptosis with a poorly formed lid crease who undergo levator resection or levator advancement, creation of a lid crease by suturing the incised skin to the levator aponeurosis can result in crease formation and also resolve the eyelash ptosis.
- Asian patients with poorly defined lid crease and/or prolapse of orbital fat with resultant eyelash ptosis who undergo repair or double eyelid surgery with creation of a lid fold often have resolution of their eyelash ptosis.
- Cicatricial entropion or frank trichiasis should be addressed with appropriate margin rotation techniques or follicle excision or ablation. In severe cases of cicatricial entropion or even isolated eyelash ptosis from severe destructive pathology (i.e., leprosy), the anterior lamella at the lid margin can be resected and the posterior lamella advanced.

35.8.1 Instruments Needed

- Surgical marking pen and calipers.
- Local anesthesia such as a 50:50 mixture of 2% lidocaine with 1:100,000 U epinephrine and bupivacaine 0.75% (4 cc).
- Castroviejo needle holder.
- Fine forceps such as 0.3 mm forceps or Paufique forceps.
- Bipolar or monopolar cautery with a Colorado needle tip.
- Westcott or iris scissors.
- 2 prong skin hook retractor.
- Cotton tip applicators and soft 4 by 4 sponges.
- Sutures for eyelash rotation.
  - Absorbable: 6–0 double-armed Polyglactin or PDS.
  - Nonabsorbable: 7–0 nylon or Prolene sutures.
- Sutures for primary procedure (i.e., skin closure, levator advancement sutures, wedge resection, or tarsal strip closure sutures).

35.8.2 Preoperative Checklist

- Informed consent.
- Instrumentation on hand.
- Preoperative photographic documentation with frontal and side views in repose and with the lashes elevated showing clearance of the visual axis.
- Preoperative assessment of corneal breakdown from lash-corneal touch.
- Preoperative assessment describes symptoms and signs of visual field obstruction.

35.8.3 Operative Technique

Isolated eyelash rotation or in conjunction with blepharoplasty, horizontal tightening or levator advancement can be done under local, monitored, or general anesthesia in an appropriate setting. As eyelash ptosis repair and/or levator advancement surgery cannot be adjusted intraoperatively if done under general anesthesia, the author prefers light-monitored anesthesia care with avoidance of any narcotic or benzodiazepines which might limit adjustment (i.e., Propofol only).

- A lid crease and/or blepharoplasty incision is marked in the upright position. If a lid crease is not present, the patient can be given a handheld mirror and a bent paperclip can be used to find their desired crease height.
- After sedation, if used, local anesthesia is injected and a period of 8 minutes or more is left to pass to achieve hemostasis. No more than 2 cc of local should be used as this can affect adjustment.
- An incision is made with a #15 blade and any excess skin is removed.
- The curved portion of the Westcott scissors is placed along the inferior edge of the skin incision and a 2- to 3-mm strip of pretarsal orbicularis is removed. This exposes the septum safely.
  - In cases with a well-formed lid crease, the insertion of the levator aponeurosis–septal complex on the tarsal plate is well visualized.
  - In congenital ptosis patients with a poorly formed lid crease or in Asian patients with a low septal insertion, the septum might be thin and low-lying orbital fat or frank tarsal plate may already be seen (▶ Fig. 35.2 and ▶ Fig. 35.3).

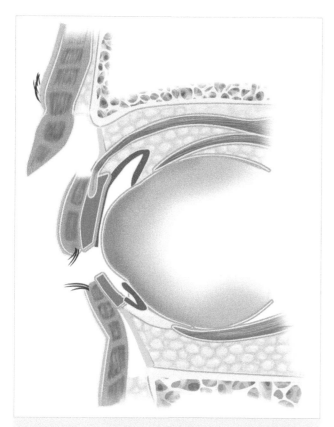

Fig. 35.2 Dissection is taken under orbicularis oculi to expose the orbital septum. Alternatively, some orbicularis muscle can be removed.

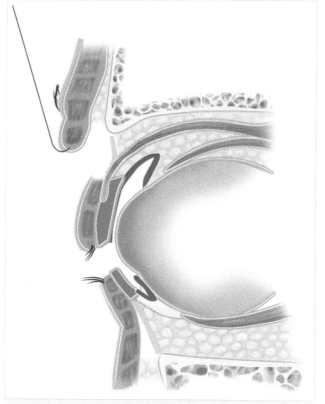

Fig. 35.3 The orbicularis muscle is retracted.

- Any ptosis repair or horizontal tightening with tarsal strip is performed.
- If eyelash ptosis persists, it can be addressed directly as follows:
  - For mild, more focal segmental lash ptosis, a suture can be passed at the lash line entering through the skin among the lashes and running internally anterior to pretarsal orbicularis and out the wound. A double-armed suture is used and the second needle is placed through the same needle hole to bury the suture material. The two sutures diverge from each other and are then passed into either the levator aponeurosis or the levator-septal complex. Between two and four of these sutures should be used. Either absorbable or nonabsorbable sutures can be used (▶ Fig. 35.4, ▶ Fig. 35.5, and ▶ Fig. 35.6).
  - For more pronounced, diffuse lash ptosis, dissection should be performed subcutaneously in the inferior direction for 2 mm toward the lashes. Three to five nonabsorbable sutures, such as a 7–0 nylon, are then placed along the wound passing within the anterior pretarsal orbicularis muscle in a horizontal mattress manner. Each pass should reach toward the anterior lash line and then be secured to the superior edge of the tarsal plate in a partial thickness pass (▶ Fig. 35.7).
  - In all cases, further elevation of the lashes can be achieved with sharper lid crease formation. The subdermal tissue at the inferior incision edge should be secured to the levator aponeurosis (or the superior tarsal plate) as in any lid crease formation suture technique. The author recommends 7–0 nylon be used in four or five locations.
- The wound is closed per routine.

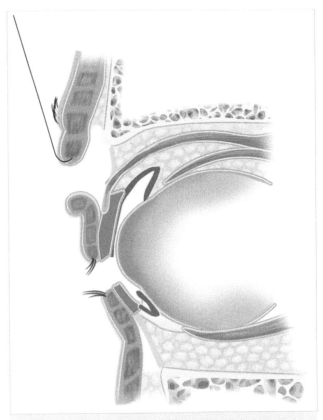

Fig. 35.5 Dissection is taken inferiorly on the anterior surface of the tarsal plate. This will release any partially dehisced levator aponeurosis fibers.

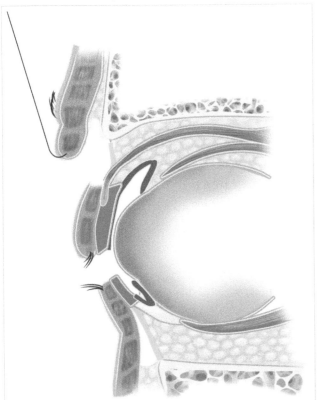

Fig. 35.4 The septum is freed from the levator aponeurosis and any dehiscence is identified.

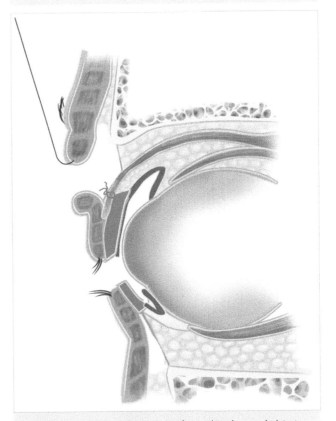

Fig. 35.6 The levator aponeurosis is advanced to the tarsal plate to correct ptosis if needed.

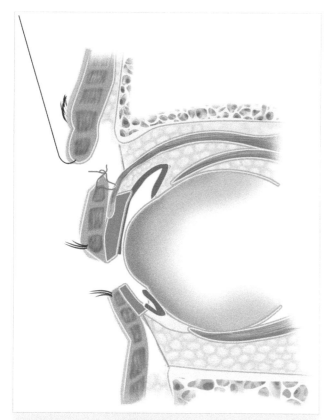

Fig. 35.7 To correct mild eyelash ptosis, an additional suture such as 6–0 polyglactin or 7–0 nylon is placed in addition to the ptosis-correcting sutures to advance orbicularis at the lid crease incision to a superior position on the levator aponeurosis. This can be done in an interrupted or horizontal mattress fashion in anywhere from one to six locations across the lid.

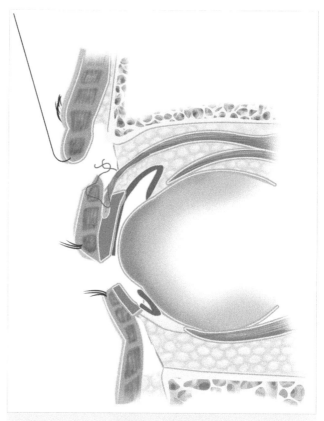

Fig. 35.8 More severe lash ptosis can be corrected by additionally incorporating the tarsal plate and/or the deep dermis.

35.8.4 Expert Tips/Pearls/Suggestions

- It is very useful to assess the effect after placing two or three sutures by sitting the patient up and asking them to open their eyes and look up and down.
- Horizontal tightening for floppy eyelid syndrome can worsen or improve lash ptosis, unfortunately not always predictably.
  - Mild blepharoptosis and eyelash ptosis can be corrected in the moderately floppy eyelid with a lateral wedge resection only.
  - Moderate blepharoptosis and eyelash ptosis with mild floppy eyelid will do best with a levator advancement and lateral tarsal strip.
  - A tarsal strip alone for moderate floppy eyelid will often worsen lash ptosis.
- Congenital ptosis repair is often difficult laterally and requires removal of the stiff septum more thoroughly. This may lead to eyelash ptosis that was not present preoperatively and should be anticipated (see ▶ Fig. 35.8 and ▶ Fig. 35.9).

35.8.5 Postoperative Care Checklist

- Apply antibiotic ointment with or without steroids and a nonsticking gauze such as Xeroform and begin ice therapy.

- Patients should use ice 20 minutes of every hour while awake for the first 36 hours then apply ice 20 minutes four times a day with 5 minute hot-wet washcloth soaks beforehand.
- Patients may shower in 24 hours and should avoid heavy lifting or vigorous activity for 7 days.
- The patient is advised to sleep with the head of the bed elevated.

35.9 Complications and Their Management

Pain, bruising, bleeding, and scarring are expected. Vision loss, dry eye, double vision, numbness are rare and not more or less of an issue than in routine oculoplastic surgeries.

The most common specific complication is failure to elevate or maintain elevation of the eyelashes and asymmetry. In cases where focal eyelash ptosis recurs, sutures have either absorbed or broken. If diffuse lash ptosis is noted, there should be concern that adequate horizontal tightening has not been performed. Depending on the techniques used for tightening, ptosis repair or double eyelid surgery, an escalation or combination of techniques should be used to achieve the desired result.

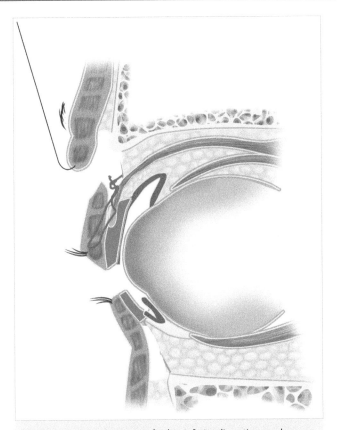

Fig. 35.9 In very severe cases, further inferior dissection can be performed to free orbicularis from the tarsal plate (or may already be naturally found) and sutures can reach into the tissue surrounding the superior eyelash follicle. This can be performed as diagramed or alternatively with a double-armed taper needle that enters to the skin externally in a double-armed manner with each skin pass entering through the same needle hole and then grasping the tarsal plate and levator aponeurosis.

References

[1] Kaur S, Mahajan BB. Eyelash Trichomegaly. Indian J Dermatol. 2015; 60(4): 378–380

[2] Thibaut S, De Becker E, Caisey L, et al. Human eyelash characterization. Br J Dermatol. 2010; 162(2):304–310

[3] Elder MJ. Anatomy and physiology of eyelash follicles: relevance to lash ablation procedures. Ophthal Plast Reconstr Surg. 1997; 13(1):21–25

[4] Langford JD, Linberg JV. A new physical finding in floppy eyelid syndrome. Ophthalmology. 1998; 105(1):165–169

[5] Schlötzer-Schrehardt U, Stojkovic M, Hofmann-Rummelt C, Cursiefen C, Kruse FE, Holbach LM. The Pathogenesis of floppy eyelid syndrome: involvement of matrix metalloproteinases in elastic fiber degradation. Ophthalmology. 2005; 112(4):694–704

[6] Malik KJ, Lee MS, Park DJ, Harrison AR. Lash ptosis in congenital and acquired blepharoptosis. Arch Ophthalmol. 2007; 125(12):1613–1615

[7] Lee TE, Lee JM, Lee H, Park M, Kim KH, Baek S. Lash ptosis and associated factors in Asians. Ann Plast Surg. 2010; 65(4):407–410

36 Blepharoptosis Reoperation

Michael A. Burnstine

Abstract

Eyelid ptosis surgery may require reoperation to obtain an excellent symmetric result and a satisfied patient. The purpose of reoperation is to address an undercorrection or overcorrection of eyelid height and contour or to correct eyelid crease or fold asymmetries. In an eyelid that has had many surgeries or a large dissection in primary repair, scar formation and distorted anatomy may make reoperation difficult. Posterior or anterior revisions with tarsectomy can be performed to correct undercorrected margin reflex distances (MRD). In this chapter, I discuss segmental tarsectomy, first described by Henry Baylis, to address residual contour abnormalities and undercorrected eyelid ptosis. The tarsoconjunctival Müller's muscle resection (Fasanella-Servat) is another useful procedure for ptosis reoperation and has been described in detail in Chapter 23.

Keywords: revision eyelid surgery, full-thickness eyelid resection, tarsectomy

36.1 Introduction

Over the course of a career, ptosis revision is unavoidable. While there are no definitive data on the incidence of ptosis reoperation, Bernice Brown surveyed expert eye plastic surgeons and found the rate of revision to be between 12 and 18%.[1] The goal of this surgery is to provide eyelid symmetry with adequate eye protection to the unhappy patient.

Depending on the ptosis type, the appropriate method of surgical correction may vary (▶ Table 36.1). In eyelids that have consecutive eyelid retraction (overcorrection), recession of the levator may be performed. In the patient who has not had many eyelid surgeries with minimal middle lamellar scarring, revision ptosis surgery can be performed through an anterior or posterior approach.[2–7]

This chapter focuses on ptosis reoperation in patients who are undercorrected, and in whom multiple eyelid surgeries has resulted in significant full-thickness scarring. Frequently, the anterior, middle, and posterior lamellar layers are scarred-down. The levator muscle and aponeurosis and Müller's muscle may be difficult to identify. In this type of blepharoptosis revision surgery, segmental tarsectomy offers a reliable, reproducible result for minimal to moderate eyelid height and contour deformities.[4–7]

36.2 Anatomical Considerations

In an eyelid that has had many previous surgeries with removal of skin, subcutaneous tissue, muscle, and orbital fat in conjunction with levator advancement or Müller's muscle conjunctiva resection, it may be difficult to separate the eyelid layers. Scar tissue may exist between anterior, middle, and posterior lamellae. In these eyelids, it is nearly impossible to re-advance the levator and correct eyelid height deficiencies. Posterior approaches tend to be more effective. Gladstone, Bassin, and Putterman have described a posterior approach to address contour abnormalities.[5,6] Reoperation with Fasanella-Servat has also been described.[7,8] Here, I discuss segmental tarsal resection, first described by Henry Baylis,[4] and historically employed in primary blepharoptosis surgery.[9,10]

Table 36.1 Methods of surgical correction

Ptosis type	LE	Primary procedure	Overcorrection	Undercorrection
Aponeurotic	>10 mm	MMCR	Levator recession	MMCR/ELA/T
		ELA	Levator recession	MMCR/ELA/T
Myogenic				
A. Static/congenital	0–4 mm	FS	Loosen sling	Tighten or repeat sling
	4–10 mm	LR	Levator recession	Repeat LR or T
	>10 mm	MMCR/ELA/FS	Levator recession	MMCR/ELA/T
B. Progressive	0–4 mm	FS or SB	Loosen sling	Tighten or repeat sling
	4–10 mm	LR or SB	Levator recession	Repeat LR or T
	>10 mm	ELA/LR	Levator recession	MMCR/ELA/T
Mechanical	>10 mm	Blepharoplasty	Skin grafting	Revision blepharoplasty
		Brow elevation	Botox to forehead	Revision brow surgery

Abbreviations: ELA, external levator advancement; FS, frontalis sling; LE, levator excursion (mm); LR, levator resection; MMCR, Müller's muscle–conjunctival resection; SB, supramaximal blepharoplasty; T, tarsectomy, anterior or posterior approach.

36.3 Goals of Intervention/ Indications

The main goal of revision upper eyelid ptosis surgery is to create symmetry and meet the patient's ideal outcome, which includes:

- Improvement in the superior field of vision.
- Enhancement of the face by creating a more aesthetically pleasing vertical palpebral fissure.
- Equalization of the margin crease and fold positions.

36.4 Risks of the Procedure

- Bleeding.
- Infection.
- Failure to achieve the desired result with persistent asymmetry in the MRD1 and palpebral fissure.
- Asymmetric eyelid crease and fold distances.
- Increased eyelid lagophthalmos on downgaze (increased palpebral fissure on downgaze).
- Postoperative lagophthalmos and exposure keratopathy.
- Exacerbation of preexisting dry eye disease.

36.5 Benefits of the Procedure

- Improvement of superior field of vision.
- Symmetric eyelid height and contour.
- Aesthetic enhancement of the upper face, including widened vertical palpebral fissure.

36.6 Informed Consent

- Include risks and benefits (as described above).
- Discuss the need for enhancement to equalize the eyelid crease and folds if a resultant asymmetry occurs.
- Explain risk of lagophthalmos and exposure keratopathy.
- Warn the patient about worsening dry eye disease.

36.7 Contraindications

- Severe dry eye disease and preexisting corneal keratopathy.
- Patients with a poor Bell's phenomenon which would place the corneal surface at significant risk.

36.8 Procedure

The procedure described can be done in an outpatient surgery center or in an office-based setting.

36.8.1 Instruments Needed (▶ Fig. 36.1)

- Surgical marking pen.
- Ruler.
- Local anesthesia (10 cc for a bilateral case):
  - Lidocaine 2% with 1:100,000 U epinephrine (5 cc).
  - Marcaine 0.75% (4 cc).
  - Sodium bicarbonate 8.4% (1 cc).

- Vitrase 150 USP units/mL (0.5 cc).
- Castroviejo needle holder.
- Bishop Harmon forceps.
- Colorado needle tip with monopolar cautery.
- Protective scleral contact lenses.
- Hemostat.
- Sutures:
  - 6–0 Vicryl (polyglactin), S-14 needle for reapproximating scarred tissue (tarsus, levator complex).
  - 6–0 Prolene (polypropylene) for wound closure.

36.8.2 Preoperative Checklist

- Informed consent.
- Instrumentation on hand.
- Clear discussion with the patient on the desired eyelid crease and fold positions.
- Preoperative photographic documentation.

36.8.3 Operative Technique

This procedure can be performed under local, monitored, or general anesthesia in an office-based procedure room, ambulatory operating room, or hospital-based setting.

- Premedication with lorazepam 1 mg and acetaminophen-hydrocodone 5 mg/325 mg may be given 30 minutes before the procedure.
- The upper eyelid incisions are marked. This is the most important step!
  - The eyelid crease is set following discussion of the patient's wishes and the surgeon's judgment, usually matching the fellow side (▶ Fig. 36.2).
  - A decision is made as to how much eyelid skin will show (margin fold distance), almost always matching the fellow side.
  - The resection amount is determined prior to the procedure. It is 1 mm of tarsus to 1 mm of contour or height undercorrection.

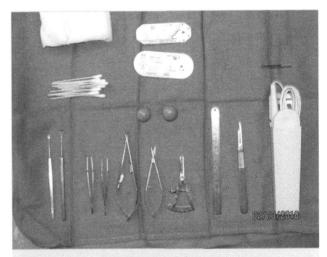

Fig. 36.1 Surgical instruments needed to perform tarsectomy for residual ptosis.

- Local anesthesia is injected and massaged into place, waiting 5 to 10 minutes for the full anesthetic and hemostatic effect (▸ Fig. 36.3).
  - Hyaluronidase is used to help spread the local anesthetic with minimal injection sites.
- A 4–0 silk traction suture or similar suture may or may not be placed at the upper eyelid margin, according to surgeon's preference.
- An incision is made along the marking with a #15 blade or diamond knife (▸ Fig. 36.4).
- With a corneal protector in place, a full-thickness blepharotomy is performed through skin, subcutaneous tissue, orbicularis muscle, levator aponeurosis, Müller's muscle, and conjunctiva using the Colorado needle tip, Westcott scissors, or diamond blade (▸ Fig. 36.5).
- A wedge of full-thickness eyelid tissue is then removed from the crease incision inferiorly (including tarsus). Typically, a rectangular or elliptical shape of tissue is removed to correct the deformity (▸ Fig. 36.6).
  - Determination of how much tissue to remove is driven by the amount of residual ptosis as well as eyelid crease and fold asymmetries.
  - Tarsus is usually removed.
- After removing tissue and obtaining hemostasis, the scarred tissue is closed with partial thickness, buried, interrupted 6–0 Vicryl sutures, re-approximating the freshly created tissue ends (▸ Fig. 36.7).
- The skin wound is closed with a running 6–0 Prolene suture. (▸ Fig. 36.8).

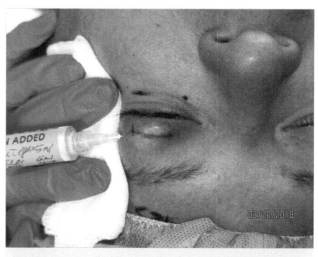

Fig. 36.3 Injection of local anesthesia which consists of lidocaine with 1:100,000 U epinephrine, hyaluronidase, Marcaine, and sodium bicarbonate.

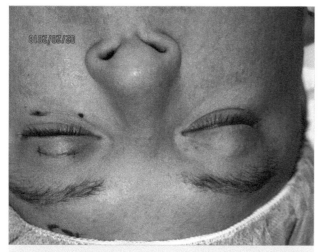

Fig. 36.2 Marking the eyelid crease to mirror the contralateral side.

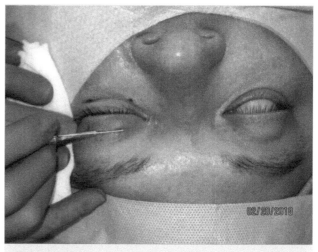

Fig. 36.4 The incision is made with a #15 blade.

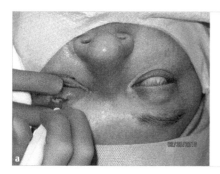
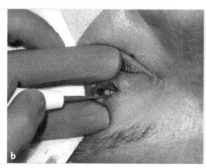

Fig. 36.5 Dissection through partial **(a)** to full-thickness eyelid **(b)** with a monopolar cautery device with a fine Colorado needle tip.

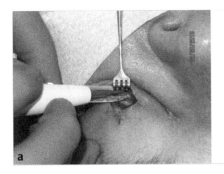
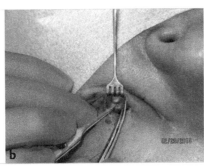

Fig. 36.6 After marking the amount of tarsus to be removed with a caliper (a), tarsectomy is performed (b). The ratio of tarsal removal to eyelid elevation is 1:1.

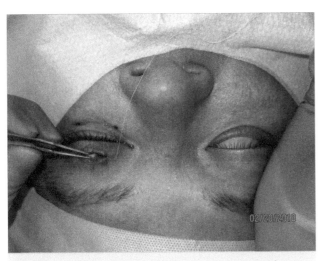

Fig. 36.7 Wound closure with a 6–0 Vicryl suture from partial thickness tarsus to the levator complex.

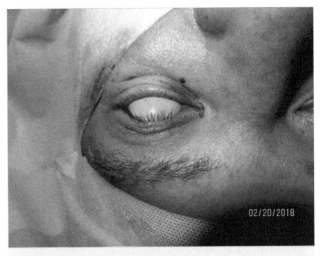

Fig. 36.8 Skin closure with a running 6–0 Prolene suture.

36.8.4 Expert Tips/Pearls/Suggestions

- Ensure no other conditions exist prior to performing the ptosis revision, including eyebrow ptosis, lash ptosis, or asymmetric margin crease and folds.
- The line of the blepharoplasty incision will determine the height and contour of the newly formed upper eyelid crease.
- The eyelid resection (tarsus or full-thickness eyelid) is determined preoperatively based on how much eyelid elevation is needed and how much skin must be removed.
- Segmental resections can be performed for segmental contour abnormalities.
- In general, most women prefer a higher eyelid crease than men. A clear discussion must be had before the procedure.
- Measure twice and cut once.

36.8.5 Postoperative Care Checklist

- Ice is applied to the operative sites for 48 hours, 15 minutes on/15 minutes off while awake.
- The patient is advised to sleep with the head of the bed elevated.
- The patient may shower the next day.
- The wound should be kept clean with tepid water, and the bacitracin eye ointment applied four times daily.
- Postoperative medications are given:
  - Antibiotic eye ointment (bacitracin preferred) to the wounds.

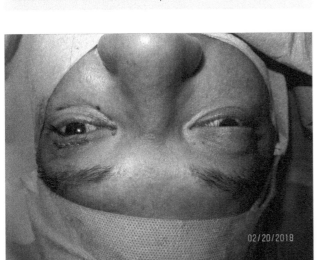

Fig. 36.9 Typical postoperative eyelid opening after scleral contact lens removal.

- Frequently, there will be a small amount of lagophthalmos postoperatively.
- The eyelids will typically be symmetric on the operating room table (▶ Fig. 36.9) and postoperatively (▶ Fig. 36.10).

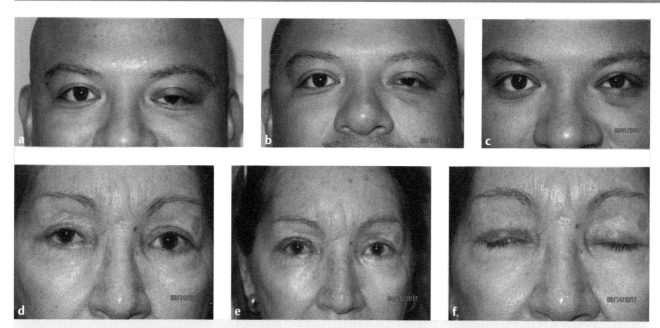

Fig. 36.10 Typical pre- and postoperative results after surgery. Initial photograph (**a**), postoperative residual ptosis (**b**), and final result (**c**) after tarsectomy. An additional patient referred after 5 upper eyelid surgeries with residual right upper blepharoptosis (**d**), status post tarsectomy (**e**), and postoperative lagophthalmos (**f**).

○ Oral pain medication, typically acetaminophen/
hydrocodone, 5 mg/325 mg.
• Workouts and strenuous exercise should be avoided for 1 week if considered acceptable from a medical standpoint.
• Blood thinners such as aspirin and nonsteroidals should be avoided for 1 week.
• No eye or eyelid exercises are needed to maintain the created eyelid height and contour.
• Suture removal is performed at week 1.

36.9 Complications and Their Management

Operating on small amounts of residual blepharoptosis after levator surgery, using either an anterior or posterior approach, is nuanced. Complications that may result include upper eyelid ectropion, lagophthalmos, increased palpebral fissure on downgaze, and worsening dry eye. The ectropion can be managed with massage. Postoperative lagophthalmos and dry eye exacerbation can typically be managed with artificial tears and lubricating ointment. In the event of dry eye decompensation and severe corneal exposure keratopathy, a PROSE lens may be prescribed or eyelid recession may be performed.[11],[12]

References

[1] Brown BZ. Ptosis revision. Int Ophthalmol Clin. 1989; 29(4):217–218
[2] Dortzbach RK, Kronish JW. Early revision in the office for adults after unsatisfactory blepharoptosis correction. Am J Ophthalmol. 1993; 115(1):68–75
[3] Shore JW, Bergin DJ, Garrett SN. Results of blepharoptosis surgery with early postoperative adjustment. Ophthalmology. 1990; 97(11):1502–1511
[4] Baylis HI, Shorr N. Anterior tarsectomy reoperation for upper eyelid blepharoptosis or contour abnormalities. Am J Ophthalmol. 1977; 84(1):67–71
[5] Gladstone GJ, Putterman AM. Internal vertical shortening for the correction of diffuse or segmental postoperative blepharoptosis. Am J Ophthalmol. 1985; 99(4):429–436
[6] Bassin RE, Putterman AM. Full-thickness eyelid resection in the treatment of secondary ptosis. Ophthal Plast Reconstr Surg. 2009; 25(2):85–89
[7] Liu F, Ma Y, Luo X, Yang J. Bleparoptosis reoperation with combining excision of tarsus and levator muscle. Ann Plast Surg. 2015; 75(6):591–595
[8] Pang NK, Newsom RW, Oestreicher JH, Chung HT, Harvey JT. Fasanella-Servat procedure: indications, efficacy, and complications. Can J Ophthalmol. 2008; 43(1):84–88
[9] Beard C. Ptosis. St. Louis, C.V. Mosby 1976
[10] Fasanella RM, Servat J. Levator resection for minimal ptosis: another simplified operation. Arch Ophthalmol. 1961; 65:493–496
[11] Chahal JS, Heur M, Chiu GB. Prosthetic replacement of the ocular surface ecosystem. Scleral lens therapy for exposure keratopathy. Eye Contact Lens. 2017; 43(4):240–244
[12] Samimi DB, Chiu GB, Burnstine MA. PROSE scleral lens: a novel aid for staged eyelid reconstruction. Ophthal Plast Reconstr Surg. 2014; 30(5):e119–e121

37 Nonsurgical Management of Ptosis

Christine Greer, Michael A. Burnstine

Abstract

Nonsurgical treatments of ptosis benefit patients who are poor surgical candidates. This includes patients with progressive ptosis and poor Bell's phenomenon as seen in chronic progressive external ophthalmoplegia (CPEO), myotonic dystrophy, and patients with variable ptosis secondary to myasthenia gravis. The eyelid may be elevated mechanically or pharmacologically.

Keywords: nonsurgical ptosis management, eyelid crutches, eyelid taping, haptic contact lens, prop contact lens, pharmacologic eyelid elevation

37.1 Introduction

In most cases, definitive treatment for blepharoptosis is surgical. However, in patients who are poor surgical candidates or who do not desire surgery, other options exist. Patients with progressive ptosis and poor Bell's phenomenon as seen in chronic progressive external ophthalmoplegia (CPEO) and myotonic dystrophy are poor surgical candidates owing to their risk of corneal exposure and keratopathy. These patients, similar to patients with myasthenia gravis, have a variable or progressive degree of ptosis, making the optimal change in eyelid position a moving target. Nonsurgical elevation of the eyelid may be mechanical or pharmacologic. Mechanical elevation of the lid can be achieved with devices such as eyelid crutches, tape, or contact lenses. Pharmacologic options include alpha-2 agonists such as brimonidine and apraclonidine, which activate the sympathetically innervated Müller's muscle and can improve eyelid position about 1 to 2 mm. Botulinum toxin can be used to elevate the eyelid by paralyzing the muscles of eyelid protraction, indirectly improving eyelid position. In this chapter these treatments are described in detail.

37.2 Mechanical Eyelid Elevation

37.2.1 Eyelid Crutches

An eyelid crutch is a bar that is placed along the inside of an eyeglasses frame to support the eyelid (▶ Fig. 37.1). These devices are made of metal wire and custom-designed to accommodate the shape and contour of the eye and eyelid. The crutch is positioned at or just above the eyelid crease, applying backward and upward pressure against the upper eyelid which tucks the eyelid and raises the margin above the pupil. There are two types of eyelid crutches: adjustable for mild amounts of ptosis, and reinforced for moderate to severe ptosis.[1] An adjustable crutch attaches to the lens frame typically on the nasal side of the frame, and can be adjusted based on the degree of ptosis. This type of crutch is ideal in patients suffering from conditions in which the ptosis fluctuates. This type of crutch often migrates and needs to be readjusted due to weakening of the metal from its pivot point on the spectacle.[1] Reinforced crutches are secured at both ends to the lens frame. Thus, they have the disadvantage of not being adjustable, but the advantage of not migrating.

Eyelid crutches are ideal for patients who are poor surgical candidates or those with temporary or fluctuating symptoms. Limitations include discomfort, especially if improperly fitted, restricted blink, the requisite cleaning regimen, and risk of damage to the globe in an accident. Glasses fitted with eyelid crutches should not be used for extended duration as restricted blink may lead to drying of the eye.

37.2.2 Eyelid Taping

Similar to the eyelid crutch, eyelid taping can be used as a temporary measure to elevate the eyelid (▶ Fig. 37.2). Various types of disposable, adhesive tapes may be used, and the method is safe, inexpensive, and easy to use. Though not routinely used, one study has demonstrated efficacy of octyl-2-cyanoacrylate liquid bandage for severe ptosis.[2] The disadvantage of eyelid taping is that the tape must be applied daily, and efficacy is largely user-dependent. In patients with a poor Bell's phenomenon, eyelid taping should be used for small time periods to ensure corneal protection.

37.2.3 Haptic Contact Lens

Ptosis crutches and eyelid taping may not elevate the lid satisfactorily and can cause severe dry eye symptoms. These aids restrict the natural blink reflex, and as such they should be avoided in

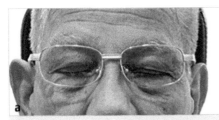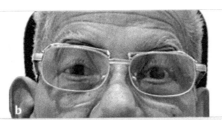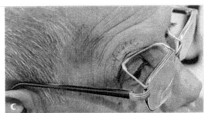

Fig. 37.1 Patient with blepharoptosis with corrective lenses (**a**) and after fitting with eyelid ptosis crutches on glasses frames (**b, c**). (Used with permission of Ray Favella at worldoptics.com.)

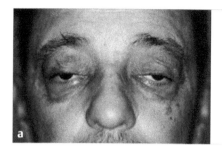
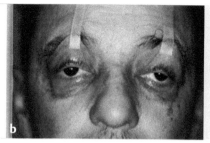

Fig. 37.2 A patient with chronic progressive external ophthalmoplegia managed with eyelid taping. Pretaping (a) with poor margin reflex distance 1 (MRD1) and posttaping (b), clearing the visual axis.

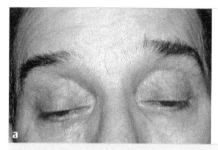
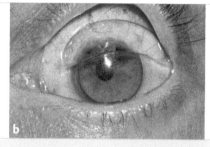
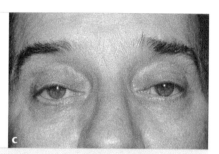

Fig. 37.3 Severe myopathic blepharoptosis before "prop" haptic lens (a), with fitting of the "prop" lens (b), and ptosis improvement with the haptic contact lens in place (c). (Used with permission from Collin JRO, Tyers AG, eds. Color Atlas of Ophthalmic Plastic Surgery. 3rd ed. Elsevier; 2017:208.)

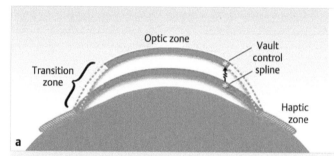
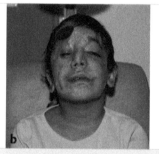
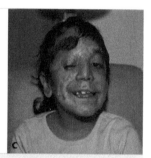

Fig. 37.4 A vaulted PROSE contact lens (a) fit in a 12-year-old girl after a severe motor vehicle accident causing bilateral paralytic ptosis, status post multiple ocular surgeries, and eyelid reconstructions for a paralytic ptosis in the sighted left eye. Note the chin up posture pretreatment (b) and the improved chin position and margin reflex distance 1 (MRD1) posttreatment (c). (Images courtesy of Karen G. Carrasquillo, OD, PhD, FAOO, FSLS, at BostonSight.)

cases of dry eye, exposure keratopathy, and in patients at risk for exposure keratopathy. In such cases, a "prop" or haptic contact lens is an option. A haptic contact lens is a scleral contact lens equipped with a shelf on which the margin of the upper eyelid rests (▶ Fig. 37.3). As an alternative, a vaulted PROSE lens may be used (▶ Fig. 37.4). The lens traps tears to protect the cornea, creating a prosthetic ocular surface environment. This option is particularly useful in patients with myotonic dystrophy and other types of ptosis accompanied by poor orbicularis function.[3] The major benefit of haptic contact lens use is superior protection of the corneal surface. Limitations are the potential for discomfort and the need for meticulous lens hygiene.

37.3 Pharmacologic Eyelid Elevation

37.3.1 Topical Therapy

Sympathomimetic eye drops such as apraclonidine and brimonidine provide a temporary lift of the upper eyelid.

Apraclonidine (0.5%) and brimonidine (0.1 or 0.2%) are alpha-2-adrenergic agonists, which cause Müller muscle contraction. This results in upper eyelid elevation of about 1 to 2 mm, though experimental studies support elevation closer to 1 mm.[4,5] Topical sympathomimetics are most commonly used in cases of inadvertent ptosis after botulinum toxin effect deep to the orbicularis muscle. The botulinum toxin migrates to the levator palpebrae superioris muscle inducing an upper eyelid ptosis. Studies have found that apraclonidine has a peak onset at 30 to 45 minutes after drop instillation.[4,6] The effect is not long lasting. There have been no studies evaluating the efficacy of apraclonidine or brimonidine in the setting of neurotoxin-related ptosis and there are currently no established dosing regimens for this use. We suggest a dosing schedule of one drop placed into the affected eye two to three times daily. Apraclonidine and brimonidine are associated with follicular conjunctivitis and contact dermatitis[7] with documented rates as high as 36% and 15%, respectively.[8] If these reactions are encountered, topical therapy should be discontinued.

37.3.2 Neurotoxin Injections

In patients with ptosis, compensatory use of the frontalis muscle to elevate the eyelid often occurs secondarily, resulting in muscle strain. The relationship between the protractors and retractors can be targeted pharmacologically with botulinum toxin in cases where surgical management is not an option. Treatment of the eyelid protractors (corrugator, procerus, and orbicularis oculi muscles) reduces protractor activity, thus decreasing the level of ptosis and allowing antagonistic levator and frontalis muscles to compensate with less patient effort.[9,10] (▶ Fig. 37.5). Use of botulinum toxin for ptosis in CPEO and asymmetric ptosis secondary to blepharospasm has also been described.[9,10] Patients in whom exposure is of significant concern may benefit from such treatment, but careful titration is necessary as overtreatment may compromise the lacrimal pump and may lead to exposure keratopathy. Further studies assessing botulinum toxin's clinical utility in the treatment of ptosis are necessary.

37.4 Management of Ptosis in the Anophthalmic Patient

In anophthalmic patients or patients with phthisis bulbi, blepharoptosis may be managed by altering the size and shape of the ocular prosthesis (▶ Fig. 37.6). Frequently, a ptosis shelf is added to create symmetry between both orbits (▶ Fig. 37.7).

37.5 Management of Pseudoptosis with Filler Injection

Pseudoptosis created by asymmetries in margin crease and fold may be addressed by botulinum to lower brows and create margin crease and margin fold symmetry (▶ Fig. 37.8). Alternatively, hyaluronic filler may be added to a deflated orbit to create symmetry (▶ Fig. 37.9).[11-13] Adverse side effects of this treatment with fat or hyaluronic gels may include vision loss, upper eyelid edema, or an irregular eyelid appearance.[14]

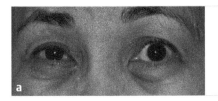
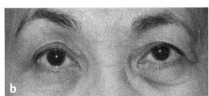

Fig. 37.5 Nonsurgical ptosis management with botulinum toxin for right hemifacial spasm, before **(a)** and after treatment **(b)**.

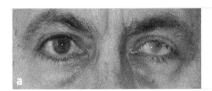
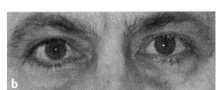

Fig. 37.6 A patient with phthisis bulbi **(a)** fit with an ocular prosthetic to create symmetry between sides **(b)**. (Images courtesy of Stephen Haddad, BCO, Los Angeles, CA.)

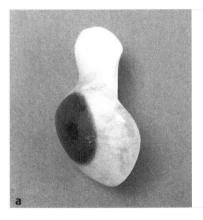
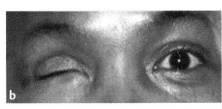

Fig. 37.7 A ptosis shelf **(a)** fabricated to address blepharoptosis in an anophthalmic patient. Preplacement **(b)** and postplacement **(c)**. (Images courtesy of Stephen Haddad, BCO, Los Angeles, CA.)

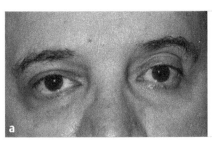
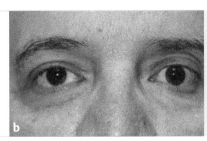

Fig. 37.8 Botulinum toxin added above the left eyebrow to create eyelid crease and fold symmetry. Preneurotoxin **(a)** and postneurotoxin **(b)**.

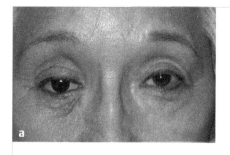
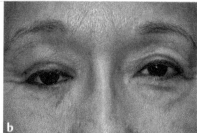
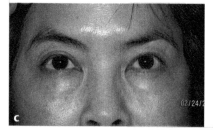
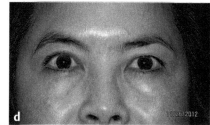

Fig. 37.9 Juvederm added to the brow and superior orbit to create volume and symmetry in an anophthalmic patient (**a, b**) and sighted patient (**c, d**).

References

[1] Eye crutches - ptosis crutch. Zenttech.com. Available at zenntech.com/alter-eyewear-sunglass-eyeglass-modify-glasses/ptosis-eye-crutches.php. Updated 2017. Accessed August 4, 2017

[2] Osaki TH, Osaki MH, Belfort R, Jr, Osaki T, Sant'anna AE, Haraguchi DK. Management of progressive myopathic blepharoptosis with daily application of octyl-2-cyanoacrylate liquid bandage. Ophthal Plast Reconstr Surg. 2009; 25 (4):264–266

[3] Tyers AG, Collin JRO. Colour atlas of ophthalmic plastic surgery. 3rd ed. Philadelphia, Pa: Butterworth Heinemann, Elsevier; 2008

[4] Munden PM, Kardon RH, Denison CE, Carter KD. Palpebral fissure responses to topical adrenergic drugs. Am J Ophthalmol. 1991; 111(6):706–710

[5] Wijemanne S, Vijayakumar D, Jankovic J. Apraclonidine in the treatment of ptosis. J Neurol Sci. 2017; 376:129–132

[6] Kirkpatrick CA, Shriver EM, Clark TJE, Kardon RH. Upper eyelid response to topical 0.5% apraclonidine. Ophthal Plast Reconstr Surg. 2018; 34(1):13–19

[7] Girkin CA, Bhorade AM, Giaconi JA, et al. Medical management in glaucoma. In: Cantor LB, Rapuano CJ, Gioffi GA, eds. Basic and Clinical Science Course (BCSC) Section 10: Orbit, Eyelids, and Lacrimal System. San Francisco, CA: American Academy of Ophthalmology (AAO); 2016

[8] Gordon RN, Liebmann JM, Greenfield DS, Lama P, Ritch R. Lack of cross-reactive allergic response to brimonidine in patients with known apraclonidine allergy. Eye (Lond). 1998; 12(Pt 4):697–700

[9] Putterman AM. Botox enhancing eyebrow elevation in external ophthalmoplegia ptosis. Ophthal Plast Reconstr Surg. 2014; 30(5):444–445

[10] Fagien S. Temporary management of upper lid ptosis, lid malposition, and eyelid fissure asymmetry with botulinum toxin type A. Plast Reconstr Surg. 2004; 114(7):1892–1902

[11] Moon HS, Ahn B, Lee JH, Rah DK, Park TH. Rejuvenation of the deep superior sulcus in the eyelid. J Cosmet Dermatol. 2016; 15(4):458–468

[12] Romeo F. Upper eyelid filling with or without surgical treatment. Aesthetic Plast Surg. 2016; 40(2):223–235

[13] Morley AM, Taban M, Malhotra R, Goldberg RA. Use of hyaluronic acid gel for upper eyelid filling and contouring. Ophthal Plast Reconstr Surg. 2009; 25(6): 440–444

[14] Khan TT, Woodward JA. Retained dermal filler in the upper eyelid masquerading as periorbital edema. Dermatol Surg. 2015; 41(10):1182–1184

38 Unique Considerations in Upper Facial Surgery

Margaret L. Pfeiffer, Jessica R. Chang

Abstract

This chapter addresses particular preoperative, intraoperative, and postoperative considerations that arise with the upper facial surgery techniques reviewed in this book. Available evidence and consensus guidelines are summarized to provide a framework for the surgeon to answer questions such as whether and when to stop blood-thinning medications, what kind of perioperative antibiotics are indicated, and how to safely use electrosurgical and other energy-based devices. Certain patient comorbidities that may impact surgical planning are also presented.

Keywords: anticoagulation medications, antiplatelet medications, antibiotics, cautery, ointment

38.1 Introduction

When should anticoagulants or antiplatelet agents be held before surgery? Are perioperative antibiotics necessary? What form of cautery is safest with patients who have implanted electronic devices? In the course of appropriate preoperative evaluation and surgical planning, these and many other questions arise.

The evidence for holding or prescribing perioperative medications is reviewed in the following sections, focusing on drugs that may exacerbate bleeding and on infection prevention. The final section reviews safety considerations with various energy-based devices used in plastic surgery. Common perioperative issues that arise for the upper facial surgeon are reviewed to raise awareness of potentially serious risks for certain patients and to summarize the existing evidence and guidelines to help clinicians assess and manage these risks. Treatment should always be tailored to the individual patient.

38.2 Perioperative Medications

In this section, we review perioperative blood thinner and antibiotic medication use.

38.2.1 Blood-Thinner Considerations

Antithrombotic medications increase the risk of bleeding, which may lead to increased operative time, intraoperative complications, postoperative bruising, and poor postoperative cosmesis; rarely, orbital compartment syndrome and significant vision loss occur. One study at a large oculofacial plastic surgery practice found that 40% of patients used at least one antithrombotic agent.[1] Given the aging population and recommendations for aspirin as prevention for cardiovascular disease, this proportion will continue to increase; although recent recommendations suggest aspirin may not be as beneficial, it will likely take years for this to take effect.[1]

There are no randomized controlled trials on perioperative management of antithrombotic medications in oculofacial surgery. Management is guided largely by retrospective studies and trials in other surgical fields. The oculoplastic surgeon must balance the potentially life-threatening risk of thromboembolic events with the risk of bleeding complications, such as orbital

compartment syndrome, and, rarely, the need for blood transfusion. Understanding when to stop and restart these agents is critical to perioperative management.

38.2.2 Classes of Blood Thinners

There are three main classes of blood thinners currently approved by the Food and Drug Administration (FDA) for use in the United States: (1) antiplatelet agents, (2) anticoagulants, and (3) direct oral anticoagulants.

Antiplatelet Agents

The antiplatelet agents inhibit platelet aggregation and thrombus formation. Antiplatelet agents include aspirin, clopidogrel (Plavix), ticagrelor (Brilinta), cilostazol (Pletal), dipyridamole (in Aggrenox), and prasugrel (Effient). The two most commonly used antiplatelet agents are aspirin and clopidogrel. Aspirin is indicated for both primary and secondary prevention of cardiovascular disease, though many patients use it for analgesia unrelated to cardiovascular disease. Because it is easily obtained over-the-counter, many patients forget to include aspirin when reporting a medication list, particularly if it is a low dose (e.g., 81 mg or "baby" aspirin).[1] In contrast, clopidogrel is used as secondary prevention in patients with prior thromboembolic event, prior myocardial infarction, or an implanted device such as a cardiac stent. Aspirin and clopidogrel may be used synergistically (termed dual antiplatelet therapy) in patients at high risk for thromboembolic event. These patients tend to bleed more than patients on a single agent.[2]

Nonsteroidal anti-inflammatory drugs (NSAIDs) also inhibit platelet activity, though the effect is usually of shorter duration. NSAIDs may be nonselective (e.g., ibuprofen, indomethacin, or naproxen) or selective (e.g., celecoxib). The effect of nonselective NSAIDs on intra- or postoperative bleeding complications is unclear; some studies suggest increased risk, while others suggest there is no increased risk of bleeding complications.[3,4] There is evidence that the selective COX-2 inhibitor celecoxib (Celebrex) does not significantly affect platelet function or intraoperative bleeding.[5] Other NSAIDs that affect COX-2 more than COX-1, such as meloxicam and etodolac, have also been shown to have little impact on bleeding risk.[6,7] For postsurgical pain, the intravenous NSAID ketorolac (Toradol) is often offered by the anesthesiologists as an alternative to narcotics, but there have been conflicting studies over whether this may cause increased risk of postoperative bleeding.[8] A study in patients undergoing endoscopic sinus surgery comparing ketorolac to fentanyl showed no increase in postoperative hemorrhage and equal analgesia.[9] A recent randomized controlled trial of 100 patients undergoing levator advancement surgery found better analgesia scores with IV ketorolac compared to usual care, and no patients had significant postoperative hemorrhage.[10]

Anticoagulants

The anticoagulants directly inhibit clotting factors in the coagulation cascade and are indicated in patients with prior pulmonary or venous thromboembolism, or prophylactically in the setting of atrial fibrillation, prosthetic heart valves, and rheumatic heart disease. Warfarin (Coumadin) is the most commonly used oral anticoagulant. Heparin is delivered intravenously, but its derivative called fractionated or low-molecular-weight heparin is available by subcutaneous injection.

Warfarin inhibits the production of vitamin K-dependent clotting factors. It acts on the extrinsic pathway of the coagulation cascade and is monitored by prothrombin time (PT) or its derivative, the international normalized ratio (INR). In contrast, heparin primarily affects the intrinsic pathway and is monitored by the partial thromboplastin time (PTT). These values essentially quantify the amount of anticoagulant effect of the particular agent. Warfarin is a complicated medication, with many food and drug interactions, a narrow therapeutic index, and frequent monitoring for dose titration. In the event of emergency surgery or uncontrolled intraoperative or postoperative hemorrhage, the anticoagulation effect of warfarin is reversible with vitamin K and fresh frozen plasma.

There are several low-molecular-weight heparin agents available, the most common of which is enoxaparin (Lovenox). The oculofacial surgeon may encounter enoxaparin for it use as a bridging agent in patients on warfarin. Essentially, in select patients, the warfarin is held preoperatively and the patient is started on subcutaneous injections of enoxaparin instead for a brief period before and after surgery. The enoxaparin is a shorter-acting agent whose dose can be held immediately prior to surgery with the goal of mitigating intraoperative bleeding while allowing for appropriate perioperative reduction in thromboembolic risk. A meta-analysis on bridging therapy in moderate-risk patients with atrial fibrillation on warfarin showed, however, that bridging therapy increased bleeding risk without decreasing thromboembolism risk, calling into question the utility of bridging therapy.[11,12]

Direct Oral Anticoagulants

The direct oral anticoagulants (DOACs), sometimes referred to as new oral anticoagulants (NOACs), were invented as an alternative to warfarin. Their advantage lies in the fact that they have a more predictable pharmacologic profile, fewer food and drug interactions, and require no regular monitoring. They have a more rapid onset of action (average 2–3 hours vs. 3–4 days) and a shorter half-life (average 12 hours vs. 20–60 hours) compared to warfarin.[13] However, their disadvantage is that they lack a reversal agent, and lab tests for monitoring their effect are less readily available. The currently available DOACs are apixaban (Eliquis), dabigatran (Pradaxa), and rivaroxaban (Xarelto). All are indicated in patients with atrial fibrillation, and dabigatran and rivaroxaban are also FDA-approved for pulmonary embolus and deep venous thrombosis.

38.2.3 Balancing Thrombotic Risks and Bleeding Risks

The decision to cease or continue blood thinners prior to surgery requires a careful understanding of risk. In the oculoplastic literature, the risk of major hemorrhage intraoperatively or postoperatively is less than 1%,[14] and the risk of vision loss from retrobulbar hemorrhage after blepharoplasty is even lower

(0.0045% from survey data).[15] The data on bleeding risk in oculofacial surgery with and without blood thinners are sparse without randomized trials in eyelid, lacrimal, or orbital surgery. A prospective study by Custer et al of 1,500 oculoplastic procedures reported an overall rate of severe hemorrhage of 0.4%.[14] The authors found that patients who continued antiplatelets and anticoagulants had no increased risk of intraoperative bleeding, postoperative bruising, or severe bleeding complications compared to controls; however, they noted "troublesome bleeding" prolonging 9% of surgeries.[14]

Recommendations in the facial plastics and dermatologic literature suggest continuation of blood thinners is associated with low rates of severe hemorrhagic complications.[16-19] Importantly, intraoperative and postoperative hemorrhages in oculofacial surgery carry special risk compared to facial plastic or dermatologic surgery because of the potential for orbital compartment syndrome and vision loss. Therefore, although these fields have larger, more robust studies on perioperative blood thinner use, it is difficult to extrapolate their findings.

Bleeding risks must be balanced with the risk of thrombotic event should blood thinners be held. No randomized trials exist that report the rate of thrombotic event in patients who discontinued blood thinners for surgery. In patients who have warfarin stopped for any reason, including perioperatively, there is an approximately 1% risk of a thromboembolic event within 30 days.[20] This risk increases fourfold in patients with mechanical heart valves.[21] One meta-analysis estimated the additional risk of any vascular event of withholding aspirin for 7 days perioperatively at roughly 1 cardiac event to 1.4 cardiac events per 1,000 patients.[22] Therefore, the upper facial surgeon must weigh a 1% or greater risk of thromboembolic events with the less than 1% risk of a severe hemorrhagic surgical complication.

The American College of Chest Physicians has released evidence-based guidelines for patients on blood thinners undergoing elective procedures. This requires risk-stratification of patients for perioperative thromboembolism (► Table 38.1) and of procedures for bleeding (► Table 38.2). Reconstructive plastic surgery falls within the high bleeding risk category, defined as greater than or equal to 2% 2-day risk of major bleed.[23] Eyelid and brow oculoplastic procedures likely do not require categorization in this group, but one could classify orbital and sinus cases as high-risk bleeding procedures. These guidelines are patient-driven: in high-risk patients, guidelines recommend stopping DOACs and warfarin and bridging with low-molecular-weight heparin; low-risk patients should also stop these medications, but do not require bridging. High-risk patients should continue antiplatelet agents when possible, and low-risk patients may stop antiplatelet agents.[24]

Patients with recent cardiac stents are particularly high risk, and recent guidelines state that "elective noncardiac surgery should not be performed within 30 days of bare metal stent or 12 months of drug-eluting stent implantation because of in-stent thrombosis as well as bleeding risk from dual antiplatelet therapy during surgery."[25]

38.2.4 Time to Stop Blood Thinners Preoperatively

Recommendations in the literature vary on appropriate timing to stop blood thinners preoperatively. Platelet function takes

Table 38.1 Suggested risk stratification for perioperative thromboembolism[28]

Risk stratum	Indication for VKA therapy		
	Mechanical heart valve	Atrial fibrillation	Venous thromboembolism
High	• Any mitral valve prosthesis • Any caged-ball or tilting disc aortic valve prosthesis • Recent (within 6 mo) stroke or TIA	• CHADS$_2$ score of 5 or 6 • Recent (within 3 mo) stroke or TIA • Rheumatic valvular heart disease	• Recent (within 3 mo) VTE • Severe thrombophilia (e.g., deficiency in protein C, protein S, or antithrombin; antiphospholipid antibodies; multiple abnormalities)
Moderate	• Bileaflet aortic valve prosthesis and one or more of the following: atrial fibrillation, prior stroke or TIA, hypertension, diabetes, congestive heart failure, age > 75 years	• CHADS$_2$ score of 3 or 4	• VTE within the past 3–12 mo • Nonsevere thrombophilia (e.g., heterozygous favor V Leiden or prothrombin gene mutation) • Recurrent VTE • Active cancer (treated within 6 mo or palliative)
Low	• Bileaflet aortic valve prosthesis without atrial fibrillation and no other risk factors for stroke	• CHADS$_2$ score of 0–2 (assuming no prior stroke or TIA)	• VTE > 12 mo previous and no other risk factors

Abbreviations: CHADS$_2$, congestive heart failure, hypertension, age ≥ 75 years, diabetes mellitus, and stroke or TIA; TIA, transient ischemic attack; VKA, vitamin K agonist; VTE venous thromboembolism.

Table 38.2 Suggested overall periprocedural anticoagulant and bridging management for patients receiving chronic oral anticoagulants (including vitamin K antagonists and direct oral anticoagulants [DOACs]) based on thromboembolic and procedural bleeding risk[23]

	High-risk bleeding procedures	Low-risk bleeding procedures	Minimal-risk bleeding procedures
High-thromboembolic risk	• DOAC users: Interrupt DOAC therapy; bridging with LMWH not suggested for DOACs • Warfarin users: Interrupt warfarin therapy with LMWH bridging suggested on the basis of clinician judgment and the most current evidence[a,b]	• DOAC users: Interrupt DOAC therapy; bridging with LMWH not suggested for DOACs • Warfarin users: Interrupt warfarin therapy with LMWH bridging suggested on the basis of clinician judgment and the most current evidence[a]	• Do not interrupt anticoagulant therapy[c]
Intermediate-thromboembolic risk	• DOAC users: Interrupt DOAC therapy; bridging with LMWH not suggested for DOACs • Warfarin users: Consider interrupting warfarin therapy without LMWH bridging suggested on the basis of clinician judgment and the most current evidence[a,b]	• DOAC users: Interrupt DOAC therapy; bridging with LMWH not suggested for DOACs • Warfarin users: Consider interrupting warfarin therapy without LMWH bridging suggested on the basis of clinician judgment and the most current evidence[a]	• Do not interrupt anticoagulant therapy[c]
Low-thromboembolic risk	• DOAC users: Interrupt DOAC therapy; bridging with LMWH not suggested for DOACs • Warfarin users: Interrupt warfarin therapy; bridging with LMWH not necessary	• DOAC users: Interrupt DOAC therapy; bridging with LMWH not suggested for DOACs • Warfarin users: Interrupt warfarin therapy; bridging with LMWH not necessary	• Do not interrupt anticoagulant therapy[c]

Abbreviations: DOAC, direct oral anticoagulant; LMWH, low-molecular-weight heparin.
[a]Atrial fibrillation: bridging not recommended on the basis of Level 1 evidence, but evidence in a few high-risk CHADS$_2$ patients (scores of 5 and 6). Mechanical heart valve and venous thromboembolism: retrospective studies suggest that bridging increases bleeding risk without reducing thrombosis.
[b]May administer prophylactic low-dose LMWH for venous thromboembolism (VTE) prevention in patients undergoing high bleeding risk procedures or major surgeries that confer a high risk of VTE.
[c]May consider interrupting DOAC therapy on the day of the procedure.

Table 38.3 When to discontinue blood thinners before surgery

Class	Agent	Half-life of effect	Recommended to stop before surgery	
Antiplatelets	Aspirin	1 wk	7–14 d	Irreversible inhibition of platelets
	Clopidogrel	1 wk	5 d	
Anticoagulants	Warfarin	20–60 h	3–5 d	
	LMWH	12 h	24 h	
DOACs	Dabigatran	13–18 h	2–4 d	Depending on renal function
	Apixaban	12 h	48 h	
	Rivaroxaban	5–9 h	24–48 h	

Abbreviation: LMWH, low-molecular-weight heparin.

Table 38.4 Dietary supplements that potentially influence risk of hemorrhage

Supplements that may increase bleeding risk		Supplements to decrease bleeding/ bruising risk
Some evidence	*Not well studied*	*Little evidence of efficacy*
Vitamin E	Dong quai	Arnica
Fish oil/Omega 3	Lycopene	Rhododendron
Ginger	L-Arginine	
Ginseng	Taurine	
Ginkgo biloba	Passion flower	
Garlic	Chamomile	
Selenium	Cinnamon	
	Cayenne pepper	
	Curcumin	
	Feverfew	
	Tree ear mushrooms	
	Grape seed extract	
	Echinacea	
	Green tea extract	
	Glucosamine	
	Chondroitin sulfate	
	Coenzyme Q10	
	Policosanol	
	Turmeric	
	Magnesium	

longer to recover than anticoagulant effect, so the antiplatelet agents require stopping the soonest before surgery than other classes. As most of the antiplatelets irreversibly inhibit platelet function, generation of new platelets must occur to regain clotting effect. Generally, most sources recommend stopping aspirin and prasugrel 7 days prior to surgery and clopidogrel and ticagrelor 5 days prior.[26,27] Warfarin can be stopped 5 days prior to surgery. The DOACs can be stopped 2 days before surgery, except in the context of renal dysfunction, which alters the clearance rate of dabigatran because it is cleared by the kidneys (▶ Table 38.3). All agents can be restarted the day after surgery.

38.2.5 Supplements and Other Considerations

Many supplements have been shown to have anticoagulant effect including but not limited to garlic, Ginkgo biloba, ginger, ginseng, fish oil, vitamin E, and selenium (▶ Table 38.4). These all affect the coagulation cascade at different points and are well reviewed in a recent article.[29] There are anecdotal reports of bleeding episodes on many of these agents, yet more detailed studies have shown mostly equivocal bleeding risk at normal doses but potentially increased risk when used in combination with blood thinners. Perhaps the most well studied is vitamin E, which inhibits platelet aggregation in a dose-dependent manner at doses higher than 400 IU/day and was found clinically to be linked to hemorrhagic events in atrial fibrillation patients on warfarin.[30]

Arnica Montana is a herb available in topical and oral formulations marketed for its ability to reduce postoperative bruising, widely recommended by surgeons postoperatively. It has also been studied also for its effect on postoperative pain and edema. One prospective, placebo-controlled study in men undergoing sequential upper blepharoplasty found no difference in ecchymosis or patient comfort in patients on oral Arnica.[31] Arnica has been found, however, to reduce edema but not ecchymosis after rhinoplasty and to reduce ecchymosis compared to placebo after facelifting.[32]

Finally, thrombocytopenia ($< 150 \times 10^9$/L platelets) may result from various medical conditions and carries significantly higher risk for severe bleeding complications with upper facial plastic surgery. No guidelines specifically address eyelid surgery, but a minimum platelet level of 100×10^9/L has been recommended for eye and brain surgery, and a minimum level of 50×10^9/L platelets is recommended for other major surgeries.[33] Patients with thrombocytopenia or specific bleeding disorders should be managed in conjunction with a hematologist to reduce bleeding risk prior to surgery.

38.3 Perioperative Antibiotic Considerations

Recommendations for antibiotic prophylaxis in other surgical fields such as dermatologic surgery are well established, yet no formalized evidence-based recommendations exist for oculofacial plastic surgery. When discussing antibiotics and surgical procedures, there are several points at which antibiotics may be given. "Preoperative antibiotics" refers to those given days prior to a procedure, which is not a common practice. "Perioperative antibiotics" refers to medication given on the day of surgery, typically intravenously and prior to incision. "Postoperative antibiotics" are prescribed for the days after surgery and are usually oral or topical.

Systemic prophylactic antibiotic use in blepharoplasty has increased over 200% from 1985 to 2000 in a survey of plastic surgeons[34] and increased from 1992 to 2018 in surveys of members of the American Society of Ophthalmic Plastic and Reconstructive Surgery (ASOPRS).[35,36] Increased use of antibiotics is not without risk, from systemic complications to the patient such as allergy, anaphylaxis, or gastrointestinal infection to public health concerns such as promoting antibiotic resistance.

38.3.1 Current Practice Patterns in Oculofacial Plastic Surgery

There is a lack of high-quality evidence and standardized recommendations from oculofacial plastic societies, allowing for wide variability in practice patterns. A survey of 728 oculoplastic surgeons from 43 countries found that practice patterns varied widely across countries.[37] Overall, 14% of respondents gave intravenous antibiotics at the time of routine eyelid surgery, 24% gave oral antibiotics after surgery, and 88% gave topical antibiotics after surgery. The frequency of postoperative oral antibiotic use varied most and was country-dependent, ranging from 0 to 20% in countries such as the United States, Canada, Chile, and much of Europe to 80 to 100% in India, Bolivia, and Venezuela. Respondents stated that their choices in prescribing antibiotic were largely dictated by personal experience and training as opposed to being data-driven. A recent survey of ASOPRS members showed similar results: 89% of respondents prescribed a topical antibiotic after blepharoplasty and 14% prescribed an oral antibiotic after blepharoplasty, most commonly cephalexin.[36]

38.3.2 Patterns and Rates of Surgical Site Infection

The rate of surgical site infection has been shown to increase in patients older than 70 years, with diabetes mellitus, poor nutritional or immunocompromised status, smoking, and increased body mass index,[38–40] and to be higher in longer procedures and those with skin grafts and flaps compared to simple excisions.[40,41] Large studies have calculated the rate of surgical site infection in cutaneous surgery to range from 1 to 3%.[38]

Postoperative infection following eyelid surgery is even more rare, ranging from 0.04% in a study of over 2,000 patients undergoing a variety of eyelid procedures[42] to 0.2% in a study of over 1,600 patients undergoing blepharoplasty.[43] Carter et al reported a slightly higher rate of 0.4% in blepharoplasty patients undergoing concurrent CO_2 laser resurfacing.[43] Severe infectious complications have been reported after blepharoplasty, including orbital cellulitis, no light perception vision,[44] and necrotizing

fasciitis.[45–47] Chronic cutaneous infection with mycobacterium species is also reported yet rare after eyelid surgery.[48,49] The rarity of postoperative infection after blepharoplasty has led many authors to advocate against systemic antibiotic use,[43,50,51] but topical antibiotic use remains common.

38.3.3 Preoperative Recommendations

Preoperative antibiotics are very infrequently used in the setting of upper facial surgery.

38.3.4 Perioperative Recommendations

There are specific surgical and patient factors that require single dose oral or intravenous antibiotic prophylaxis 60 minutes prior to surgical incision.

Studies in dermatologic surgery have identified procedures involving skin grafting, wedge excision or flaps on the ear or nose, and procedures in the groin or below the knee as higher risk for surgical site infection that warrant perioperative antibiotics.[38,41]

The American Heart Association recommends systemic antibiotic prophylaxis in patients at high risk for infective endocarditis (prosthetic heart valves, history of infective endocarditis, transplanted hearts with valvulopathy, unrepaired congenital heart defects, cardiac valve repairs in the past 6 months).[38,52] The American Dental Association/American Academy of Orthopedic Surgery recommend systemic antibiotic prophylaxis in those at high risk for joint infection (joint replacement within 2 years, history of prosthetic joint infection, immunosuppression, or other higher risk patient factors listed earlier).[38,52]

The recommended perioperative antibiotics of choice are first-generation cephalosporins (most commonly cephalexin 2 gm by mouth) or penicillinase-resistant penicillins in procedures in which the nasal or oral mucosa is left intact. If penicillin-allergic, clindamycin 600 mg is preferred.

In the plastic surgery literature, a meta-analysis found that routine antibiotic prophylaxis in clean procedures is controversial and not routinely recommended.[53] However, in high-risk clean and clean-contaminated procedures, for example those high-risk patient factors listed above or procedures in which the nasal or oral mucosa is encountered, the authors recommend prophylactic antibiotics. These were found to decrease the rate of surgical site infection compared to placebo by almost 50%.[53]

38.3.5 Postoperative Recommendations

In dermatologic surgery on clean and clean-contaminated wounds, the use of a prophylactic topical antibiotic is not recommended.[54] Large prospective studies have shown no significant difference in infection rates after dermatologic surgery using antibacterial or non-antibacterial ointment or no ointment altogether.[55]

In the limited oculoplastic literature on the topic, a prophylactic topical antibiotic ointment is recommended. In 542 consecutive patients undergoing upper blepharoplasty, one surgeon evaluated twice daily bacitracin ointment use versus Refresh PM ointment and found a statistically significant decrease in wound infection in the bacitracin group (0.26 vs. 6.3%), so much so that the Refresh PM arm of the study was discontinued prematurely.[56] Further studies are needed by oculoplastic surgeons on postoperative ointment regimens to validate this finding.

There are no specific studies that address postoperative oral antibiotic use.

38.4 Energy Devices

Several different instruments are routinely used to cut/incise and to aid in hemostasis in upper facial plastic surgery. This section briefly reviews the following types: electrocautery, electrosurgery, and CO_2 laser, and their respective safety considerations. A primary safety consideration with electrosurgery is electromagnetic interference (EMI) with implanted devices, including cardiac pacemakers and defibrillators but also cochlear implants, deep brain stimulators, peripheral nerve stimulators, and other devices. Intraoperative fire or inadvertent burns are concerns with all of the devices listed above, and the risk of fire may be elevated in upper facial surgery due to the proximity to supplemental oxygen. Finally, the smoke plume from all of these devices is carcinogenic, and while smoke evacuators are mandated for laser devices, good ventilation or even suction/evacuation should be employed with the other cautery devices as well.

38.4.1 Types of Devices

"Electrocautery" is often inaccurately used to describe "electrosurgery." Electrocautery specifically refers to the use of an electric current through a resistor to create heat which is then applied to tissue to stop bleeding.[57] The disposable battery-operated handheld thermal cautery devices are examples of electrocautery widely used in upper facial plastic surgery. The tip becomes very hot but no electric current passes through the patient tissue.

"Electrosurgery" differs from electrocautery in that the tip of the device handpiece, whether bipolar or monopolar, is not heated but conducts an electric current to the tissue to effect cutting, coagulation (desiccation), or fulguration (spray coagulation). All devices have two electrodes, but with the monopolar handpiece the dispersive pad (often referred to as the "grounding pad" although this is an inaccurate term carried forward from older devices that are no longer used) is the second electrode, while with the bipolar handpiece the electrodes are much closer together. The control unit for the electrosurgery device converts power line current (50–60 Hz) into alternating current from 300,000–4,000,000 Hz; this higher frequency is in the range of radio waves and is thus the electrosurgery control unit is sometimes called a radiofrequency generator.[57] The term "radiosurgery" describes electrosurgery at higher frequencies (3–4 MHz) but works by the same principles.[58]

CO_2 laser is used by some surgeons for both incisions and cautery, and there are international consensus standards for training for safe use in health care.[59] Thermal cauterization is used to stop bleeding without causing electrical current in the patient.

Electromagnetic Interference

A large and growing number of patients have cardiac implanted electronic devices (CIED) and other implanted electronic devices that may be disrupted by the interference generated by electrosurgical devices, causing adverse effects ranging from patient discomfort to device damage to potentially life-threatening events.[60–62] It is the responsibility of the surgeon to inquire about such devices and take appropriate precautions. Guidelines from the American Society of Anesthesiologists and the American College of Cardiology/American Heart Association are updated regularly and provide an excellent resource when questions arise about CIEDs.[63,64] To summarize current recommendations: monopolar electrosurgery should be avoided whenever possible in patients with implanted electronic devices; "Coagulation" is a higher-voltage setting than "Cut" and causes more interference; and finally, if monopolar electrosurgery must be used, the dispersive pad should be placed near the site of surgery and away from the device (e.g., for a cardiac device, the dispersive pad should be placed on the right shoulder such that less of the current from the monopolar tip being used on the face passes through the region of the cardiac device).[57,62,65,66]

Furthermore, a cardiologist should evaluate the CIED postoperatively whenever monopolar electrosurgery is used, and ideally preoperatively to determine whether the device should be deactivated or re-programmed, or whether a magnet or alternative/external pacing or defibrillation devices should be available to improve intraoperative safety.[62,65] Using metallic forceps and touching the monopolar electrode to them is not safer.[62] Electrosurgery with a bipolar handpiece has much lower risk of interference, as the current is limited to the tissue in the very small region between the tips, but a low-intensity electromagnetic field is still created with an approximate 15 cm diameter.[62] Thermal devices such as high-temperature electrocautery or CO_2 laser are safest with respect to electronic implants as the patient is not exposed to any electric current.[60]

Left ventricular assist devices (LVAD) are increasingly implanted in patients with severe heart failure. There are a variety of LVAD products, some of which are more susceptible to EMI from electrosurgery than others. Similar to prosthetic valves, they also require blood thinners, although some require anticoagulants and heparin bridging while others are used with antiplatelet agents alone.[67] Perioperative management requires coordination with a specialized LVAD team.

Noncardiac Devices

It is recommended that monopolar electrosurgery be avoided with cochlear implants, and even bipolar handpieces should be used at least 1 cm from the device.[57] Similar precautions should be taken with brain stimulators, and ideally one should consult with the physician who implanted the device and/or the device manufacturer.[67] Although there is no evidence of damage related to inert patient implants such as hip or knee replacements, it is advised to avoid placing the dispersive pad near these implants.[69] A growing variety of electronic devices are being implanted in patients as technology advances, and several of these may be in close proximity to the upper face, therefore it behooves the surgeon to inquire about all devices preoperatively.

38.4.2 Fire Risk and the Triad

The triad of ignition source, fuel, and oxidizer are needed for a fire to develop. Operating on the upper face poses a few unique conditions for fire hazard, mostly related to the proximity of supplemental oxygen, although fire may occur even without the use of supplemental oxygen with any of the cauterizing devices discussed in this chapter. A recent survey of ASOPRS members reported that 32% had experienced at least one operating room fire.[70] For many upper facial surgeries, monitored sedation anesthesia with supplemental oxygen via nasal cannula is used, as opposed to general anesthesia with endotracheal tubes. Nasal cannulas create an oxygen-rich environment in the area of surgery (the face). When drapes expose only the upper face, there is still risk that high concentrations of oxygen may build up under drapes and escape suddenly into the surgical field, creating a fire hazard; leaving the entire face open may actually help excess O_2 dissipate and reduce fire risk.[70] Even when the entire face is exposed, fires may occur more readily with higher O_2 flow rate and higher cautery settings including fulguration or "spray" that allows for wider dispersion of the electric spark. It is a good habit to communicate with the anesthesia team when cautery is needed so that supplemental oxygen can be turned off temporarily, but one must realize that the higher concentration of O_2 does not dissipate immediately. Patient skin and hair were the most common fuel sources in a survey of ASOPRS members.[70] Additional fuel for fire includes false lashes and their adhesives,[71] as well as the alcohol from gut suture packets.[69]

In addition to flash fires, unintended electrosurgery burns may result from the dispersive pad not being fully or uniformly secured to the patient. The size of the dispersive pad provides a low-resistance pathway but if not properly attached to the patient, or if the patient is in contact with an alternate conductive surface, such as the metal railing of the surgery bed or metallic jewelry, the current may pass through this location instead, causing a burn. Current may also arc when a monopolar handpiece is activated in proximity to a conductive material, such as a metal retractor, resulting in tissue burns along the area contacted by the retractor. This is called capacitive coupling, and risk can be reduced by not activating the handpiece until contacting the tissue of interest and using lower power. When one deliberately uses the monopolar handpiece to cauterize a vessel clamped by a forcep, it is important to ensure the forcep is not touching other tissue, and to have dry gloves.[69]

CO_2 lasers are used for incision, cautery, and resurfacing. CO_2 lasers are used as scalpels and as cautery, and for resurfacing broad areas of skin, depending on the settings used. These lasers do not carry risk of EMI because the mechanism of cutting and cauterizing is thermal. They still pose a serious fire risk, however, and require specific precautions such as soaking drapes in saline, using flame-retardant endotracheal tubes, and avoiding certain anesthetic gases. There are standardized guidelines for safe use and maintenance of lasers for medical use.[59]

38.4.3 Effects of the Plume

Similar to cigarette or any other smoke, surgical smoke contains carcinogens; it may also contain live cellular and viral material that is potentially hazardous.[57] Laser thermal disruption of viable human cells similarly creates a plume containing carbon particles, virus, bacteria, DNA, and over 40 toxic gases.[72]

Smoke evacuators are required for laser plume, with recommended filters that remove particulates down to 0.1 microns to capture most viruses, known as ultra-low particulate air (ULPA)

filters.[72] For electrosurgery, local ventilation with high-efficiency particulate air (HEPA) filters are recommended by the National Institute for Occupational Safety and Health, but these only remove particles above 0.3 microns, which does not capture viruses.[57] Wall-suction may be used, with filter canisters, at a suggested distance within 2 cm of the source of the plume. Finally, high-filtration surgical masks are also recommended, but these alone are insufficient protection.[72]

38.5 Conclusions

There is wide variability in current practice patterns regarding blood-thinner use, antibiotic use, and energy-based devices used for cauterization in upper facial plastic surgery. Guidelines from related medical specialties provide evidence-based or expert recommendations that may help inform surgeons regarding perioperative blood-thinner management to balance the risk of vision-threatening hemorrhage against a potentially life-threatening thromboembolic event. There are new blood-thinning medications emerging that are difficult to monitor or reverse, and each agent has its own pharmacokinetics. Fortunately, there are regularly updated consensus guidelines for blood-thinner management in surgery that may be applied to upper facial surgery. Beyond these guidelines, the surgeon may be aided by the internist, cardiologist, hematologist, and anesthesiologist to carefully tailor blood-thinner management to each patient's individual risk.

The available literature pertaining to antibiotic use before or after surgery is clearer: the evidence favors limited, judicious use of perioperative antibiotics. Current practice patterns in oculofacial surgery vary widely, however, and as with blood-thinner management individual patient risk must always be considered.

When it comes to energy-based devices used in surgery, one of the most important considerations is EMI with electrosurgery devices and implanted electronic devices. Monopolar electrosurgery devices are widely used but facilities do not always have guidelines to regulate their use, and a range of newer devices may have different names (such as "radiosurgery") but operate on similar principles and carry similar risks. Furthermore, a wide variety of implanted electronic devices are increasingly common, and one must assess for these prior to using electrosurgical cautery. Finally, all energy devices reviewed in this chapter pose a fire risk, especially when supplemental oxygen is used, and all devices create a plume of potentially hazardous smoke. Care must be taken to mitigate fire and plume effects for the patient and operating room staff, respectively.

References

[1] Kent TL, Custer PL. Bleeding complications in both anticoagulated and nonanticoagulated surgical patients. Ophthalmic Plast Reconstr Surg. 2013;29 (2):113–117

[2] Huang Y, Li M, Li JY, et al. The efficacy and adverse reaction of bleeding of clopidogrel plus aspirin as compared to aspirin alone after stroke or TIA: a systematic review. PloS One. 2013;8(6):e65754

[3] Gobble RM, Hoang HL, Kachniarz B, Orgill DP. Ketorolac does not increase perioperative bleeding: a meta-analysis of randomized controlled trials. Plast Reconstr Surg. 2014;133(3):741–755

[4] Kelley BP, Bennett KG, Chung KC, Kozlow JH. Ibuprofen may not increase bleeding risk in plastic surgery: a systematic review and meta-analysis. Plastic Reconstr Surg. 2016;137(4):1309–1316

[5] Teerawattananon C, Tantayakom P, Suwanawiboon B, Katchamart W. Risk of perioperative bleeding related to highly selective cyclooxygenase-2 inhibitors: a systematic review and meta-analysis. Semin Arthritis Rheum. 2017;46 (4):520–528

[6] Warner TD, Giuliano F, Vojnovic I, Bukasa A, Mitchell JA, Vane JR. Nonsteroid drug selectivities for cyclo-oxygenase-1 rather than cyclo-oxygenase-2 are associated with human gastrointestinal toxicity: a full in vitro analysis. Proc Natl Acad Sci U S A. 1999;96(13):7563–7568.

[7] Van Ryn J, Kink-Eiband M, Kuritsch I, et al. Meloxicam does not affect the antiplatelet effect of aspirin in healthy male and female volunteers. J Clin Pharmacol. 2004;44(7):777–784

[8] Chan DK, Parikh SR. Perioperative ketorolac increases post-tonsillectomy hemorrhage in adults but not children. Laryngoscope. 2014;124(8):1789–1793

[9] Moeller C, Pawlowski J, Pappas AL, Fargo K, Welch K. The safety and efficacy of intravenous ketorolac in patients undergoing primary endoscopic sinus surgery: a randomized, double-blinded clinical trial. Int Forum Allergy Rhinol. 2012;2(4):342–347

[10] Wladis EJ, Dennett KV, Chen VH, De A. Preoperative Intravenous Ketorolac Safely Reduces Postoperative Pain in Levator Advancement Surgery. Ophthalmic Plast Reconstr Surg. 2019;35(4):357–359

[11] Regan DW, Kashiwagi D, Dougan B, Sundsted K, Mauck K. Update in perioperative medicine: practice changing evidence published in 2016. Hosp Pract (1995). 2017; 45(4):158–164

[12] Ayoub K, Nairooz R, Almomani A, Marji M, Paydak H, Maskoun W. Perioperative heparin bridging in atrial fibrillation patients requiring temporary interruption of anticoagulation: evidence from meta-analysis. J Stroke Cerebrovasc Dis. 2016; 25(9):2215–2221

[13] Esparaz ES, Sobel RK. Perioperative management of anticoagulants and antiplatelet agents in oculoplastic surgery. Curr Opin Ophthalmol. 2015; 26(5):422–428

[14] Custer PL, Trinkaus KM. Hemorrhagic complications of oculoplastic surgery. Ophthal Plast Reconstr Surg. 2002; 18(6):409–415

[15] Hass AN, Penne RB, Stefanyszyn MA, Flanagan JC. Incidence of postblepharoplasty orbital hemorrhage and associated visual loss. Ophthal Plast Reconstr Surg. 2004; 20(6):426–432

[16] Bordeaux JS, Martires KJ, Goldberg D, Pattee SF, Fu P, Maloney ME. Prospective evaluation of dermatologic surgery complications including patients on multiple antiplatelet and anticoagulant medications. J Am Acad Dermatol. 2011; 65(3):576–583

[17] Alcalay J, Alkalay R. Controversies in perioperative management of blood thinners in dermatologic surgery: continue or discontinue? Dermatol Surg. 2004; 30(8):1091–1094, discussion 1094

[18] Callahan S, Goldsberry A, Kim G, Yoo S. The management of antithrombotic medication in skin surgery. Dermatol Surg. 2012; 38(9):1417–1426

[19] Kraft CT, Bellile E, Baker SR, Kim JC, Moyer JS. Anticoagulant complications in facial plastic and reconstructive surgery. JAMA Facial Plast Surg. 2015; 17(2):103–107

[20] Garcia DA, Regan S, Henault LE, et al. Risk of thromboembolism with short-term interruption of warfarin therapy. Arch Intern Med. 2008;168(1):63–69

[21] Cannegieter SC, Rosendaal FR, Briet E. Thromboembolic and bleeding complications in patients with mechanical heart valve prostheses. Circulation. 1994;89(2):635–641

[22] Burger W, Chemnitius JM, Kneissl GD, Rucker G. Low-dose aspirin for secondary cardiovascular prevention - cardiovascular risks after its perioperative withdrawal versus bleeding risks with its continuation - review and meta-analysis. J Intern Med. 2005;257(5):399–414

[23] Spyropoulos AC, Al-Badri A, Sherwood MW, Douketis JD. Periprocedural management of patients receiving a vitamin K antagonist or a direct oral anticoagulant requiring an elective procedure or surgery. J Thrombosis Haemost. 2016;14(5):875–885

[24] Darvish-Kazem S, Gandhi M, Marcucci M, Douketis JD. Perioperative management of antiplatelet therapy in patients with a coronary stent who need noncardiac surgery: a systematic review of clinical practice guidelines. Chest. 2013; 144(6):1848–1856

[25] Ghadimi K, Thompson A. Update on perioperative care of the cardiac patient for noncardiac surgery. Curr Opin Anaesthesiol 2015;28(3):342–348

[26] Bonhomme F, Hafezi F, Boehlen F, Habre W. Management of antithrombotic therapies in patients scheduled for eye surgery. Eur J Anaesthesiol. 2013; 30 (8):449–454

[27] McClellan AJ, Flynn HW, Jr, Smiddy WE, Gayer SI. The use of perioperative antithrombotics in posterior segment ocular surgery. Am J Ophthalmol. 2014; 158(5):858–859

[28] Douketis JD, Spyropoulos AC, Spencer FA, et al. Perioperative management of antithrombotic therapy: Antithrombotic Therapy and Prevention of Thrombosis, 9th ed: American College of Chest Physicians Evidence-Based Clinical Practice Guidelines. Chest. 2012;141(2 Suppl):e326S–e50S

[29] Stanger MJ, Thompson LA, Young AJ, Lieberman HR. Anticoagulant activity of select dietary supplements. Nutr Rev. 2012; 70(2):107–117

[30] Pastori D, Carnevale R, Cangemi R, et al. Vitamin E serum levels and bleeding risk in patients receiving oral anticoagulant therapy: a retrospective cohort study. J Am Heart Assoc. 2013; 2(6):e000364

[31] Kotlus BS, Heringer DM, Dryden RM. Evaluation of homeopathic Arnica montana for ecchymosis after upper blepharoplasty: a placebo-controlled, randomized, double-blind study. Ophthal Plast Reconstr Surg. 2010; 26(6):395–397

[32] Iannitti T, Morales-Medina JC, Bellavite P, Rottigni V, Palmieri B. Effectiveness and safety of arnica montana in post-surgical setting, pain and inflammation. Am J Ther. 2016; 23(1):e184–e197

[33] Estcourt LJ, Malouf R, Doree C, Trivella M, Hopewell S, Birchall J. Prophylactic platelet transfusions prior to surgery for people with a low platelet count. Cochrane Database Syst Rev. 2018; 9:CD012779

[34] Lyle WG, Outlaw K, Krizek TJ, Koss N, Payne WG, Robson MC. Prophylactic antibiotics in plastic surgery: trends of use over 25 years of an evolving specialty. Aesthet Surg J. 2003; 23(3):177–183

[35] Hurley LD, Westfall CT, Shore JW. Prophylactic use of antibiotics in oculoplastic surgery. Int Ophthalmol Clin. 1992; 32(3):165–178

[36] Kossler AL, Peng GL, Yoo DB, Azizzadeh B, Massry GG. Current trends in upper and lower eyelid blepharoplasty among American Society of Ophthalmic Plastic and Reconstructive Surgery Members. Ophthal Plast Reconstr Surg. 2018; 34(1):37–42

[37] Fay A, Nallasamy N, Bernardini F, et al. multinational comparison of prophylactic antibiotic use for eyelid surgery. JAMA Ophthalmol. 2015; 133(7):778–784

[38] Rosengren H, Dixon A. Antibacterial prophylaxis in dermatologic surgery: an evidence-based review. Am J Clin Dermatol. 2010; 11(1):35–44

[39] Li X, Nylander W, Smith T, Han S, Gunnar W. Risk factors and predictive model development of thirty-day post-operative surgical site infection in the veterans administration surgical population. Surg Infect (Larchmt). 2018; 19 (3):278–285

[40] Saleh K, Schmidtchen A. Surgical site infections in dermatologic surgery: etiology, pathogenesis, and current preventative measures. Dermatol Surg. 2015; 41(5):537–549

[41] Dixon AJ, Dixon MP, Askew DA, Wilkinson D. Prospective study of wound infections in dermatologic surgery in the absence of prophylactic antibiotics. Dermatol Surg. 2006; 32(6):819–826, discussion 826–827

[42] Lee EW, Holtebeck AC, Harrison AR. Infection rates in outpatient eyelid surgery. Ophthal Plast Reconstr Surg. 2009; 25(2):109–110

[43] Carter SR, Stewart JM, Khan J, et al. Infection after blepharoplasty with and without carbon dioxide laser resurfacing. Ophthalmology. 2003; 110(7):1430–1432

[44] Morgan SC. Orbital cellulitis and blindness following a blepharoplasty. Plast Reconstr Surg. 1979; 64(6):823–826

[45] Goldberg RA, Li TG. Postoperative infection with group A beta-hemolytic Streptococcus after blepharoplasty. Am J Ophthalmol. 2002; 134(6):908–910

[46] Suñer IJ, Meldrum ML, Johnson TE, Tse DT. Necrotizing fasciitis after cosmetic blepharoplasty. Am J Ophthalmol. 1999; 128(3):367–368

[47] Jordan DR, Mawn L, Marshall DH. Necrotizing fasciitis caused by group A streptococcus infection after laser blepharoplasty. Am J Ophthalmol. 1998; 125(2):265–266

[48] Crosswell EG, Leyngold IM. Atypical mycobacterial infection following upper eyelid blepharoplasty. Ophthal Plast Reconstr Surg. 2016; 32(5):e116–e118

[49] Mauriello JA, Jr, Atypical Mycobacterial Study Group. Atypical mycobacterial infection of the periocular region after periocular and facial surgery. Ophthal Plast Reconstr Surg. 2003; 19(3):182–188

[50] González-Castro J, Lighthall JG. Antibiotic use in facial plastic surgery. Facial Plast Surg Clin North Am. 2016; 24(3):347–356

[51] Ferneini EM, Halepas S, Aronin SI. Antibiotic prophylaxis in blepharoplasty: review of the current literature. J Oral Maxillofac Surg. 2017; 75(7):1477–1481

[52] Rossi AM, Mariwalla K. Prophylactic and empiric use of antibiotics in dermatologic surgery: a review of the literature and practical considerations. Dermatol Surg. 2012; 38(12):1898–1921

[53] Zhang Y, Dong J, Qiao Y, He J, Wang T, Ma S. Efficacy and safety profile of antibiotic prophylaxis usage in clean and clean-contaminated plastic and reconstructive surgery: a meta-analysis of randomized controlled trials. Ann Plast Surg. 2014; 72(1):121–130

[54] Levender MM, Davis SA, Kwatra SG, Williford PM, Feldman SR. Use of topical antibiotics as prophylaxis in clean dermatologic procedures. J Am Acad Dermatol. 2012; 66(3):445–451

[55] Dixon AJ, Dixon MP, Dixon JB. Randomized clinical trial of the effect of applying ointment to surgical wounds before occlusive dressing. Br J Surg. 2006; 93(8):937–943

[56] Alford M. Infection rates comparing topical antibiotic versus antibiotic-free ointment in blepharoplasty surgery. Am J Cosmet Surg. 2015; 32:149–153

[57] Smith TL, Smith JM. Electrosurgery in otolaryngology-head and neck surgery: principles, advances, and complications. Laryngoscope. 2001; 111(5):769–780

[58] Taheri A, Mansoori P, Sandoval LF, Feldman SR, Pearce D, Williford PM. Electrosurgery: part I. Basics and principles. J Am Acad Dermatol. 2014; 70(4):591.e1–591.e14

[59] Brahmavar SM, Hetzel F. Medical Lasers: Quality Control, Safety Standards, and Regulations. AAPM General Medical Physics Committee and American College of Medical Physics; Madison, WI: 2001. Available at https://www.aapm.org/pubs/reports/rpt_73.PDF

[60] Blandford AD, Wiggins NB, Ansari W, Hwang CJ, Wilkoff BL, Perry JD. Cautery selection for oculofacial plastic surgery in patients with implantable electronic devices. Eur J Ophthalmol. 2018; Jul 1:1120672118787440

[61] Howe N, Cherpelis B. Obtaining rapid and effective hemostasis: part II. Electrosurgery in patients with implantable cardiac devices. J Am Acad Dermatol. 2013; 69(5):677.e1–677.e9

[62] Dawes JC, Mahabir RC, Hillier K, Cassidy M, de Haas W, Gillis AM. Electrosurgery in patients with pacemakers/implanted cardioverter defibrillators. Ann Plast Surg. 2006; 57(1):33–36

[63] American Society of Anesthesiologists. Practice advisory for the perioperative management of patients with cardiac implantable electronic devices: pacemakers and implantable cardioverter-defibrillators: an updated report by the American Society of Anesthesiologists task force on perioperative management of patients with cardiac implantable electronic devices. Anesthesiology. 2011; 114(2):247–261

[64] Fleisher LA, Fleischmann KE, Auerbach AD, et al. 2014 ACC/AHA guideline on perioperative cardiovascular evaluation and management of patients undergoing noncardiac surgery: executive summary: a report of the American College of Cardiology/American Heart Association Task Force on Practice Guidelines. Circulation. 2014; 130(24):2215–2245

[65] Rozner MA. Corrections to electrosurgery in patients with cardiac pacemakers or implanted cardioverter defibrillators. Ann Plast Surg. 2007; 58(2):226–227

[66] Jones DB, Brunt LM, Feldman LS, Mikami DJ, Robinson TN, Jones SB. Safe energy use in the operating room. Curr Probl Surg. 2015; 52(11):447–468

[67] Nicolosi AC, Pagel PS. Perioperative considerations in the patient with a left ventricular assist device. Anesthesiology. 2003; 98(2):565–570

[68] Weaver J, Kim SJ, Lee MH, Torres A. Cutaneous electrosurgery in a patient with a deep brain stimulator. Dermatol Surg. 1999; 25(5):415–417

[69] Committee AEaPS. AST Standards of Practice for Use of Electrosurgery: Association of Surgical Technologists; 2012:25

[70] Maamari RN, Custer PL. Operating room fires in oculoplastic surgery. Ophthal Plast Reconstr Surg. 2018; 34(2):114–122

[71] Michaels JP, Macdonald P. Ignition of eyelash extensions during routine minor eyelid surgery. Ophthal Plast Reconstr Surg. 2014; 30(3):e61–e62

[72] Smalley PJ. Laser safety: risks, hazards, and control measures. Laser Ther. 2011; 20(2):95–106

39 Staying Out of Trouble: Strategies Based on Recent OMIC Oculofacial Plastic Surgery Claims

Robert G. Fante

Abstract

Every treatment or surgery has the risk of failing to accomplish the intended objective of improving patients' condition or appearance. Hence, every physician must learn to manage this disappointing outcome and help patients move forward with acceptance or additional treatment. Breakdown in the physician–patient relationship can contribute to the likelihood of medical malpractice claims against the physician. This chapter discusses the causes for common problems and suggests strategies to avoid malpractice claims.

Keywords: malpractice, liability, claim, indemnity, informed consent, standard of care, plaintiff, defendant, negligence

39.1 Introduction

In the United States, there are approximately 1,600 ophthalmologists who self-identify as specialists in oculofacial plastic surgery according to the American Academy of Ophthalmology (AAO). Among these are the nearly 800 members of the American Society of Ophthalmic Plastic and Reconstructive Surgery (ASOPRS). In addition, there are numerous surgeons from related disciplines such as otolaryngology, plastic surgery, and dermatology who also frequently perform oculofacial plastic surgical procedures.

The Ophthalmic Mutual Insurance Company (OMIC) provides medical liability insurance (malpractice insurance) for the largest segment of U.S. ophthalmologists, with approximately 5,000 member physicians as of 2018. Using OMIC's internal database of over 4,500 closed claims since 1987, lessons can be learned regarding the problems and issues that arise in the practice of oculofacial plastic surgery. Approximately 20 to 25% of all claims will end in an indemnity payment to the claimant or plaintiff, typically a settlement (or more rarely, jury verdict award). Indemnity payments for oculofacial plastic surgery are generally lower than those for many higher risk medical specialties such as neurosurgery and obstetrics, but average about $215,000. For comparison, recent indemnity payments for all branches of ophthalmology averaged about $280,000 based on a study from 20 U.S. medical liability carriers.[1]

Laws governing the practice of medicine are state-dependent, and the 50 U.S. states vary considerably. Physicians must become familiar with the laws of the states in which they practice, but certain concepts are universal. The *standard of care* is an important concept that is defined as the level and type of care that would be provided by a reasonably competent and skilled physician with a similar background in the same medical community. The standard of care is determined on a case-by-case basis by the medical experts who testify about the care. While practicing medicine at the standard of care does not necessarily protect against dissatisfied patients and potential malpractice claims, practicing below the standard of care is

definitely associated with successful claims against doctors. In a recent OMIC study, in cases for which the medical care provided in oculofacial plastic surgery cases was judged by physician reviewers to be below the standard of care, an indemnity settlement was made in 84% of claims. Conversely, for cases with alleged patient harm due to complications that are well-recognized in the medical literature, but with medical care at the standard of care, indemnity settlements were made in only 10% of claims.[2] Circumspect judgment, timely referrals to colleagues for assistance when needed, and continuing education are among the most useful tactics to maintain the standard of care.

Lawsuits for medical malpractice are *civil*, not *criminal*, legal actions and are thus governed by *tort law*: allegedly injured patients must show that the physician acted negligently in rendering care *and* that the negligence resulted in injury. Typically, four legal elements must be established: (1) that the physician had a professional duty owed to the patient, (2) that the physician breached that duty, (3) that an injury was caused by the breach, and (4) that there were resulting damages, which are economic (lost wages, cost of health care) and noneconomic ("pain and suffering").

Although trends and past experience will not necessarily predict the future medicolegal climate, this chapter will summarize some of the most useful lessons learned from recent claims.

39.2 Particular Problem Areas in the Practice of Upper Facial Plastic Surgery

Cosmetic dissatisfaction with the results of blepharoplasty (or other surgery) is the single most common reason for a claim against the surgeon; however, such claims rarely result in a financial settlement or other indemnity payment.[2] When loss of function occurs from surgery, there is a higher risk that a claim will result in an indemnity award to the patient.

39.2.1 Blepharoplasty and Ptosis Repair

Blepharoplasty is the surgery most frequently associated with a malpractice claim for this specialty. This is not surprising since blepharoplasty is the single most common oculofacial plastic procedure. Large settlements ranging from $300,000 to $1,300,000 have been negotiated by OMIC for permanent visual loss due to retrobulbar hemorrhage after blepharoplasty, most commonly from failure of the surgeon to promptly and adequately address the situation. Smaller settlements of $150,000 to $430,000 have been negotiated for other complications, including lagophthalmos, corneal damage, and worsened dry eye. Similar settlements are associated with ptosis repair. Practice patterns that avoid or aggressively manage these problems are recommended to prevent malpractice settlements.

39.2.2 Brow Lifting

Most other types of oculofacial plastic surgery care are less commonly associated with claims, although claims related to orbital, lacrimal, trauma, and periocular reconstruction have all occurred. Brow lifting is rarely associated with successful claims; only one has resulted in indemnity (under $30,000) in the past 20 years for OMIC. The majority of brow lifting claims have been cosmetic, resulting in no indemnity payment.

39.2.3 Invasive Skin Treatments

Laser and chemical peel skin treatments for actinic damage and/or facial aging such as rhytids and dyschromias are also common oculofacial plastic procedures performed in many practices, often by the physician and sometimes by ancillary staff. In OMIC's experience, skin scarring with periocular deformity (e.g., ectropion) and/or perioral and cheek deformities have led to multiple settlements with indemnity payments ranging from $125,000 to $900,000. Conservative planning, careful training and supervision of ancillary staff, and close postprocedure management are each reasonable tactics to prevent scarring and subsequent liability claims.

39.3 Fillers and Autologous Fat

While there have been no claims related to autologous fat grafting or hyaluronic acid fillers in the recent OMIC database, there have been several claims associated with adverse outcomes from Radiesse hydroxylapatite facial filler in the upper face.[2] Of these, two claims alleged unsatisfactory cosmetic appearance, while the third alleged infection. It is recommended that careful informed consent be obtained regarding the potential complications with Radiesse (and fat) including the relative difficulty in removing either material in the event of a problem.

39.4 Goals for the Upper Facial Surgeon

The goal of every upper facial surgeon should be to meet the needs of the patient. To do this, the surgeon must establish the correct diagnosis, know when to say no to surgery, communicate effectively with the patient, obtain a good informed consent with the risks/benefits/alternatives to the treatment, execute the surgical plan, follow-up with the patient, and manage complications.

39.4.1 Establishing the Correct Diagnosis

In many published series of malpractice cases against internists and general surgeons, the most common paid claim has been *failure to diagnose* or *failure to treat* a serious medical problem to the local standard of care. Although this type of claim is much less common for oculofacial plastic surgery, several large settlements have resulted from these claims. For example, a claim for alleged failure to diagnose squamous cell carcinoma that resulted in enucleation and maxillectomy led to a $975,000

indemnity payment, and another claim for alleged failure to diagnose glaucoma for a patient who was left on topical loteprednol for months after blepharoplasty resulted in a $400,000 indemnity payment. Physician clinical vigilance during routine patient care is the best defense to avoid similar claims and indemnities. For unusual or difficult situations, it may be helpful to arrange re-evaluation on an additional visit, or referral for a second opinion.

39.4.2 Knowing When to Say No to Treatment

There is a complex interplay between the patient's anatomy, pathology, and coexistent medical, psychological, and social factors that may affect surgical decision-making and outcome. Not every patient is a good candidate for treatment, nor is the evident pathology always amenable to successful treatment. Consider saying "No, I am unable to help you" to new or existing patients if:

- Multiple prior surgeries for the same (or similar) problems have been unsuccessful. Particular caution may be exercised if no records are available, or if the records show that the previous failed plans are similar to the ones you propose.
- Substantial anger at a previous surgeon is detected or the patient describes social isolation as a result of previous treatment. Listen and avoid patients who share phrases such as "My life is ruined" or "I can't go out."
- A patient treats your staff with disrespect, violence, or consistent rudeness.
- A patient pushes you to cut corners or create a new procedure just for him/her.
- Magical or utopian thinking is detected, for example "My husband will love me again" or "This surgery will help me get a promotion at work."
- Your trusted staff tells you the patient seems "crazy" or extraordinarily demanding.

39.4.3 Effective Communication

Controlling for the difference in the number of male- and female-insured ophthalmologists in the United States, it has been reported that male ophthalmologists had 1.54 times more claims against them than females.[3] Even within oculofacial plastic surgery, male physicians had 1.25 times more claims than females. While the etiologies for this disparity are complex, differences in gender communication styles have been studied and may play an important role: female physicians generally engage in more "active partnership, positive and emotionally focused talk, and psychosocial counseling." Although the correlation between the quality of patient–doctor relationships and malpractice claims is also complex, both male and female physicians can work to communicate interest, empathy, and availability for all patients. In cases of potential medical error, communication of an honest explanation is important. Understanding the patient perspective about their concerns and medical issues is critical. Taking time to listen to stories and patient feelings about "Mom's skin cancer" or "Dad's eye complication" may be helpful in establishing trust to improve the patient–doctor relationship, and assist in decision-making.

Do the Right Procedure for the Right Patient

Previous chapters have outlined the details of correctly choosing which upper facial or eyelid procedure(s) is most likely to improve your patient's condition. It is incumbent upon the surgeon to explain the nature of the pathology, details of the proposed treatment, and expected outcome at a level of complexity and language the patient can understand.

Informed Consent

Informed consent is an oral agreement reached after a conversation between the treating physician and the patient about the condition, proposed procedure, and its risks, benefits, and alternatives. The record of that consent must be documented electronically or on paper. The discussion and documentation must be detailed enough to identify the risks and potential complications that are commonly encountered or which are rare but severe enough that a reasonable person would want to know they are possible (such as blindness). The process must have allowed the patient an opportunity to ask questions and confirm understanding of the issues involved. Inadequate evidence of informed consent is a major problem in a malpractice claim, even if the standard of care was otherwise met. The likelihood of an indemnity payment is far higher if informed consent cannot be established; in fact, recent OMIC experience shows that the majority of such claims resulted in an indemnity payment. On the other hand, complications that occur during or after surgery that were clearly discussed preoperatively are typically less likely to be seen as a mistake by the patient or to result in a claim. Plain language consent forms in English and Spanish for common oculofacial plastic surgery procedures are freely available for download at https://www.omic.com/risk-management/

consent-forms/ Copies for blepharoplasty and ptosis repair are included in Appendix A.

For cosmetic patients, a separate Cosmetic Financial Consent can help alleviate conflicts regarding payment for "touch-ups" and can reinforce the idea that a guarantee of 100% satisfaction cannot be made (Appendix B). Always strive to clarify surgeon and patient expectations of treatment.

39.4.4 Surgical Plan and Execution

A written surgical plan should be documented at a preoperative visit, and the informed consent document should match the plan. If conditions are found in surgery that alter the plan so that it is executed differently, the reasons should be clearly explained in the operative report or noted elsewhere in the patient's medical record on the day of surgery. Any deviation from the surgical plan should also be carefully explained to the patient and/or family on the day of surgery.

39.4.5 Patient Follow-up

Follow-up should be scheduled and documented based on the underlying condition, the surgical procedures performed, coexistent medical conditions, and any unintended complications seen. Referral to other specialists should be sought for any unstable or new condition. In addition, if treatment includes a planned hiatus from anticoagulant therapy, it is imperative that the surgeon ensures that the patient follows up with the treating physician for resumption of anticoagulation.

At each posttreatment visit, the results should be observed and communicated to the patient with openness and honesty. Anticipate patient concerns. It may be appropriate to explain

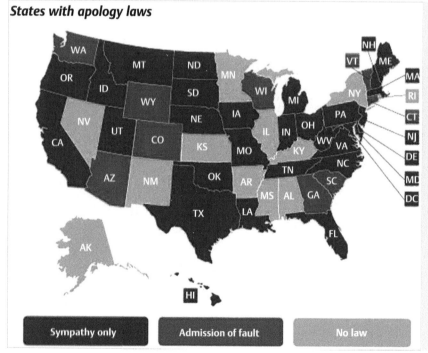

Fig. 39.1 36 of the 50 U.S. states have apology laws that are intended to improve physician–patient communication and defuse complex situations. Statements by physicians to patients or family that express sympathy, and sometimes even culpability (fault), are not admissible in legal proceedings in these states as marked. (The image is provided courtesy of Annals of Internal Medicine; various news reports.)

the natural course of wound healing, and the patient's variance from average. Communicate complications if they arise. Clear instructions regarding home care and medications must always be provided. Finally, communicate in an open and honest way your assessment of the final result, while also listening to the patient's assessment.

39.4.6 Actively Manage Complications

If any complications occur during surgery, or if complications arise during the posttreatment course, it is best to candidly explain the situation and actively manage the problems. Patients usually appreciate the opportunity to directly contact the surgeon, and it may be helpful to establish greater trust and alliance by providing a cell phone number, or other contact information.

39.4.7 Revisit Patient Expectations Frequently

Whether the posttreatment course is simple or complex, it is also valuable to revisit patient expectations frequently. Reminding patients of their pretreatment condition, often with the use of photographs, can be very helpful to engender acceptance of minor posttreatment imperfections.

39.5 The Unhappy Patient: Cosmetic Dissatisfaction and Patient Expectations

The single most common reason for claims against oculofacial plastic surgeons is cosmetic dissatisfaction, but these claims are also the least likely to lead to an indemnity payment. Most surgeons have worked with patients who can be difficult to please, and even expertly performed surgery will not always provide the intended outcome. As a consequence, most surgeons will have the occasional patient who is unhappy with his or her postoperative appearance despite having achieved the preoperative goals without complications. For these patients, there has been no breach of the standard of care, and, by definition, there are no functional problems. These cosmetically dissatisfied patients can be separated into two groups: (1) those who have one or more minor asymmetries or contour abnormalities that the surgeon can see and possibly correct, and (2) those who have an ideal of potential, future beauty that can be difficult for the surgeon to appreciate, or is based on much earlier versions of themselves, or is impossible to achieve. The surgeon may choose to offer additional treatment to someone in the first group, while for those in the second group additional treatment can be problematic. In both cases, there is no malpractice by declining to offer further treatment since there is neither duty nor harm. Open communication is critical in both situations.

In practical terms, this dual strategy—fixing small problems when possible and declining when appropriate—translates into fewer successful malpractice claims based solely on cosmetic dissatisfaction against upper facial surgeons. The first group can often be satisfied with a minor revision, while the second group

will usually have little foundation for a claim. In the OMIC series, only 2.7% of such claims resulted in an indemnity payment and the payments were small, averaging $13,500.[2] Although the risk of indemnity claims appears minor, it should also be understood that cosmetic dissatisfaction is the single most common reason that claims have been filed against oculofacial plastic surgeons. The nuisance factor for physicians is substantial. Fortunately there are several tactics that can help reduce the likelihood of a claim.

39.5.1 Refunds

For some unhappy patients, it may be sensible to consider offering or agreeing to a refund if that will satisfy them and there are no concerns about the quality of your care. Details matter here, for example a verbal discussion with the patient (regardless of who initiated it) that leads to a refund is not reportable to state medical boards, malpractice insurance carriers, or the National Practitioner Data Bank (NPDB). However, a written demand for money (even if only a refund) falls under the definition of a claim and should be discussed with the claims department of your insurance carrier. The claims representative can help you determine if reporting the written demand is required to your state. In any case, no refund can exceed the amount the patient originally paid without being considered an indemnity payment that may be reportable to state boards and the NPDB. It is advisable that surgeons request a release of liability from the patient in exchange for a refund. A valid release of liability should be written by a qualified medical liability attorney in your state, but note that asking for such a release may raise questions in the patient's (or family's) mind about possible medical error.

39.5.2 I'm Sorry Laws

In order to promote better communication in difficult situations, 38 states have laws that make an expression of sympathy or culpability by a physician to the patient or family inadmissible as evidence of negligence or an admission of liability (▶ Fig. 39.1). Apologizing for the more difficult path experienced by the patient with a suboptimal outcome or a complication may make the physician appear less arrogant, help to defuse anger, and prevent a lawsuit or claim. Saying "I'm sorry" also makes it easier to disclose information about an adverse event. Since all states consistently uphold the duty of physicians to be honest health advocates for the patient, disclosure is ethical and necessary. As several institutions have moved to early communication of errors with the patient and family, including full disclosure and apology when errors occur, dramatic reductions in claims, lawsuits, settlement, legal expenses, and total liability costs have been reported.[4-6] When confronted with a patient who has had an adverse event, physicians in large institutions or small private practices will generally find that empathetic care, full disclosure, and some expression of regret are helpful in defusing anger and avoiding claims. Among the resources that may be helpful when responding to difficult situations is an OMIC online guide: Responding to unanticipated outcomes (www.omic.com/unanticipated-outcomes-steps-for-responding/). When in doubt, get help for these discussions from your professional liability carrier.

39.6 Expert Tips/Pearls/Suggestions

- Know when to say NO (Section 39.4.2).
- Make sure that every patient completes a cosmetic financial agreement (Appendix B) before the first surgery that details the practice's policies and charges for revisions. Even if you choose to waive any charges, it is better that the patient knows the policies beforehand.
- When surgery has been completed and problems arise:
  - When low-risk and simple interventions are possible, it may be sensible to actively help the patient by taking action (e.g., injecting filler or revising a scar to subtly improve blepharoplasty results).
  - Avoid defensiveness or silence, which do not communicate the caring attitude that patients seek.
  - Show empathy and say you are sorry that things are working out this way—make them feel that you are their ally in the struggle for a good result.
- Make problem patients feel like very important persons (VIPs) by seeing them often until minor issues are resolved, while subtly adjusting their expectations toward realistic possibilities. At times, regular phone communication until the issue is resolved can be helpful.
- Take professional quality preoperative photographs and offer copies to the patient so that the positive effects of your treatment can be readily remembered.
- If concerns about outcome arise, discuss your concerns confidentially with the risk-management hotline of your medical liability insurance carrier.

Wise surgeons will tell you that they never regretted saying no to someone, but they may certainly have regretted saying yes.

39.7 Coping with the Process of a Malpractice Claim

It is a very distressing when a claim is served on a physician or a patient makes it clear that he will be making one. It has been estimated that by age 65, 99% of physicians in high-risk specialties and 75% of those in low-risk specialties, including ophthalmology, can expect to have had a medical professional liability claim against them; 71% and 19% will have made an indemnity payment, respectively.[7]

It is likely that an oculofacial plastic surgeon will eventually have to face a malpractice claim. The physician will naturally have a cascade of reactions including panic, defensiveness, and anger; many malpractice insurance companies offer programs and resources to help physicians cope with these feelings. The physician should contact the malpractice insurance claims department promptly, and the patient's chart should be immediately sequestered. Deletions or alterations to the medical record must be completely avoided, as they most often make a

claim indefensible. Office staff should be informed about the confidential nature of the claim, and given instructions about how to manage contact from the patient or her representatives.

For most claims, there will be a process of *discovery*, in which the plaintiff attorney representing the allegedly injured patient and the defense attorney representing the physician will collect information about the claim. For the physician, questions asked by the plaintiff attorney in a *deposition* (statement under oath) will be among the more stressful parts of discovery. The defense legal team will guide the physician in the best strategies for answering questions in a deposition. Both sides may also seek expert opinions from peer physicians regarding details of the medical/surgical management and the standard of care.

After discovery, the defense legal team and the malpractice insurer may have informed opinions regarding the likely outcome of a claim, but the decision about whether to negotiate a settlement or to steadfastly fight the claim ultimately rests with the physician. In some states, settlements or other indemnity payments below a certain threshold (e.g., $30,000) are not permanently listed with one's medical license; as a consequence, physicians should request details regarding state regulations. However, the NPDB lists any and all indemnity payments.

39.8 Conclusions

The goal of all upper facial surgeons should be to have patients who are satisfied with their final outcome and each episode of care. Unfortunately, that goal does not always translate into each patient care experience and malpractice claims are part of the practice of medicine in America. Upper facial surgeons can learn strategies to reduce the risk of medical error for their patient and mitigate the risk of medical liability claims. The risk management departments of malpractice insurers can often provide confidential guidance about the details of a particular case and general guidelines about patient communication, standards of care, and medical record keeping.

References

[1] Thompson AC, Parikh PD, Lad EM. Review of ophthalmology medical professional liability claims in the United States from 2006 through 2015. Ophthalmology. 2018; 125(5):631–641

[2] Fante RG, Bucsi R, Wynkoop K. Medical professional liability claims: experience in oculofacial plastic surgery. Ophthalmology. 2018; 125(12):1996–1998

[3] Fountain TR. Ophthalmic malpractice and physician gender: a claims data analysis (an American Ophthalmological Society thesis). Trans Am Ophthalmol Soc. 2014; 112:38–49

[4] Lambert BL, Centomani NM, Smith KM, et al. The "seven pillars" response to patient safety incidents: effects on medical liability processes and outcomes. Health Serv Res. 2016; 51 Suppl 3:2491–2515

[5] McDonald TB, Helmchen LA, Smith KM, et al. Responding to patient safety incidents: the "seven pillars". Qual Saf Health Care. 2010; 19(6):e11

[6] Mazor KM, Reed GW, Yood RA, Fischer MA, Baril J, Gurwitz JH. Disclosure of medical errors: what factors influence how patients respond? J Gen Intern Med. 2006; 21(7):704–710

[7] Jena AB, Seabury S, Lakdawalla D, Chandra A. Malpractice risk according to physician specialty. N Engl J Med. 2011; 365(7):629–636

39.9 Appendix A

Place letterhead here and remove note. Change font for large print

Note: These forms are intended as a sample only of the information you as the surgeon should personally discuss with the patient. Please review and modify to fit your actual practice.

It is important to document and explain the etiology of the condition causing the droopy eyelid and how that condition might affect the results of surgery.

Give the patient a copy.

39.9.1 Informed Consent for Ptosis Surgery (Droopy Eyelid Surgery)

What Is Ptosis and How Is It Corrected?

Ptosis is a condition that occurs when one or both upper eyelids droop and the edge of the upper eyelid falls toward or over the pupil. Ptosis is usually caused by stretching or thinning of the tendon between the muscle that raises the eyelid and the eyelid itself. With stretching or thinning, the muscle that normally raises the eyelid has to work harder to lift it. This leads to symptoms of eyelid and forehead muscle fatigue, and eyelid heaviness. Other, less common causes of ptosis are nerve or muscle damage from any cause, various types of eyelid surgery, infection, muscle weakness, and systemic diseases such as stroke and tumors behind the eye, myasthenia, hypertension, thyroid disorders, and diabetes. Children can be born with congenital ptosis; the muscle is abnormally stiff and does not function well. This condition usually lasts until it is surgically corrected. Ptosis surgery is not the procedure of choice for removing excess fat and skin in the upper eyelid. Under certain circumstances it can be combined with the operation known as blepharoplasty when fat and skin removal is an added goal of surgery.

To correct ptosis, the surgeon needs to make an incision or cut the skin of the upper eyelid in order to reach the muscles and tendons. The surgeon chooses where to make the incision based upon what treatment the eyelid needs. With the *front* or *anterior* approach, the surgeon makes an incision in the skin in the upper eyelid crease or fold in order to reach the muscle and tendon; if there is no eyelid fold, one can be created when the incision is made. The anterior approach allows the surgeon to trim excess skin and fatty tissue from the upper eyelid if needed during the surgery. If no skin or fat needs to be removed, the surgeon can raise the eyelid through an *inside* approach by placing the incision on the inside or moist part of the upper eyelid; with this approach, there is no cosmetic scarring. If the muscle is not strong enough to lift the eyelid, the surgeon must create a "sling" by connecting the moving eyelid to the frontalis muscle in the forehead.

How Will Ptosis Surgery Affect My Vision and Appearance?

The droopy eyelid is like a curtain that blocks the view. Patients with ptosis frequently notice that they have less peripheral or side vision, particularly when looking up. The more ptosis, the greater the peripheral vision loss. When the eyelid is raised, either manually by hand or surgically through one of the approaches described above, the blockage is removed and the eye can see. Ptosis surgery only corrects vision loss due to droopy eyelids. It does not improve blurred vision caused by problems inside the eye or by visual loss caused by neurological disease behind the eye. To prevent amblyopia or poor visual development in children born with congenital ptosis, the surgery needs to be done early in life.

Patients with ptosis report that droopy eyelids make them look and feel "tired." When the eyelid is raised in ptosis surgery, patients usually prefer the new eyelid position, and feel it improves their appearance as well as their peripheral vision. When only one eyelid is raised, it may affect how the eyelid on the other side looks. If this happens, ptosis surgery on the other side may be needed. If the position and shape of the eyelids do not match, additional surgery may be needed.

What Are the Major Risks of Ptosis Surgery?

Risks of ptosis surgery, like most eyelid surgical procedures include, but are not limited to, bleeding, infection, an asymmetric or unbalanced appearance, scarring, difficulty closing the eyes (which may cause damage to the underlying corneal surface), a "wide-eyed" or "open" appearance, difficulty with or inability to wear contact lenses, double vision, tearing, or dry eye problems, numbness and/or tingling in the operated eyelid, near the eye, or on the face, and in rare cases, loss of vision. While ptosis correction is usually permanent, the condition can recur. If it does, you may need to have repeat surgery.

The result of ptosis surgery cannot be guaranteed. Ptosis correction involves surgery on the tendon and/or muscle inside the eyelid, which can make the results unpredictable. At times, the surgeon may need to adjust the position and shape of the eyelid after ptosis surgery. The adjustments can be done early (within the first 10 days) after surgery, or later on if asymmetry of the eyelid position or shape occur. The final result depends upon your anatomy, your body's wound healing response, and the underlying cause of the ptosis. Some patients have difficulty adjusting to changes to their appearance. Some patients have unrealistic expectations about how changes in appearance will impact their lives. Carefully evaluate your goals, expectations and your ability to deal with changes to your appearance and the possible need for repeat surgery before agreeing to this surgery.

What Are the Alternatives to Ptosis Surgery?

Patients can live with ptosis and blocked or reduced peripheral vision; however, there is no reliable method to correct ptosis on a permanent basis without surgery. Patients who are too sick to have surgery may find relief by lifting their eyelid with their fingers or tape in order to see. Obviously, the eyelid droops again as soon as this temporary lifting is stopped.

What Type of Anesthesia Is Used and What Are Its Risks?

In children, general anesthesia is necessary. In teenagers and adults, ptosis surgery is usually performed on an outpatient basis under local anesthesia. The patient must be able to cooperate to some degree. Ptosis surgery with minimal (oral) sedation is desired in most cases. Some cases require sedation from a needle placed into a vein in patient's arm before surgery.

Fortunately, even with no sedation, most patients do not find the operation to be very painful, and it only takes a short period of time. Risks of anesthesia, when administered, include but are not limited to damage to the eye and surrounding tissues and structures, loss of vision, breathing problems, and, in extremely rare circumstances, stroke or death.

Patient's Acceptance of Risks

I have read the above information and have discussed it with my physician. I understand that it is impossible for the physician to inform me of every possible complication that may occur. My physician has told me that results cannot be guaranteed and that adjustments and more surgery may be necessary. By signing below, I agree that my physician has answered all of my questions and that I understand and accept the risks, benefits, and alternatives of ptosis correction.

I consent to ptosis surgery on:

_____ Right eye _____ Left eye _____ Both eyes

_____ _____
Patient (or person authorized to sign for patient) Date

Blepharoplasty Consent Form

As you age, the skin and muscles of your eyelids and eyebrows may sag and droop. You may get a lump in the eyelid due to normal fat around your eye that begins to show under the skin. These changes can lead to other problems. For example:

- Excess skin on your upper eyelid can block your central vision (what you see in the middle when you look straight ahead) and your peripheral vision (what you see on the sides when you look straight ahead). Your forehead might get tired from trying to keep your eyelids open. The skin on your upper eyelid may get irritated.
- Loose skin and fat in the lower lid can create "bags" under the eyes that are accentuated by drooping of your cheeks with age. Many people think these bags look unattractive and make them seem older or chronically tired.

Upper or lower blepharoplasty (eyelid surgery) can help correct these problems. Patients often refer to this surgery as an "eyelid tuck" or "eyelid lift." Please know that the eyelid itself may not be lifted during this type of surgery, but instead the heaviness of the upper eyelids and/or puffiness of the lower eyelids are usually improved.

Ophthalmologists (eye surgeons) call this surgery "blepharoplasty." The ophthalmologist may remove or change the position of skin, muscle, and fat. Surgery may be on your upper eyelid, lower eyelid, or both eyelids. The ophthalmologist will put sutures (stitches) in your eyelid to close the incision (cut).

- For the upper lid, the doctor makes an incision in your eyelid's natural crease.
- For the lower lid, the doctor makes an incision either through the skin just below your lashes, or in the conjunctiva (moist inside surface of your lid) where you can't see it.

There are several options for anesthesia to make you comfortable during surgery. Blepharoplasty is sometimes done with just local anesthesia (medicine injected around your eye to numb the area). You may also be sedated (relaxed or put to sleep) by medi-cine from a needle in your arm or pills taken before surgery. Less commonly, or if eyelid surgery is combined with other surgery, you may be given a deeper type of anesthesia that makes you unconscious for the surgery (general anesthesia). Your ophthalmologist will discuss which type of anesthesia seems right for you, and an anesthesia specialist may be involved.

Many people find that blepharoplasty helps correct their eyelid problems. But how much it helps depends on factors that include your symptoms, eyelid structure, appearance, goals, and ability to adapt to changes. Here are some common ways that blepharoplasty can help:

- Improved peripheral vision (to the sides) and when looking up. You may be able to relax your forehead since you will not rely as much on those muscles to keep your eyes open.
- Many people with bags under their eyes feel that blepharoplasty of the lower eyelid improves how they look and makes them feel younger or less tired. But this is cosmetic surgery and some people are disappointed. Talk with your ophthalmologist about what you can expect from blepharoplasty.
- Blepharoplasty does not correct all vision problems. For instance, you will not be able to read printed words more clearly just because you had blepharoplasty. Talk with your ophthalmologist about other ways to improve vision such as with eyeglasses, contact lenses, cataract surgery, or LASIK surgery.

It is your choice whether to have blepharoplasty. Here are some other options:

- You may decide to do nothing. Excess skin, muscle, and fat around your eye will not go away, but might not bother you enough to do something about it.
- You may be able to have a different type of surgery that will lift your eyebrows. Talk with your ophthalmologist about other surgery options.
- There are other treatments and procedures to improve the appearance of lower eyelids. For instance, you could have Botox injections, filler injections, laser treatment, or a chemical peel. Talk with your ophthalmologist about these and other choices.

As with all surgery, there are risks (problems that can happen) with blepharoplasty. Here are some of the most common or serious:

- Bleeding, infection, or numbness. Temporary numbness of the eyelashes is common for the first month or two.
- Changes in how you look such as bruising, scarring, or asymmetric appearance (one side of your face not matching the other).
- Eye problems. These can include trouble closing your eyes (which can damage the cornea—the part of your eye where a contact lens sits), inability to wear contact lenses, tearing, or dry eye. Temporary dryness is common for the first few weeks.
- Vision changes such as double vision, vision loss, or in very rare cases, blindness.
- Anesthesia problems. Local anesthesia injections can damage the eye, area around the eye, or cause vision loss. General anesthesia has its own risks that you would discuss with an anesthesiology specialist.

- Your eyelids may not look or feel as perfect after surgery as you had hoped. There are no guarantees about how your eyes will look, how good your peripheral vision will be, or how you will feel after blepharoplasty surgery. This is because people differ in eyelid structure, response to surgery, how well they heal, and expectations about how surgery will help. Gradual improvement in minor issues usually occurs with continued healing over the first 6 months after blepharoplasty.
- You may need more treatment or surgery to take care of problems that happen after blepharoplasty. You may have to pay more since this extra treatment or surgery might not be included in the fee for blepharoplasty.

Consent. By signing below, you consent (agree) that:
- You read this informed consent form, or someone read it to you.
- You understand the information in this informed consent form.
- The ophthalmologist or staff answered your questions about blepharoplasty surgery.
- The ophthalmologist or staff offered you a copy of this informed consent form.
- You accept that blepharoplasty can change how your eyes or eyelids look.
- You understand that there may be additional costs if you need more surgery or other treatment.

I Consent to Have Blepharoplasty Surgery on (Circle Your Choices):

Upper lid: Right Left Both
 Lower lid: Right Left Both
 Patient (or person authorized to sign for patient) Date
 Place letterhead here and remove note. Change font for large print
 Note: This form is intended as a sample only of the information you as the surgeon should personally discuss with the patient. Please review it and modify to fit your actual practice. Give the patient a copy.

Consent for Use of Hyaluronic Acid Fillers

Indications

HYALURONIC ACID injectable gels are injected into areas of facial tissue where moderate to severe facial wrinkles and folds occur. It temporarily adds volume to the skin and subcutaneous tissues, may give the appearance of a smoother skin surface and may help smooth moderate to severe facial wrinkles and folds.

Correction is temporary; therefore, touch-up injections as well as repeat injections are usually needed to maintain optimal correction. Less material (about half the amount) is usually needed for repeat injections. Most patients need one or possibly two treatments to achieve optimal wrinkle smoothing. The results may last as long as 9 months to 1 year.

Alternatives

Other treatments for soft-tissue augmentation include, but are not limited to, products such as Radiesse and autologous fat. Aside from these treatments, additional options for the correc-tion of lines and wrinkles do exist, including facial creams, botulinum toxin Type A, chemical peels, and laser skin surface treatments, and surgery. Other options not mentioned here may exist. All options should be discussed with your physician.

Side Effects and Complications

Most side effects are mild or moderate in nature, and their duration is short lasting (7 days or less). The most common side effects include, but are not limited to, temporary injection-site reactions such as redness, pain/tenderness, firmness, swelling, lumps/bumps, bruising, itching, infection, and discoloration.

In the first 24 hours after injection, you should avoid strenuous exercise, extensive sun or heat exposure, and alcoholic beverages. Exposure to any of the above may cause temporary redness, swelling, and/or itching at the injection sites. If there is swelling, you may need to place an ice pack over the swollen area. You should ask your physician when makeup may be applied after your treatment.

Be sure to report any redness and/or visible swelling that lasts for more than a few days, or any other symptoms that cause you concern.

Contraindications

HYALURONIC ACID injectable gel should not be used if you have:
- Severe allergies marked by a history of anaphylaxis or history or presence of multiple severe allergies.
- A history of allergies to gram-positive bacterial proteins.

The following are important treatment considerations for you to discuss with us and understand in order to help avoid unsatisfactory results and complications:
- **Please inform us prior to treatment:** If you are using substances that can prolong bleeding, such as aspirin or ibuprofen, as with any injection, may experience increased bruising or bleeding at the injection site.
- **Please inform us prior to treatment:** If you are on immunosuppressive or therapy used to decrease the body's immune response, as there may be an increased risk of infection.
- **Please inform us prior to treatment**: If you are pregnant or breastfeeding.
- **Please inform us prior to treatment**: If you have history of excessive scarring (e.g., hypertrophic scarring and keloid formations) and pigmentation disorders.

If laser treatment, chemical peeling, or any other procedure based on active dermal response is considered after treatment with hyaluronic acid injectable gel, there is a possible risk of an inflammatory reaction at the treatment site.

The safety and effectiveness of HYALURONIC ACID injectable gel for the treatment of areas other than facial wrinkles and folds (such as lips) have not been established in controlled clinical studies. Use in patients under 18 years has not been established.

Patient's Acceptance of Risks

I have read the above information and have discussed it with my physician. I understand that it is impossible for the doctor to inform me of every possible complication that may occur. No guarantees about results have been made. By signing below, I agree that my doctor has answered all of my questions and that I understand and accept the risks, benefits, and alternatives of HYALURONIC ACID.

_____

_____

Patient Signature Date

39.10 Appendix B

39.10.1 Patient Cosmetic Surgical Agreement

Patient Name: _____

Date of Surgery: _____

Patient Responsibilities

I have listed all known allergies, all of the medications, vitamins, and herbals I am using, all my prior operations, as well as all illnesses and medical conditions on my patient information form.

I have reviewed the surgical consent form and agree to follow my surgeon's instructions and postoperative care plan. I also agree to keep my surgeon informed of my permanent address so that s/he may contact me regarding any late findings or developments. I also agree to follow all postoperative instructions given to me.

Payment Policies

A scheduling deposit equal to 25% of the total fee is due at the time a surgery date is chosen and a commitment is made to me. This deposit is refundable until 2 weeks prior to the scheduled date of surgery. Less than 2 weeks from the scheduled date of surgery, the deposit is nonrefundable.

Surgeon fees, payable to my surgeon, are due in full 2 weeks prior to surgery. VISA, MC, personal or cashier's check, money orders, or cash are accepted. This payment is to include the entire balance, which is the remaining 75% of the surgeon's fee. This entire amount (25% plus 75% balance) is nonrefundable.

Facility fees and anesthesia fees are payable directly to the providers. Each has its own policy regarding time and method of payment.

Extra Expenses

I understand that the fees quoted to me by the staff of my surgeon are solely for the anticipated procedure, as described on the Cosmetic Surgery Quote. I understand that there is a very small possibility that there might be additional expenses due to complications. I agree that I am solely responsible if there are any such additional expenses.

I understand that there is no guarantee that I will be 100% satisfied with the results of my cosmetic surgery. However, after healing is essentially complete, if my surgeon and I both agree that the procedure(s) did not substantially accomplish the results which could be reasonably expected under all of the circumstances, and if we both agree that a surgical revision could be expected to significantly improve the results of the initial procedure(s), then my surgeon agrees to provide the surgery at no charge. This agreed upon revision must be performed within 1 year following the original surgery. If, however, my surgeon is performing surgery in any area in which another surgeon has previously performed surgery, there will be a charge for any surgical revisions performed. I understand that I am responsible for all other charges that may be associated with any revision, such as facility and anesthesia fees, laboratory tests, prescription drugs, etc.

_____

_____

Patient/Responsible Party Surgeon's Signature

_____

Date

Index